Jeng-Shyang Pan, Hsiang-Cheh Huang, Lakhmi C. Jain and Wai-Chi Fang (Eds.)

Intelligent Multimedia Data Hiding

Studies in Computational Intelligence, Volume 58

Editor-in-chief
Prof. Janusz Kacprzyk
Systems Research Institute
Polish Academy of Sciences
ul. Newelska 6
01-447 Warsaw
Poland
E-mail: kacprzyk@ibspan.waw.pl

Further volumes of this series
can be found on our homepage:
springer.com

Vol. 34. Ajith Abraham, Crina Grosan, Vitorino Ramos (Eds.)
Swarm Intelligence in Data Mining, 2006
ISBN 978-3-540-34955-6

Vol. 35. Ke Chen, Lipo Wang (Eds.)
Trends in Neural Computation, 2007
ISBN 978-3-540-36121-3

Vol. 36. Ildar Batyrshin, Janusz Kacprzyk, Leonid Sheremetor, Lotfi A. Zadeh (Eds.)
Preception-based Data Mining and Decision Making in Economics and Finance, 2006
ISBN 978-3-540-36244-9

Vol. 37. Jie Lu, Da Ruan, Guangquan Zhang (Eds.)
E-Service Intelligence, 2007
ISBN 978-3-540-37015-4

Vol. 38. Art Lew, Holger Mauch
Dynamic Programming, 2007
ISBN 978-3-540-37013-0

Vol. 39. Gregory Levitin (Ed.)
Computational Intelligence in Reliability Engineering, 2007
ISBN 978-3-540-37367-4

Vol. 40. Gregory Levitin (Ed.)
Computational Intelligence in Reliability Engineering, 2007
ISBN 978-3-540-37371-1

Vol. 41. Mukesh Khare, S.M. Shiva Nagendra (Eds.)
Artificial Neural Networks in Vehicular Pollution Modelling, 2007
ISBN 978-3-540-37417-6

Vol. 42. Bernd J. Krämer, Wolfgang A. Halang (Eds.)
Contributions to Ubiquitous Computing, 2007
ISBN 978-3-540-44909-6

Vol. 43. Fabrice Guillet, Howard J. Hamilton (Eds.)
Quality Measures in Data Mining, 2007
ISBN 978-3-540-44911-9

Vol. 44. Nadia Nedjah, Luiza de Macedo Mourelle, Mario Neto Borges, Nival Nunes de Almeida (Eds.)
Intelligent Educational Machines, 2007
ISBN 978-3-540-44920-1

Vol. 45. Vladimir G. Ivancevic, Tijana T. Ivancevic
Neuro-Fuzzy Associative Machinery for Comprehensive Brain and Cognition Modeling, 2007
ISBN 978-3-540-47463-0

Vol. 46. Valentina Zharkova, Lakhmi C. Jain
Artificial Intelligence in Recognition and Classification of Astrophysical and Medical Images, 2007
ISBN 978-3-540-47511-8

Vol. 47. S. Sumathi, S. Esakkirajan
Fundamentals of Relational Database Management Systems, 2007
ISBN 978-3-540-48397-7

Vol. 48. H. Yoshida (Ed.)
Advanced Computational Intelligence Paradigms in Healthcare, 2007
ISBN 978-3-540-47523-1

Vol. 49. Keshav P. Dahal, Kay Chen Tan, Peter I. Cowling (Eds.)
Evolutionary Scheduling, 2007
ISBN 978-3-540-48582-7

Vol. 50. Nadia Nedjah, Leandro dos Santos Coelho, Luiza de Macedo Mourelle (Eds.)
Mobile Robots: The Evolutionary Approach, 2007
ISBN 978-3-540-49719-6

Vol. 51. Shengxiang Yang, Yew Soon Ong, Yaochu Jin Honda (Eds.)
Evolutionary Computation in Dynamic and Uncertain Environment, 2007
ISBN 978-3-540-49772-1

Vol. 52. Abraham Kandel, Horst Bunke, Mark Last (Eds.)
Applied Graph Theory in Computer Vision and Pattern Recognition, 2007
ISBN 978-3-540-68019-2

Vol. 53. Huajin Tang, Kay Chen Tan, Zhang Yi
Neural Networks: Computational Models and Applications, 2007
ISBN 978-3-540-69225-6

Vol. 54. Fernando G. Lobo, Cláudio F. Lima and Zbigniew Michalewicz (Eds.)
Parameter Setting in Evolutionary Algorithms, 2007
ISBN 978-3-540-69431-1

Vol. 55. Xianyi Zeng, Yi Li, Da Ruan and Ludovic Koehl (Eds.)
Computational Textile, 2007
ISBN 978-3-540-70656-4

Vol. 56. Akira Namatame, Satoshi Kurihara and Hideyuki Nakashima (Eds.)
Emergent Intelligence of Networked Agents, 2007
ISBN 978-3-540-71073-8

Vol. 57. Nadia Nedjah, Ajith Abraham and Luiza de Macedo Mourella (Eds.)
Computational Intelligence in Information Assurance and Security, 2007
ISBN 978-3-540-71077-6

Vol. 58. Jeng-Shyang Pan, Hsiang-Cheh Huang, Lakhmi C. Jain and Wai-Chi Fang (Eds.)
Intelligent Multimedia Data Hiding, 2007
ISBN 978-3-540-71168-1

Jeng-Shyang Pan
Hsiang-Cheh Huang
Lakhmi C. Jain
Wai-Chi Fang
(Eds.)

Intelligent Multimedia Data Hiding

New Directions

With 207 Figures and 27 Tables

Springer

Jeng-Shyang Pan
Professor of Department
of Electronic Engineering
National Kaohsiung University
of Applied Sciences
415 Chien-Kung Road
Kaohsiung 807
Taiwan
E-mail: jspan@cc.kuas.edu.tw

Hsiang-Cheh Huang
Assistant Professor of Department
of Electrical Engineering
National University of Kaohsiung
700 University Road
Kaohsiung 811
Taiwan
E-mail: huang.hc@gmail.com

Lakhmi C. Jain
Professor of Knowledge-Based
Engineering
Founding Director of the KES Centre
University of South Australia
Adelaide
Mawson Lakes Campus
South Australia
SA 5095
Australia
E-mail: Lakhmi.jain@unisa.edu.au

(Winston) Wai-Chi Fang, IEEE Fellow
Senior Engineer/Manager
NASA's Jet Propulsion Laboratory
California Institute of Technology
4800 Oak Grove Drive
Pasadena, CA 91109-8099
USA
E-mail: wai-chi.fang@jpl.nasa.gov

ISSN print edition: 1860-949X
ISSN electronic edition: 1860-9503
ISBN-10 3-642-42922-X Springer Berlin Heidelberg New York
ISBN-13 978-3-642-42922-4 Springer Berlin Heidelberg New York

Springer is a part of Springer Science+Business Media
springer.com

Cover design: deblik, Berlin
Typesetting by the editors using a Springer LaTeX macro package
Printed on acid-free paper SPIN: 11544234 89/SPi 5 4 3 2 1 0

Foreword

When the first watermarking papers appeared in mid 90ies, the industrial needs on copyright protection and rights management of digital media were already pressing. The music industry was already loosing large revenues due to music piracy. Watermarking was proposed as a very promising solution to combat digital piracy and illegal digital media copying. Most of the proposed techniques have been based on solid theoretical background and, thus, attracted a large interest in the scientific community. The ensuing explosive growth produced rich literature, significant theoretical results and IPR protection solutions.

Besides watermarking, which is an active technique, in the sense that a watermark must be embedded in the multimedia signal, passive techniques for IPR protection and DRM emerged recently. Such techniques (called sometimes fingerprinting or replica detection or perceptual hashing) are essentially fast retrieval/hashing techniques for broadcast/internet traffic monitoring through replica searches in copyright holder or trusted third parties databases.

Watermarking is proven to be a very good solution for intellectual property rights protection, particularly for digital images. It has also been successfully used for still image content authentication. Its use for video, audio and music IPR protection was less widespread, since the related technical and business model problems were proven to be more difficult to tackle. Fingerprinting/replica detection is still at its development phase and has found so far significant use in music copy detection. However, there are no solutions that are yet universally acceptable.

Furthermore, there are large needs related to the protection of other multimedia data types, notably digital maps, digital terrain models, 2D and 3D computer graphics and animations that have not been properly addressed so far in great detail, neither scientifically, nor in terms of introducing proper business models. These topics are widely open to scientific research.

Taking into account the explosive growth of digital media market, notably for music, still images, video content and digital maps and the persisting IPR protection problems, this market will be thirsty for new IPR/DRM solutions in the immediate future. The edited book in your hands is a very good survey of current efforts on watermarking and data hiding and will be very helpful in advancing the research for the much needed IPR/DRM solutions and tools.

Aristotle University
of Thessaloniki, Greece
22 December 2006

Director of the Artificial Intelligence
and Information Analysis Lab
Prof. Ioannis Pitas

Preface

Digital multimedia is ubiquitous in our daily lives. Due to the tremendous advances in signal processing and signal transmission techniques, it is easy to acquire and duplicate multimedia data. The wide spread use of internet in business, research and security has necessitated to protect the data and owner identity.

This book presents the latest research in the area of multimedia data hiding paradigms. The book is divided into four parts and an appendix. The first part includes chapter 1. Chapter 1 by Huang, et al. introduces multimedia signal processing and information hiding techniques. It includes multimedia representation, the need for multimedia, concepts of digital watermarking and some requirements of watermarking. Part two of this book describes the recent advances in multimedia signal processing. It contains two chapters. Chapter 2 by Pan is on digital video coding. It describes the principles of digital video compression, mainly focussing on the main techniques used in various coding standards. Chapter 3 by Peng et al. is on advances of MPEG scalable video coding standard. Two major approaches have been considered as the potential technologies. One is the wavelet-based scheme and the other is the scalable extension of MPEG-4 AVC/H.264. The latter is now chosen as the MPEG SVC standard to be finalized in 2007. This chapter presents a brief overview on the latest advances of these technologies with a focus on the MPEG standard activities. Part three of this book presents information hiding techniques including steganography, secret sharing and watermarking. It contains five chapters. Chapter 4 by Chang et al. is on a bit-level visual secret sharing scheme for multi-secret images using rotation and reversion operations. The authors have extended the concept of visual secret sharing to gray-scale image visual secret sharing. The rotation and reversion operations are applied to increase the security of the secret images. Chapter 5 by Chang et al. is on adaptive data hiding scheme for palette images applications that can offer a high embedding capacity and good image quality. The clustering technique is adopted to achieve high embedding capacity and two embedding mechanisms are used to do embedding according to the size of the cluster. The proposed scheme is a perfect balance between embedding capacity and image quality. Chapter 6 by Niu et al. is on GIS watermarking. It presents a 2D vector map data hiding for applications such as digital copyright protection, data authentication and data source tracing. Some new research directions are presented. Chapter 7 by Echizen et al. is on adapting embedding and detection for improved video watermarking. Experimental evaluations using motion pictures have demonstrated that the proposed techniques are effective for in the pixel-based watermarking maintaining picture quality and withstanding video processing. Chapter 8 by Noda et al. is on steganographic methods focussing on bit-plane complexity segmentation (BPCS) steganography. Steganography is a technique to hide secret information in some other data without leaving any apparent evidence without leaving any apparent evidence of data alteration. The authors have also presented histogram preserving JPEG steganography including experimental results.

The final part of this book includes practical applications of intelligent multimedia signal processing and data hiding systems. This part contains five chapters. Chapter 9 by Liao is on intelligent video event detection for surveillance systems. This chapter includes solutions for video-based surveillance systems in spatial and compressed domain. The techniques presented are efficient and accurate in the video retrieval process. Chapter 10 by Liu is on print-to-web linking technology using mobile phone camera and its applications in Japan. Chapter 11 by Lu et al. is on multipurpose image watermarking algorithms and applications. Chapter 12 by Huang et al. is on tabu search based multi-watermarking over lossy networks. An innovative algorithm on vector quantization based image watermarking is proposed. Experimental verification demonstrates the utility of the approach. The final chapter by Weng et al. is on reversible watermarking techniques and applications. In the appendix, authors from five chapters of this book contribute programs including source codes and/or executables related to the topics in their chapters. Interested readers are invited to use the programs. This book will be valuable to both academia and industry. This book is directed to the final year undergraduate and junior postgraduate students. Researchers and professors in the departments of electrical/electronics/communication engineering, computer science, and relating departments will find this book useful. We are indebted to the authors and the reviewers for their contribution. The editorial assistance by Springer is acknowledged.

Kaohsiung, Taiwan, December 2006	*Jeng-Shyang Pan*
Kaohsiung, Taiwan, December 2006	*Hsiang-Cheh Huang*
Adelaide, SA, Australia, December 2006	*Lakhmi C. Jain*
Pasadena, CA, USA, December 2006	*Wai-Chi Fang*

Table of Contents

Part I Fundamentals of Multimedia Signal Processing and Information Hiding

1 An Introduction to Intelligent Multimedia Data Hiding
Hsiang-Cheh Huang (National University of Kaohsiung), Jeng-Shyang Pan (National Kaohsiung University of Applied Sciences), Wai-Chi Fang (California Institute of Technology), Lakhmi C. Jain (University of South Australia) 3

Part II Advances in Multimedia Signal Processing

2 Digital Video Coding – Techniques and Standards
Feng Pan (ViXS Systems Inc.) 13

3 Advances of MPEG Scalable Video Coding Standard
Wen-Hsiao Peng (National Chiao-Tung University), Chia-Yang Tsai (National Chiao-Tung University), Tihao Chiang (National Chiao-Tung University), Hsueh-Ming Hang (National Chiao-Tung University) 55

Part III Various Data Hiding Techniques

4 A Bit-Level Visual Secret Sharing Scheme for Multi-Secret Images Using Rotation and Reversion Operations
Chin-Chen Chang (Feng Chia University), Tzu-Chuen Lu (Chaoyang University of Technology), Yi-Hsuan Fan (National Chung Cheng University) 83

5 Adaptive Data Hiding Scheme for Palette Images
Chin-Chen Chang (Feng Chia University), Yu-Zheng Wang (Academia Sinica), Yu-Chen Hu (Providence University) 103

6 GIS Watermarking: Hiding Data in 2D Vector Maps
Xia-Mu Niu (Harbin Institute of Technology), Cheng-Yong Shao (Dalian Naval Academy), Xiao-Tong Wang (Dalian Naval Academy) . . . 123

7 Adaptive Embedding and Detection for Improved Video Watermarking
Isao Echizen (Hitachi), Yasuhiro Fujii (Hitachi), Takaaki Yamada (Hitachi), Satoru Tezuka (Hitachi), Hiroshi Yoshiura (The University of Electro-Communications) 157

8 Steganographic Methods Focusing on BPCS Steganography
Hideki Noda (Kyushu Institute of Technology), Michiharu Niimi (Kyushu Institute of Technology), Eiji Kawaguchi (KIT Senior Academy) 189

Part IV Practical Applications of Intelligent Multimedia Signal Processing and Data Hiding Systems

---

9 Intelligent Video Event Detection for Surveillance Systems
Hong-Yuan Mark Liao (Academia Sinica), Duan-Yu Chen (Academia Sinica), Chih-Wen Su (Academia Sinica), Hsiao-Rong Tyan (Chung-Yuan Christian University) 233

10 Print-to-Web Linking Technology Using a Mobile Phone Camera and its Applications in Japan
Zheng Liu (C4 Technology) 261

11 Multipurpose Image Watermarking Algorithms and Applications
Zhe-Ming Lu (University of Freiburg; Harbin Institute of Technology), Hans Burkhardt (University of Freiburg), Shu-Chuan Chu (Cheng-Shiu University) 287

12 Tabu Search Based Multi-Watermarking over Lossy Networks
Hsiang-Cheh Huang (National University of Kaohsiung), Jeng-Shyang Pan (National Kaohsiung University of Applied Sciences), Chun-Yen Huang (National Kaohsiung University of Applied Sciences), Yu-Hsiu Huang (Cheng-Shiu University), Kuang-Chih Huang (Cheng-Shiu University) 325

13 Reversible Watermarking Techniques
Shao-Wei Weng (Beijing Jiao Tong University), Yao Zhao (Beijing Jiao Tong University), Jeng-Shyang Pan (National Kaohsiung University of Applied Sciences) 357

Programs Relating to Topics of This Book 391

Subject Index 393

List of Contributors

Hans Burkhardt
University of Freiburg
Freiburg, Germany
Hans.Burkhardt@informatik.uni-freiburg.de

Chin-Chen Chang
Feng Chia University
Taichung, Taiwan, R.O.C.
ccc@cs.ccu.edu.tw
http://msn.iecs.fcu.edu.tw/~ccc/

Duan-Yu Chen
Academia Sinica
Taipei, Taiwan, R.O.C.
dychen@iis.sinica.edu.tw

Tihao Chiang
National Chiao-Tung University
Hsinchu, Taiwan, R.O.C.
tchiang@mail.nctu.edu.tw

Shu-Chuan Chu
Cheng-Shiu University
Kaohsiung, Taiwan, R.O.C.
scchu@csu.edu.tw
http://home.mis.csu.edu.tw/scchu/

Isao Echizen
Systems Development Laboratory
Hitachi, Ltd.
Kawasaki, Japan
iechizen@sdl.hitachi.co.jp

Yi-Hsuan Fan
National Chung Cheng University
Chaiyi, Taiwan, R.O.C.
fyh93@cs.ccu.edu.tw

Wai-Chi Fang
NASA's Jet Propulsion Lab
California Institute of Technology
Pasadena, CA, USA
wai-chi.fang@jpl.nasa.gov

Yasuhiro Fujii
Systems Development Laboratory
Hitachi, Ltd.
Kawasaki, Japan
fujii@sdl.hitachi.co.jp

Hsueh-Ming Hang
National Chiao-Tung University
Hsinchu, Taiwan, R.O.C.
hmhang@mail.nctu.edu.tw
http://cwww.ee.nctu.edu.tw/hmhang/

Yu-Chen Hu
Providence University
Taichung, Taiwan, R.O.C.
ychu@pu.edu.tw
http://www1.pu.edu.tw/~ychu/

Chun-Yen Huang
National Kaohsiung University of Applied Sciences
Kaohsiung, Taiwan, R.O.C.
piscehuang@gmail.com

Hsiang-Cheh Huang
National University of Kaohsiung
Kaohsiung, Taiwan, R.O.C.
huang.hc@gmail.com
http://bit.kuas.edu.tw/~hchuang/

Kuang-Chih Huang
Cheng-Shiu University
Kaohsiung, Taiwan, R.O.C.
kchuang@csu.edu.tw

Yu-Hsiu Huang
Cheng-Shiu University
Kaohsiung, Taiwan, R.O.C.
yhhuang@csu.edu.tw

Lakhmi C. Jain
University of South Australia
Adelaide, SA, Australia
Lakhmi.Jain@unisa.edu.au
http://www.kes.unisa.edu.au/

Eiji Kawaguchi
KIT Senior Academy
Iizuka, Japan
e-kawagu@alto.ocn.ne.jp

Hong-Yuan Mark Liao
Academia Sinica
Taipei, Taiwan, R.O.C.
liao@iis.sinica.edu.tw
http://www.iis.sinica.edu.tw/~liao/

Zheng Liu
C4 Technology, Inc.,
Tokyo, Japan
zliu@c4t.jp
http://c4t.jp/

Tzu-Chuen Lu
Chaoyang University of Technology
Taichung, Taiwan, R.O.C.
tclu@mail.cyut.edu.tw
http://www.cyut.edu.tw/~tclu/

Zhe-Ming Lu
University of Freiburg
Freiburg, Germany;
Harbin Institute of Technology
Harbin, China
zhemingl@yahoo.com
http://dsp.hit.edu.cn/luzheming/

Michiharu Niimi
Kyushu Institute of Technology
Iizuka, Japan
niimi@mip.ces.kyutech.ac.jp

Xia-Mu Niu
Harbin Institute of Technology
Shenzhen, China
xiamu.niu@hit.edu.cn
http://isec.hitsz.edu.cn/

Hideki Noda
Kyushu Institute of Technology
Iizuka, Japan
noda@mip.ces.kyutech.ac.jp

Feng Pan
ViXS Systems Inc.
Toronto, Canada
epan@vixs.com

Jeng-Shyang Pan
National Kaohsiung University of Applied Sciences
Kaohsiung, Taiwan, R.O.C.
jspan@cc.kuas.edu.tw
http://bit.kuas.edu.tw/~jspan/

Wen-Hsiao Peng
National Chiao-Tung University
Hsinchu, Taiwan, R.O.C.
pawn@mail.si2lab.org

Cheng-Yong Shao
Dalian Naval Academy
Dalian, China
chengyong.shao@dsp.hit.edu.cn

Chih-Wen Su
Academia Sinica
Taipei, Taiwan, R.O.C.
lucas@iis.sinica.edu.tw

Satoru Tezuka
Systems Development Laboratory
Hitachi, Ltd.
Kawasaki, Japan
tezuka@sdl.hitachi.co.jp

Chia-Yang Tsai
National Chiao-Tung University
Hsinchu, Taiwan, R.O.C.
cytsai.ee90g@nctu.edu.tw

Hsiao-Rong Tyan
Chung-Yuan Christian University
Chungli, Taiwan, R.O.C.
tyan@ice.cycu.edu.tw

Xiao-Tong Wang
Dalian Naval Academy
Dalian, China
rfrm@dlut.edu.cn

Yu-Zheng Wang
Institute of Information Science,
Academia Sinica
Taipei, Taiwan, R.O.C.
wyc@iis.sinica.edu.tw

Shao-Wei Weng
Institute of Information Science,
Beijing Jiao Tong University
Beijing, China
wswweiwei@126.com

Takaaki Yamada
Systems Development Laboratory
Hitachi, Ltd.
Kawasaki, Japan
t-yamada@sdl.hitachi.co.jp

Hiroshi Yoshiura
The University of Electro-Communications
Tokyo, Japan
yoshiura@hc.uec.ac.jp

Yao Zhao
Institute of Information Science,
Beijing Jiao Tong University
Beijing, China
yzhao@center.njtu.edu.cn
http://doctor.njtu.edu.cn/zhaoy/

Part I

Fundamentals of Multimedia Signal Processing and Information Hiding

1

An Introduction to Intelligent Multimedia Data Hiding

Hsiang-Cheh Huang[1], Jeng-Shyang Pan[2], Wai-Chi Fang[3], and Lakhmi C. Jain[4]

1 Department of Electrical Engineering, National University of Kaohsiung, Kaohsiung 811, Taiwan, R.O.C.
huang.hc@gmail.com

2 Department of Electronic Engineering, National Kaohsiung University of Applied Sciences,
Kaohsiung 807, Taiwan, R.O.C.
jspan@cc.kuas.edu.tw

3 California Institute of Technology & NASA's Jet Propulsion Lab, Pasadena, CA, USA
wai-chi.fang@jpl.nasa.gov

4 University of South Australia,
Adelaide, Australia
Lakhmi.Jain@unisa.edu.au

Summary. With the widespread use of the Internet and the booming growth of the computer industry, multimedia related researches and applications have greatly increased in the last twenty years. In addition to multimedia signal processing, data hiding techniques aiming at protecting copyright-related issues are of considerable interest in academia and industry. Experts in multimedia signal processing and data hiding have been invited to contribute to this book. We hope the readers find the book of value.

1.1 Introduction to Multimedia Information

With the widespread use of Internet and the booming growth in the computer industry, multimedia related researches and applications have multiplied in the last fifteen to twenty years. Hence, we give a brief introduction to multimedia representation and the need for multimedia compression. Advanced topics will be given in Part II of this book.

1.1.1 Multimedia Representation

Multimedia involve more than one medium and including image, sound, text, video, for example, [1, 2, 3, 4]. Multiple media are simultaneously transmitted

H.-C. Huang et al.: *An Introduction to Intelligent Multimedia Data Hiding*, Studies in Computational Intelligence (SCI) **58**, 3–10 (2007)
www.springerlink.com

over the network, using the Internet or mobile channels. They can be divided into two categories. These are:

1. **Continuous media** which is a series of consecutive units of equal duration. For instance, audio, They may include video and animation.
2. **Discrete media** contains one presentation unit, which may be text, graphics on image.

Multimedia signal processing has the following goals:

(A) high quality,
(B) highly efficient compression,
(C) security-related issues,
(D) error resilient transmission, and
(E) interactivity.

Topics in the book cover the items from (A) to (D). Part II focuses on items (A) and (B), Part III and most of Part IV discuss items (A) and (C). A part of Part IV considers item (D). Item (E) mainly relates to multimedia on demand (MOD), much of this particular subject exceeds the intended scope of this book.

1.1.2 The Need for Multimedia Compression

Multimedia signals contain a great deal of data. The bit rate of the original, uncompressed data with different formats may be described as follows.

Speech:

$$8 \text{ bit/sample} \times 8 \text{ Ksample/sec} = 64 \text{ Kbit/sec}$$

CD audio: selectfont

$$16 \text{ bit/sample/channel} \times 44.1 \text{ Ksample/sec} \times 2 \text{ channel} = 1.411 \text{ Mbit/sec}$$

Digital TV:

Still picture:

$$720 \text{ pels} \times 483 \text{ lines} \times 2 \text{ byte/pixel} \times 8 \text{ bit/byte} = 5.564 \text{ Mbit/frame}$$

Motion picture:

$$5.564 \text{ Mbit/frame} \times 29.97 \text{ frame/sec} = 167 \text{ Mbit/frame}$$

Digital HDTV:

Still picture:

$$1920 \text{ pels} \times 1080 \text{ lines} \times 1.5 \text{ byte/pixel} \times 8 \text{ bit/byte} = 24.883 \text{ Mbit/frame}$$

Motion picture:

$$24.883 \text{ Mbit/frame} \times 30 \text{ frame/sec} = 746.496 \text{ Mbit/frame}$$

On account of the huge amount of multimedia data, compression is necessary for practical applications. Ways of achieving necessary multimedia compression will be described in Chapter 2. Detailed schemes with lossless compression, lossy compression, practical applications, and multimedia-related standards are discussed in Part II of this book.

1.2 Concepts and Requirements of Digital Watermarking

1.2.1 Fundamental Concepts of Digital Watermarking

Owning to the popularity of the Internet and the nature of the multimedia information that permits lossless and unlimited reproductions, the need to embed securely owner identity and other information into multimedia is urgent [5, 6, 7, 8, 9, 10, 11, 12, 13, 14]. The protection and enforcement of intellectual property rights for digital multimedia is now an important issue. Modern digital watermarking technology has a short history since 1993 [5, 15].

A typical application of digital watermarking is to identify the ownership of a multimedia object or content by embedding the owner mark. This is known as the *watermark*. Typically, most multimedia applications require an imperceptible and robust watermark. There are other demands that require perceptible or fragile watermarking. Some relevant terminology and classifications are described in Fig. 1.1.

The high level diagram of a generic watermarking scheme is shown in Fig. 1.2. Typically, a watermark insertion process is shown in Fig. 1.2(a). Here we have the original media ($\boldsymbol{X}$), which may be an image for example, and the encoder inserts a watermark ($\boldsymbol{W}$) into it. The result is the marked media $\boldsymbol{X}'$, for example, a marked image. In this embedding, process, a key may be used in order to produce a more secure watermark. This key is regarded as part of the encoding process. The dashed line in Fig. 1.2 indicates that the key may be needed for a particular design. The watermark may be extracted by use of a decoder, illustrated in Fig. 1.2(b). It may alternatively be detected using a detector. This is shown in Fig. 1.2(c). In the former process, in addition to the test media ($\boldsymbol{X}''$), the original media with or without a key may be needed. In

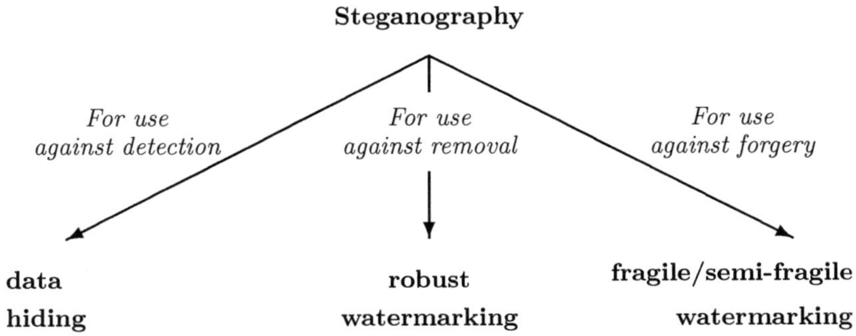

Fig. 1.1. The classification of watermarking [16].

the latter case, the inserted watermark ($\boldsymbol{W}$) is often necessary to check the identity of the watermark.

These generic models are directly applicable to the chapters dealing with data hiding topics.

Mathematical notions are also used to express the processes in Fig. 1.2. We can view the *embedding* process as a function or mapping that maps the inputs $\boldsymbol{X}$, $\boldsymbol{W}$ and/or K to the output $\boldsymbol{X}'$. That is,

$$\boldsymbol{X}' = E(\boldsymbol{X}, \boldsymbol{W}, [K]), \tag{1.1}$$

where $E(\cdot)$ denotes the embedding process, and $[K]$ indicates that K may not be included. Similarly, the *decoding* or *extraction* process, $D(\cdot)$, can be denoted by

$$\boldsymbol{W}' = D(\boldsymbol{X}'', [\boldsymbol{X}], [K]). \tag{1.2}$$

The *detection* process, $d(\cdot)$, is

$$\{\text{Yes or No}\} = d(\boldsymbol{X}'', [\boldsymbol{X}], \boldsymbol{W}, [K]). \tag{1.3}$$

Hence, $[\cdot]$ means that the element in the bracket may be optional.

1.2.2 Some Requirements of Digital Watermarking

There are many metrics used to measure the effectiveness of a watermarking algorithm. From algorithm design viewpoint, the three most critical requirements are *watermark imperceptibility*, *watermark robustness*, and *watermark capacity*. Although these three requirements are all very desirable, as pointed out in literature [17, 18, 19, 20, 21, 22], they influence, or even conflict, with each other. After fixing one dimension, the remaining two may then have conflicts between one another. Some tradeoff must then be developed [23]. The interrelationships may be threefold.

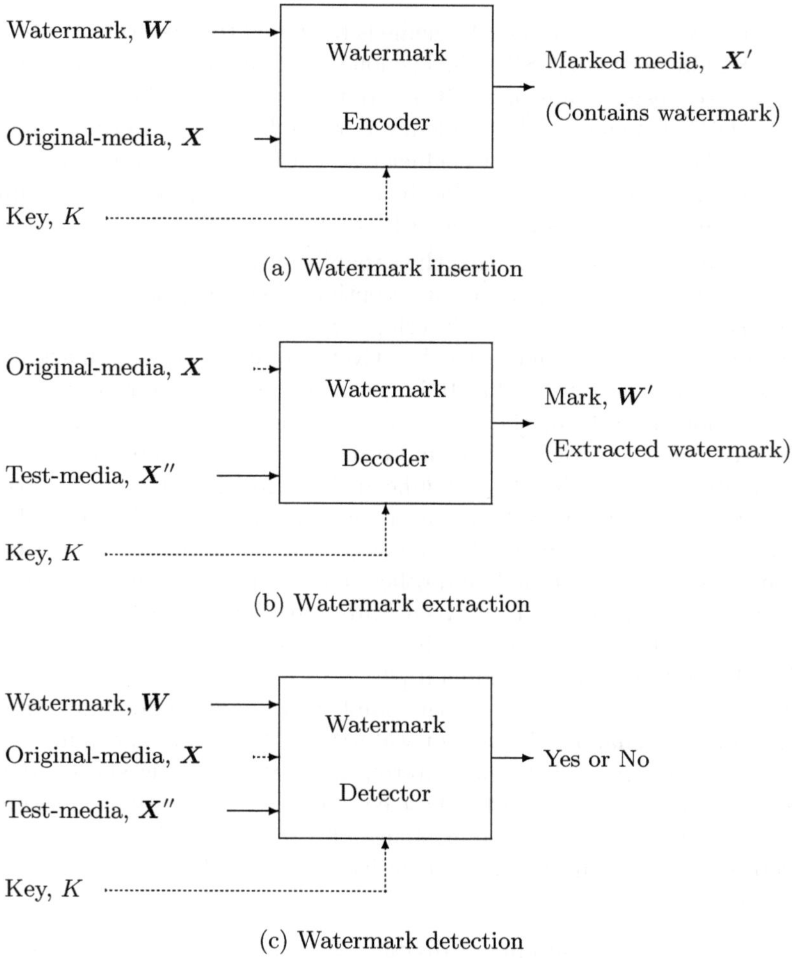

Fig. 1.2. Watermark processes.

1. Watermark imperceptibility refers to whether the viewer can see the existence of the embedded watermark or not. To make the watermark imperceptible, two situations need to be considered.
   a) The number of watermark bits embedded must be less than a particular threshold in order to make the watermark imperceptible. The theoretical bound of this threshold, or the watermark capacity described in item 3 below, is derived in literature [19]. The fewer bits embedded means a less robust watermarking algorithm.
   b) Imperceptible watermarking needs to modify the original media as little as possible. The watermarked image quality should be under the Just Noticeable Distortion (JND) region [24]. From this consideration,

the commonly employed scheme is to embed the watermark into Least Significant Bits (LSB). This is done in the frequency domain as a Discrete Cosine Transform (DCT) domain or Discrete Wavelet Transform (DWT) domain. The tendency is to embed the watermark into the higher frequency band coefficients. However, this causes the watermark to become vulnerable to common image processing techniques such as Low-Pass Filtering (LPF).

2. Watermark robustness means the capability that the watermarked media can withstand intentional or unintentional media processing, known as *attacks*. These can include filtering, transcoding, resizing, or rotation. There are also benchmarks to objectively examine the watermark robustness, such as Stirmark [25]. It is generally agreed that robustness plays an important role in the design of watermarking algorithm. To speak heuristically, in order to gain more robustness, the watermark needs to be embedded into the Most Significant Bits (MSB) in the spatial domain. Alternatively, this may be done in the lower frequency band coefficients in the transform domain. By doing so, the watermarked image quality can be seriously degraded, and others may suspect to the existence of the watermark. The tradeoff between watermark imperceptibility and watermark robustness is to embed the watermark into the "middle frequency bands" in the transform domain [26].
3. Watermark capacity refers to the number of bits embedded into the original media. That is, the size of watermark. Generally speaking, if more bits can be embedded, the watermarking algorithm is supposed to be more robust; however, under these conditions, the quality of watermarked media is degraded, and the existence of a watermark becomes more perceptible. Authors in [17, 19] have derived theoretical bounds for watermark capacity.

The fundamental concepts of digital watermarking and data hiding, may be further explored in the advanced topics relating to data hiding and applications in the subsequent chapters.

1.3 Summary

A general concept for multimedia signal processing and watermarking is presented in this chapter. Topics included in this book are also considered. In subsequent chapters, the authors will discuss the two themes of this book. These include fundamental concepts, algorithms and applications in detail. We hope readers will find them of value.

References

1. Steinmetz, R. and Nahrstedt, K. (2004): Multimedia systems. Springer Verlag, Berlin Heidelberg
2. Poynton, C.A (2003): Digital video and HDTV: algorithms and interfaces. Morgan Kaufmann Publisher, San Francisco, CA
3. Symes, P (2003): Digital video compression. Glencoe/McGraw-Hill, Columbus, OH
4. Mandal, M.K. (2002): Multimedia Signals and Systems. Kluwer Academic Publisher, Dordrecht, Netherlands
5. Pan, J.S., Huang, H.C., and Jain, L.C. (2004): Intelligent watermarking techniques. World Scientific Publishing Company, Singapore
6. Katzenbeisser, S. and Petitcolas, F. (2000): Information Hiding — Techniques for Steganography and Digital Watermarking. Artech House, Norwood, MA
7. Bloom, J., Miller, M., and Cox, I. (2001): Digital watermarking. Morgan Kaufmann Publisher, San Francisco, CA
8. Jajodia, S., Johnson, N.F., and Duric, Z. (2001): Information hiding: steganography and watermarking — attacks and countermeasures. Kluwer Academic Publisher, Dordrecht, Netherlands
9. Wayner, P. (2002): Disappearing cryptography: information hiding steganography & watermarking. Morgan Kaufmann Publisher, San Francisco, CA
10. Girod, B. and Eggers, J. (2002): Informed Watermarking. Kluwer Academic Publisher, Dordrecht, Netherlands
11. Arnold, M., Schmucker, M. and Wolthusen, S.D. (2003): Techniques and applications of digital watermarking and content protection. Artech House, Norwood, MA
12. Seitz, J. (2005): Digital watermarking for digital media. Information Science Pub., Hershey, PA
13. Perez-Gonzalez, F. and Voloshynovskiy, S. (2006): Fundamentals of digital image watermarking. John Wiley & Sons Inc., Hoboken, NJ
14. Furht, B., Muharemagic, E., and Socek D. (2005): Multimedia encryption and watermarking. Springer Verlag, Berlin Heidelberg
15. Tirkel, A.Z., Rankin, G.A., van Schyndel, R.M., Ho, W.J., Mee, N.R.A., and Osborne, C.F. (1993): Electronic water mark. Proc. Digital Image Computing Techniques and Applications '93, 666–672
16. De Vleeschouwer, C., Delaigle, J.-F., and Macq, B. (2002): Invisibility and application functionalities in perceptual watermarking — An overview. Proceedings of the IEEE, **90**, 64–77
17. Barni, M., Bartolini, F., De Rosa, A., and Piva, A. (2000): Capacity of full frame DCT image watermarks. IEEE Trans. Image Processing, **9**, 1450–1455
18. Kirovski, D. and Malvar, H.S. (2003): Spread spectrum watermarking of audio signals. IEEE Trans. Signal Processing, **51**, 1020–1033
19. Lin, C.Y. and Chang, S.F. (2001) Watermarking capacity of digital images based on domain-specific masking effects. Int'l Conf. Information Technology: Coding and Computing, 90–94
20. Macq, B., Dittmann, J., and Delp, E.J. (2004): Benchmarking of image watermarking algorithms for digital rights management. Proceedings of the IEEE, **92**, 971–984
21. Moulin, P., Mıhçak, M.K. (2002): A framework for evaluating the data-hiding capacity of image sources. IEEE Trans. Image Processing, **11**, 1029–1042

22. Wolfgang, R.B., Podilchuk, C.I., and Delp, E.J. (1999): Perceptual watermarks for digital images and video. Proceedings of IEEE, **87**, 1108–1126
23. Moskowitz, S. (2002): What is acceptable quality in the application of digital watermarking: trade-offs of security, robustness and quality. Int'l Conf. Information Technology: Coding and Computing, 80–84
24. Jayant, N.S., Johnston, J.D., and Safranek, R.J. (1993): Signal compression based on models of human perception. Proceedings of the IEEE, **81**, 1385–1422
25. Petitcolas, F.A.P. (2004): Stirmark benchmark 4.0. Available from: `http://www.petitcolas.net/fabien/watermarking/stirmark/`
26. Shieh, C.S., Huang, H.C., Wang, F.H., and Pan, J.S. (2004): Genetic watermarking based on transform domain techniques. Pattern Recognition, **37**, 555–565

Part II

Advances in Multimedia Signal Processing

2

Digital Video Coding – Techniques and Standards

Feng Pan

Video Architect, ViXS Systems Inc.,
245 Consumers Road, Toronto, M2J 1R3 Canada
epan@vixs.com

Summary. The last two decades have witnessed great advances in multimedia technologies, which allow the exchange of all sorts of audiovisual content seamlessly and pervasively. The great success of various video coding standards, such as MPEG-1 in Video CD and CDROM, MPEG-2 in digital television and DVD video, as well as H.263 in video communication, has revolutionized how we communicate and entertain. Video coding standards provide the common language that the encoder and the decoder use to communicate. It also makes the production of video compression systems possible so that the cost can be kept to an acceptable level.

In this chapter we introduce the basic principles of digital video compression, focusing on the main techniques used in various video coding standards. We also give a brief overview of the various video coding standards and their applications.

2.1 Fundamentals of Video Data Compression

The compression of digital video signal is essential as the raw RGB video is very bulky. It is difficult, if not impossible, to store or transmit uncompressed video signals in most applications. For example, according to PAL SDTV video specification, the requirements are as follows:

- in the spatial domain:
  - one frame has 704 pixels per line in width,
  - one frame has 576 lines per frame in height;
- in the temporal domain:
  - 25 frames is transmitted in 1 second;
- in the data representation:
  - one pixel is composed of 3 color components,
  - one color component has one byte,
  - one byte has 8 bits.

Thus, the data rate of a PAL SDTV video would be,

F. Pan: *Digital Video Coding – Techniques and Standards*, Studies in Computational Intelligence (SCI) **58**, 13–53 (2007)
www.springerlink.com

$$704 \text{ pixel/line} \times 576 \text{ line/frame} \times 8 \text{ bit/byte} \times 3 \text{ byte/pixel} \times 25 \text{ frame/s} = 243.3 \text{ Mbit/s}.$$

A two-hour movie of the above video signal would need 219 Gbytes of storage, which is 51 times the capacity of Digital Versatile Disk (DVD). However, after compression using MPEG-2 video coding standard, the bit rate of this video can be reduced to about 1.5 Mbits/s with no noticeable quality degradations. This is equivalent to an compression ratio of approximately 160. There exists a huge amount of redundancy in the uncompressed video signal.

2.1.1 Redundancies in Digital Video

It is known that there are very strong correlations between pixels, lines and neighboring frames of a video signal. In a typical video signal, most parts of the scenes change very slowly, or are still. This is especially true in the background area. Only the foreground objects may experience large changes. In order to effectively compress the video signal, it is important to understand the various types of redundancies in the video signal.

Statistical Redundancy

Statistical redundancy is related to the similarity, correlation and predictability of data. Digital video signal consists of still images that vary with the time, and each of these images is called a frame. Thus depending on whether it lies inside a frame or in between frames, statistical redundancy can be further classified into spatial redundancy and temporal redundancy.

Spatial Redundancy: Spatial redundancy refers to the similarities within a frame of the video signal. For example, the neighboring pixels in a frame have a similar brightness, color and saturation. Typically we can use run-length coding, predictive coding and/or transform coding to reduce the spatial redundancy.

Temporal Redundancy: Often there are only small changes between adjacent frames within a video sequence. The background may be fixed or only change very slowly while only the objects in the foreground are moving. Even when the camera pans over a scene, the change of the pixels in the scene is uniform and can be predicted. Inter frame prediction and motion compensation are an effective way of removing temporal redundancy.

Coding Redundancy

The processed video data, after predictive coding or transform coding, may show a statistically skewed distribution that can be exploited for further data compression. For example, after predictive coding, the error signal will show a biased distribution where the majority of the prediction errors are either very small or zero. Only a very small portion of the errors are of large amplitude. The error signal can be best compressed using entropy coding such as Huffman coding or arithmetic coding. The coefficients of a block based discrete cosine transform (DCT) have an energy distribution that concentrates on the top left corner of the block, and they are best represented using zigzag scanning that starts from the top left corner.

Psychovisual Redundancy

Psychovisual redundancy refers to the information that can not be perceived by the Human Vision System (HVS) or which the human vision system finds insignificant. For example, the HVS has a limited response to fine spatial detail, and is less sensitive to details near object edges or around shot-changes. Data compression can done in such a way that information that is not perceptible or of less importance is removed.

2.1.2 Evaluation of Coding Effectiveness

The effectiveness of a coding scheme can be measured by the compression ratio. This is defined as the original uncompressed file size divided by the resulting compressed file size. The higher the compression ratio, the smaller the size the compressed video signal. As the compression ratio increases, the reconstructed video signal will have bigger distortions when compared to the original. The coding quality or fidelity decreases in this case.

There are usually three ways of measuring the coding fidelity, (1) Objective Assessment. That is, to numerically compare the pixel values before and after coding; (2) Subjective Assessment, where human observers evaluate the reconstructed video focusing on aesthetic acceptability; (3) Perceptual Metrics. These are computational algorithms that could accurately predict the resulting scores of the subjective assessment. That is by comparison with the human perceptual mechanism.

Objective Assessment

The Mean Square Error (MSE) and the Peak Signal to Noise Ratio (PSNR). These are the two most commonly used objective measurements used to assess the fidelity of the compressed video. This comparison is typically done on a frame-by-frame basis. The MSE is the cumulative squared error between the compressed video frame and the original frame. The PSNR is a measure of the peak error. The MSE and PSNR are defined mathematically as,

$$\mathrm{MSE} = \frac{1}{MN} \sum_{y=0}^{M-1} \sum_{x=0}^{N-1} [I(x,y) - I'(x,y)]^2, \tag{2.1}$$

$$\mathrm{PSNR} = 20 \cdot \log_{10} \frac{255}{\sqrt{\mathrm{MSE}}}, \tag{2.2}$$

where $I(x, y)$ is the original video frame, $I'(x, y)$ is the reconstructed frame and M and N are the dimensions of the video frame. A small value of MSE means lesser error and this translates to a higher value of PSNR. This is a good quality, and a lower value represents poorer quality. Though objective assessment is simple and straight forward, the results do not correlate well with perceived picture quality. For example, similar PSNR in the texture area and the smooth area of an image will exhibit different distortions when perceived by the human eye. The HVS is less sensitive to errors in the texture area than the smooth area.

Subjective Assessment

As the ultimate observer of the compressed video is human being, it is important to use human observers concerning the quality of the video signal. During subjective assessment, a number of non-expert observers are invited to such assess the quality of the video signals. This done after the test video sequences have been shown to them for about 10 to 30 minutes in a controlled environment. These scores cover many aspects, such as blurriness, blocking, frame retention and jerkiness for example. According to the fidelity of the video signal, the score can range between 1 and 5. The value 1 indicates that the impairment is not noticeable. A value of 5 when the impairment is extremely objectionable.

It is noted that subjective assessment reflects the perceptual nature of the video signal under assessment. It is an extremely expensive process. It might not be consistent as human observers are easily affected by the circumstances which include their psychological condition, personal preferences, and viewing condition.

Perceptual Metrics

The aim of developing a perceptual metric for video quality is to find a better prediction for the human perception than the MSE/PSNR measure. There have been substantial research efforts in perceptual visual quality evaluation [1]. These perceptual metrics have a better performance than the traditional MSE/PNSR measure for some specific applications, it is difficult to find a general perceptual metric suitable for all applications. The Video Quality Experts Group (VQEG) [2] has evaluated ten perceptual metrics which have been proposed by different researchers but none of them is statistically better than the PSNR.

2.1.3 Classification of Video Coding Techniques

Many data compression techniques have been developed over the past three decades. Only a few of them are suitable for application in image or video coding. Fig. 2.1 summaries the data compression techniques that are commonly used today. Working independently, none of these data compression techniques can provide significant data compression. However, using the right combination of several techniques, very efficient data compression systems can be made. Several such combinations have been adopted as international standards. The JPEG/JPEG2000 is used for image coding. H.26x, and MPEG are used for video coding.

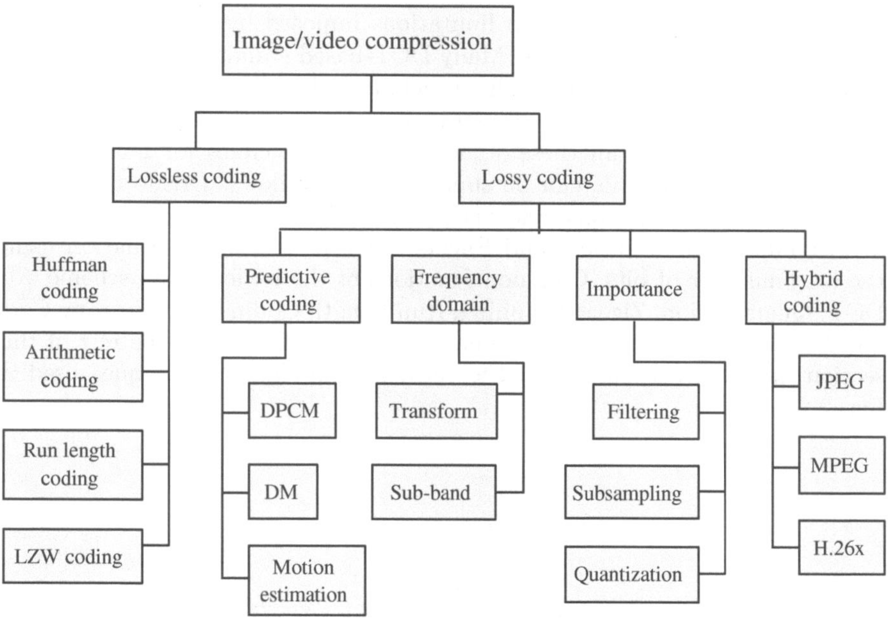

Fig. 2.1. Various image/video coding techniques.

Fig. 2.1 shows the classifications of various image and video coding techniques. If the compression scheme does not cause any information loss, but only reduces the number of bits required to describe the data, it is called Lossless Coding. Lossless Coding is a reversible process. If alternatively, in order to achieve higher compression ratio, it is permissible to have some small distortions or information loss. The scheme is called lossy coding. This is irreversible. In this chapter, the common image/video coding schemes are introduced. These are used for state of art image and video coding standards. Other techniques that are difficult to implement are not described. Examples of such schemes are known as Karhunen-Loéve Transform (KLT), Walsh-Hadamard Transform (WHT), vector quantization, and fractal transform for example. Details of the mathematics of those techniques are omitted. The principles of using them for data compression using these techniques are explained.

2.2 DCT Based Intra Frame Video Coding

A Digital Video Signal consists of a sequence of images. Video Coding has much in common with still image compression. In general, video coding consists of two parts, Still Image Compression Based Intra Coding is used to remove the spatial redundancy within an frame, and motion prediction and compensation based Inter coding is used to remove the Temporal Redundancy.

During the 1980s and 1990s, Discrete Cosine Transform (DCT) [3] which is based coding algorithms and international standards were developed. They alleviate storage and bandwidth limitations imposed by Digital Still Image and Motion Video Applications. Many DCT-based standards are now widely used and accepted worldwide. These include JPEG, H.26x, and MPEG [4]. In addition to being DCT-based, many processing functions and coding principles are common to all these standards. The principles for image coding in most of the standards can be summarized as follows: Divide the picture into 8×8 blocks, Determine relevant picture information, Discard redundant or insignificant information, and Encode relevant picture information using the least number of bits. Common functions of the basic coding scheme are, DCT, Quantization, Zigzag Scanning, Run Length Coding, and Entropy Coding. Fig. 2.2 shows a typical still image compression system. The rest of this section includes a discussion of the various compression techniques used in Fig. 2.2.

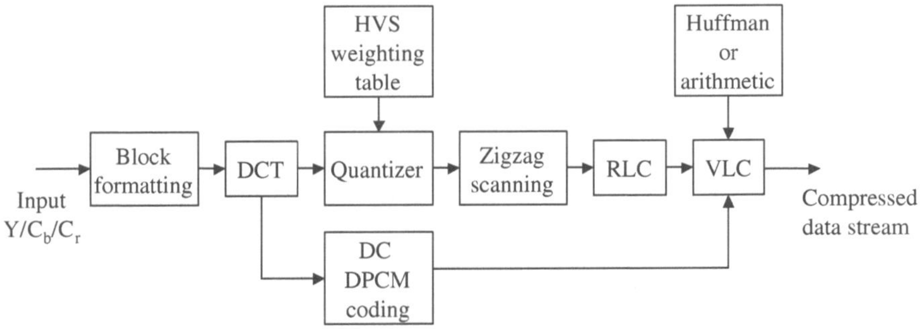

Fig. 2.2. DCT Based Image Compression Process.

2.2.1 Predictive Coding

Predictive coding [5] was known as early as 1955. In a typical image with natural scene, there usually exist many large areas with uniform colors and textures. Although the values of the neighboring pixels are not exactly the same, their differences are small when compared to that of pixel. Big differences only happen along the edges and contribute to only a very small part to the image. The chance of having small values are even higher for pixels that are co-sited in the neighboring frames. Therefore a pixel could be predicted from its neighboring pixels been coded. This is called Intra Predictive Coding. Similarly, due to high temporal redundancy, a pixel or a block of pixels can also be predicted using the pixels of the previous coded frames. This is called Inter predictive coding. Predictive coding reduces the entropy of the signal only and is lossless in principle. Further data reduction can be realized by applying a coarse quantization to the predictive error signal and entropy coding techniques are used to the resulting signal. To avoid transmission error propagation, a full value is transmitted periodically to provide an updated reference.

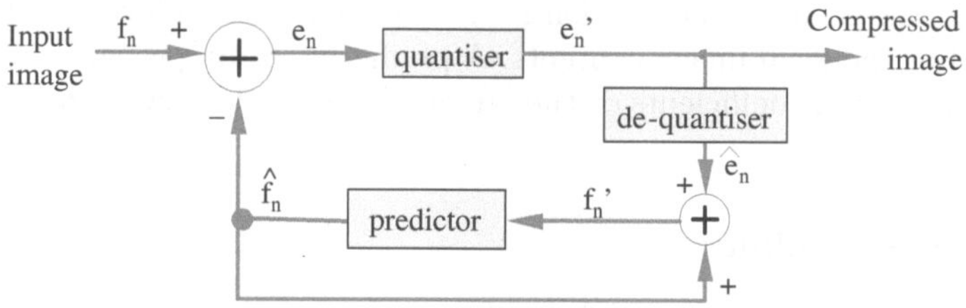

(a) Predictive encoding

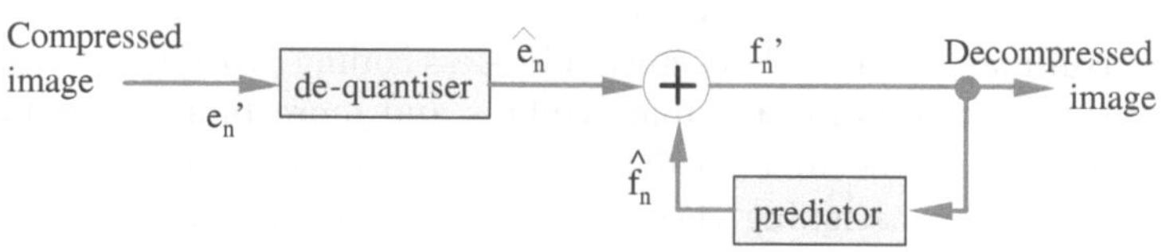

(b) Predictive decoding

Fig. 2.3. Predictive encoder and decoder.

The principle of lossy predictive coding is illustrated in Fig. 2.3. It can be seen that as each successive pixel f_n enters the predicator, it generates the anticipated value of that pixel based on past inputs,

$$\hat{f}_n = Pr(f_{n-1}, f_{n-2}, ..., f_{n-i}). \tag{2.3}$$

The prediction error is given as,

$$e_n = f_n - \hat{f}_n. \tag{2.4}$$

The above error will be quantized as e'_n to further reduce the number of bits used to describe this error signal. The quantization is a process that information loss occurs. We can design a good quantization scheme that only the information that is less important to the HVS will be suppressed.

At the decoder side, only the quantized error information, e'_n, is available. We need to then de-quantize the error, and the reconstructed signal will be,

$$f'_n = \hat{f}_n + \hat{e}_n. \tag{2.5}$$

It can be seen that, by letting $Pr(f_{n-1}, f_{n-2}, ..., f_{n-i}) = f_{n-1}$, Fig. 2.3 becomes the differential pulse code modulation (DPCM). Therefore DPCM is actually the simplified version of the predictive coding, such that it uses the previous pixel value as the prediction for the current one.

The choice of predicator determines the efficiency of the predictive coding. A good predicator will compress the data more effectively. Also we can adaptively adjust the prediction coefficients and the quantization level so that they are tailored to the local image contents. A predictive coding is called adaptive when the prediction coefficients or the quantization levels vary with the image contents.

2.2.2 Huffman Coding

Huffman coding and the arithmetic coding (to be introduced in next section) are both entropy based variable length coding, which can achieve a higher data density than fixed length code if the symbols in the signal source differ in frequency of occurrence. The length of the encoded symbol is inversely proportional to its occurring frequency.

David Huffman [6] in 1954 designed a lossless coding procedure that assigns a shorter bits to the more probable symbols and more bits to less probable symbols. He wasn't the first to discover this, but his paper presented the optimal solution for assigning these codes, which remains the most popular algorithm today and we can find it in many state-of-the-art data compression systems.

Huffman coding involves two steps, the source reduction step following by codeword construction step. During source reduction, we need firstly to sort the symbols in the order of their probability, and combine the probabilities of the lowest two probable symbols to form a parent symbol whose probability is the sum of the two child ones. This process will continue until a reduced source with only 2 parent symbols is achieved. Fig. 2.4 shows an example of Huffman coding. The top diagram shows the source reduction process, while the bottom diagram shows the code assignment process. This diagram is sometimes called a Huffman code tree.

As is in Fig. 2.4, after Huffman coding, the code length of the two least probable symbols Z and Q is 5, while for the most probable symbol S, it is coded with only one bit. We know that for a source of 6 symbols, the average code length should be $\log_2 6 \approx 3$. Using Huffman coding, the average code length for the above example can be calculated as $5 \times (0.01 + 0.02) + 4 \times 0.05 + 3 \times 0.07 + 2 \times 0.38 + 1 \times 0.47 = 1.79$ bits/symbol.

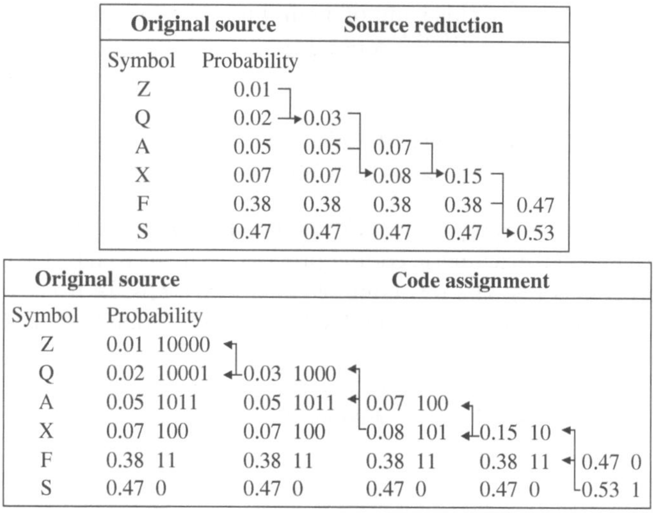

Fig. 2.4. Example of Huffman coding: source reduction and code assignment.

Thus we have achieved a compression ratio of $3/1.79 = 1.676$ without any information loss. It should be pointed out that the efficiency of Huffman coding depends on the source probability distribution. If all the symbols in a source have equal occurrence, the Huffman coding will not achieve any data reduction.

2.2.3 Arithmetic Coding

The problem with Huffman coding lies in the fact that Huffman codes have to be an integral number of bits. For example, if the probability of a character is $1/3$, the optimum number of bits to code that character is assumed to be around 1.6. The Huffman coding scheme has to assign either 1 or 2 bits to the code, and either choice leads to a longer bit length than the ideal ones.

Arithmetic coding was invented by Rissanen [7]. While Huffman coding gives a way of rounding the code words to close integer values and constructing a code with those lengths, arithmetic coding actually manages to encode symbols using non-integer numbers of bits.

In arithmetic coding, an input message of any length is represented as a real number R in the range $0 \leq R < 1$. The longer the message, the more precise is required for the number R. Assume that a signal source has M symbols, its code construction process is listed as follows:

1) Divide the interval $[0, 1)$ into segments corresponding to the M symbols; the segment of each symbol has a length proportional to its probability.
2) Choose the segment of the first symbol in the string message.

3) Divide the segment of this symbol again into M new segments with length proportional to the symbols probabilities.
4) From these new segments, choose the one corresponding to the next symbol in the message.
5) Repeat Steps 3) and 4) until the whole message is coded.
6) Represent the segment's value by a binary fraction.

Following the above steps, Fig. 2.5 has shown a source of five symbols, their probabilities and the arithmetic coding process of the message "CCODE". The decoding process is just the reversing of the above steps. In this example, any value that is between 0.03248 and 0.03280 will be decoded as "CCODE".

Symbol	Probability	Interval
C	0.2	[0, 0.2)
D	0.4	[0.2, 0.6)
A	0.1	[0.6, 0.7)
O	0.2	[0.7, 0.9)
E	0.1	[0.9, 1)

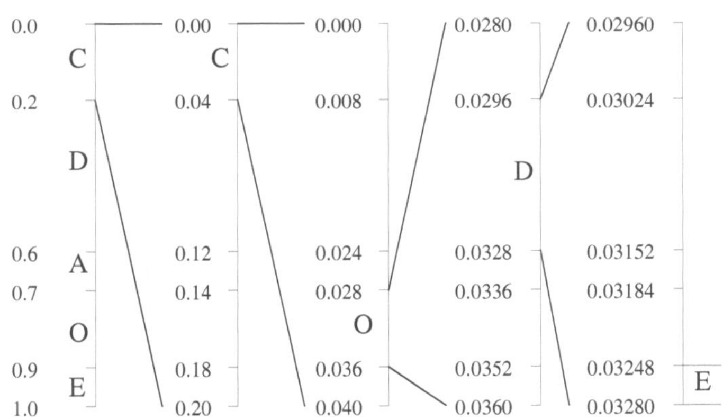

Fig. 2.5. Example of arithmetic decoding.

2.2.4 Discrete Cosine Transform

Transform coding is reversible and linear transform that maps the pixels of image into a set of transform coefficients. For natural images, the energy will be compacted at the low frequency part in the transform domain, and the high frequency coefficients will have very small magnitudes. On the other hand, the HVS is less sensitive to high frequencies thus they can be coarsely quantized or even discarded to achieve data reduction. There are many types of transform coding, such as Karhunen-Loéve Transform (KLT), Discrete Fourier Transform (DFT), Discrete Cosine Transform (DCT) and Walsh-Hadamard Transform (WHT). Compared to the others, DCT provides the good compromise between data reduction, computational complexity and minimizing blocking artifacts. DCT was first applied to image compression by Chen and Pratt [8], and is now widely used in most of image and video coding standards.

The two dimensional DCT is defined as follows,

$$F(u,v) = \frac{2C(u)C(v)}{n} \cdot \sum_{j=0}^{n-1}\sum_{k=0}^{n-1} f(j,k)\cos\left(\frac{(2j+1)u\pi}{2n}\right)\cos\left(\frac{(2k+1)v\pi}{2n}\right), \quad (2.6)$$

$$f(j,k) = \frac{2}{n}\sum_{j=0}^{n-1}\sum_{k=0}^{n-1} C(u)C(v) \cdot F(u,v)\cos\left(\frac{(2j+1)u\pi}{2n}\right)\cos\left(\frac{(2k+1)v\pi}{2n}\right); \quad (2.7)$$

$$C(u),\ C(v) = \begin{cases} \frac{1}{\sqrt{2}} & \text{if } u,v=0, \\ 1 & \text{otherwise;} \end{cases}$$

where $f(i,j), i,j = 0,...,n-1$ are the pixel values in the $n \times n$ image block, and $F(u,v), u,v = 0,...,n-1$ are its corresponding DCT coefficients. Note that Equation (2.6) is the forward transform and Equation (2.7) is the inverse transform. In most of image and video coding applications, $n = 8$. Note also that at $u = 0, v = 0$, Equation (2.6) becomes $F(0,0) = \frac{1}{8}\sum_{j=0}^{7}\sum_{k=0}^{7} f(j,k)$. It is kind of the average of the pixel values in the 8×8 image block, and is thus called the DC coefficient. The rest of $F(u,v)$ are usually referred to as AC coefficients.

It can be seen from Fig. 2.6(b) that most of the DCT coefficients are very small (dark in the image block) and only the lower frequency coefficients are having big amplitudes. The lattice of bright dots are exactly where the DC coefficients and low frequency coefficients locate for each of the 8×8 image blocks. It is also noted that in the areas where the original image have strong edges, bright dots become "brighter", indicating that there is higher entropy in those blocks, or more none zero AC coefficients. Fig. 2.6(c) shows an numerical example of one block of DCT coefficients, whose image block locates at the nose tip of Fig. 2.6(a) (the white block). We can observe that only the top left corner of the block has large values, and the rest of them are all very small.

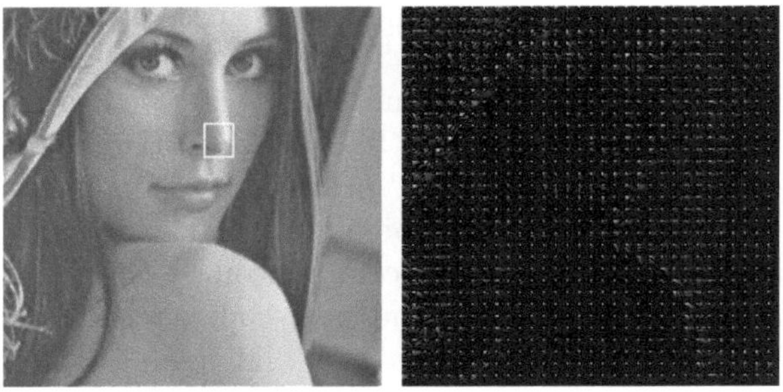

159	177	209	230	222	188	156	156
164	179	203	230	224	198	147	144
158	183	203	228	226	194	143	150
154	179	199	213	217	183	143	151
143	167	193	205	205	153	151	146
127	159	185	200	173	158	149	148
123	134	168	190	172	162	154	145
126	154	190	179	168	159	155	152

(a) Original image (b) 8×8 DCT amplitude image (c) A typical 8×8 block (nose tip)

Fig. 2.6. 8 × 8 block based DCT transform.

2.2.5 Quantization

Theoretically DCT does not result in any data reduction, as the output of DCT transform is still 64 coefficients, and even worse, the DCT coefficients have a larger dynamic range (from −255 to 255) than that of the original pixel values (0 – 255). However, as the HVS is more sensitive to lower frequencies, we can design a quantization scheme such that it has finer quantization steps for the low frequency coefficients, and a very coarse quantization steps for the high frequency coefficients.

Quantization is similar to sub-sampling in that information is discarded. During quantization, the compression is accomplished by reducing the number of bits used to describe each coefficient, rather than reducing the number of coefficients. Each coefficient is reassigned an alternative value and the number of alternate values is less than that in the original coefficients.

364	31	-181	-44	19	-12	4	-3
93	33	-39	23	20	-17	5	-6
-7	-14	7	-1	-9	12	8	-2
-17	-6	4	-11	3	12	-9	2
8	5	7	-8	-2	-6	-3	14
-3	-11	-1	4	4	1	3	-5
6	4	3	-12	-6	-4	0	-3
-2	-3	-3	1	7	3	-5	7

(a) Original DCT coefficients $F(u,v)$

16	11	10	16	24	40	51	61
12	12	14	19	26	58	60	55
14	13	16	24	40	57	69	56
14	17	22	29	51	87	80	62
18	22	37	56	68	109	103	77
24	35	55	64	81	104	113	92
49	64	78	87	103	121	120	101
72	92	95	98	112	100	103	99

(b) JPEG quantization table $Q_{lum}(u,v)$

23	3	-18	-3	1	0	0	0
8	3	-3	1	1	0	0	0
0	-1	0	0	0	0	0	0
-1	0	0	0	0	0	0	0
0	0	0	0	0	0	0	0
0	0	0	0	0	0	0	0
0	0	0	0	0	0	0	0
0	0	0	0	0	0	0	0

(c) Quantized coefficients $F^q(u,v)$

Fig. 2.7. Numerical example of quantization process.

Fig. 2.7 shows an example of original 8×8 DCT coefficients $F(u, v)$ (from Fig. 2.6), the JPEG luminance quantization table $Q_{\text{lum}}(u, v)$, and the quantized coefficients $F^q(u, v)$. Note that in Fig. 2.7, for each coefficient $F(u, v)$, its value is quantized such that $F^q(u, v) = F(u, v)/Q_{\text{lum}}(u, v)$. It is also noted that the design of the quantization table has incorporated the characteristics of the HVS, i.e., the lower frequency coefficients are fine quantized while the higher frequency coefficients are coarsely quantized. Sometimes this type of quantization is called perceptual quantization [9]. Note that it is common that different quantization tables are used for compressing luminance and chrominance separately.

Obviously, quantization is a process of approximation, and a good quantizer is one which represents the original signal with minimum perceptual loss or distortion, and thus achieves good tradeoff between the bit rate and the reconstructed video quality. In video coding, the choice of quantization value helps to regulate the bit rate such that it meets the constraints of the transmission channel. This process is usually called rate control [10].

2.2.6 Zigzag Scanning and Run Length Coding

Fig. 2.7(c) shows a very unique data structure, i.e., all the significant values are concentrated on the top left corner, and the rest are mostly zeros. Therefore we can code the coefficients in the order from low frequency coefficients to high frequency coefficients. This process is called zigzag scanning as shown in Fig. 2.8(a). After zigzag scanning, we will have a sequence of coefficients with a few nonzero in the beginning, following by a long strings of zeros. Fig. 2.8(b) shows the result of zigzag scanning. This sequence is very suitable to be coded using run length coding.

Run length coding takes advantage of the fact that, in many data streams, consecutive single tokens are often identical. In run length coding, repeated occurrence of the same value is called a run, and the number of repetition is called the length of the run. By scanning through the data stream, run length coding checks the stream for repeated occurrence of the same value and its length.

The first value of Fig. 2.8(b), 23, is called the DC coefficient of the DCT transform. It represents the average grey level of the 8×8 image block. This DC value will be coded together with DC values of the previous blocks using DPCM coding to achieve the maximum data reduction. This is based on the assumption that the neighboring blocks in an image will have similar brightness level.

The rest values in Fig. 2.8(b) are all called the AC coefficients of the DCT transform. They are run-length-coded into a number pair (L, R), such that L presents the number of zeros between the current nonzero AC value R and the previous nonzero AC value in the sequence. For example, the first pair in Fig. 2.8(c), $(0, 3)$, indicates that there is no zero between the current nonzero AC value 3, and its preceding DC value 23. Similarly, the third pair

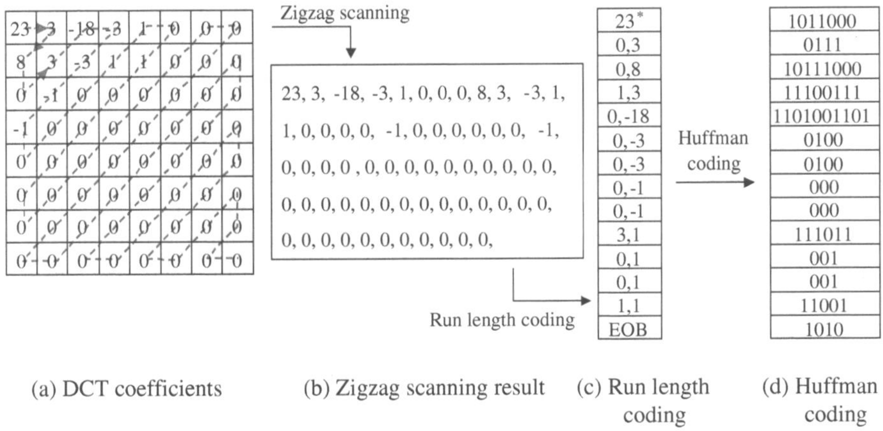

Fig. 2.8. Zigzag scanning, run length scanning and variable length coding.

in Fig. 2.8(c), (1, 3), indicates that there is one zero between the current nonzero AC value 3, and its preceding nonzero AC value 8, and so on. The last symbol, *EOB*, in Fig. 2.8(c), is the acronym of "End of the Block", indicating that there are no nonzero values in the remaining sequence of this 8×8 block. Therefore, by comparing Fig. 2.8(b) and Fig. 2.8(c), we can find that run length coding is quite effective in representing the zigzag scanned DCT coefficients.

In general, the effectiveness of run length coding depends on the number of equal values in a data stream in relation to the total number of input data. Effectiveness degrades when the input does not contain too many equal values. For example, if we apply run length coding directly to the original image block, say, Fig. 2.6(c), the result will then be disastrous as we would actually expand the data instead of compressing it.

2.2.7 Variable Length Coding in Image and Video Coding

After the run length coding, we have many different pairs of $(Length, Run)$, and the occurrences of these run length pairs are not the same. Typically the simpler pairs, such as $(0, 1)$, $(0, -1)$, $(1, 1)$ and $(1, -1)$, appear much often than the others such as $(0, -18)$. Therefore these run length pairs can be effectively compressed by entropy coding, such as Huffman coding or arithmetic coding, as we have explained in Section 2.2.2 and Section 2.2.3.

As we have mentioned previously, arithmetic coding is superior to Huffman coding in terms of speed and efficiency. Unfortunately it is patented and hence has restrictions on its use. Arithmetic coding partly gains its superiority by being "adaptive", i.e. being able to produce probability estimates on the fly. Huffman coding on the other hand is simpler and requires a set of constant probabilities for each of the symbols prior to encoding. Therefore many "old" image and video coding standards use Huffman coding, such as JPEG, H.261/3, and MPEG-1/2, MPEG-4, etc. Arithmetic coding has been used in the standards that are more recently developed, such as JPEG2000, MPEG-4 FGS or H.264.

Although Huffman coding is relatively a simpler scheme, to generate a Huffman code on the fly and send it to the decoder together with the coding results is very time consuming and will need extra bandwidth. Fortunately, in all the coding standards, the Huffman tables are generated off-line and are available for both the encoder and the decoder.

As we have discussed previously, the quantized DCT coefficients have two different types of values, i.e., the DC coefficient and the AC coefficients. The DC coefficient is similar to the average value and as such is likely to be any number within the permitted range. The AC values are likely to be close to zero, with the likelihood of being zero increasing as the coefficients near the end of the coefficient streams. These two types of information are very different so that it is worthwhile separating them and applying different methods of coding to get the optimal coding efficiency. Additionally, the luminance and chrominance components will usually have a very different data statistics, and it usually uses different code tables to be specified for each of the components, though the way to generate these quantization tables are much the same. This means that a total of four Huffman code tables are generally defined in color images or video coding, two for DC coefficients and two for AC coefficients. Obviously, if the image is monochrome, then only two tables would be required (one for DC coefficients and one AC for AC coefficients).

Fig. 2.8(d) shows the Huffman coded results for the run length pairs in Fig. 2.8(c). We can see that for an image block as complicated as in Fig. 2.6(c), we can effectively use 72 bits to describe, (*1011000 0111 10111000 11100111 1101001101 0100 0100 000 000 111011 001 001 11001 1010*). Note that the spaces are only used for readability, and are not needed in actual bit stream. Note also that the total number of bits for describing the original image block is $8 \times 8 \times 8 = 512$. This gives us the compression ratio of $\frac{512}{72} = 7.11$.

The root-mean-square (RMS) error of this image block is approximately 4.3 grey-levels. Its equivalent PSNR is 35.46 dB. The entire image has 256 such blocks, and the overall compression ratio for the entire image is 6.84 : 1 at the PSNR of 35.46 dB. Fig. 2.9 shows a comparison of the original image, the reconstructed image and the error image. It can be seen from these images that at the compression ratio of 6.84, the compressed image has almost the same perceptual quality as the original one. Note also that, in Fig. 2.9(c), the actual coding errors have been amplified 10 times in order to have a visible error image. Without this amplification we can only see a black image as the error is too small to be seen. Also the errors might be positive and negative, and this error image only shows the absolute values. By carefully examining the error image we notice that there are big errors in the high frequency portion of the image, such as the hair, the eyes or along the strong edges.

While in the flat area such as the shoulder or the face, the errors are very small. Therefore the DCT based Intra coding has successfully compressed the image by channelling the distortion to the areas that the human eye is less sensitive and difficult to detect.

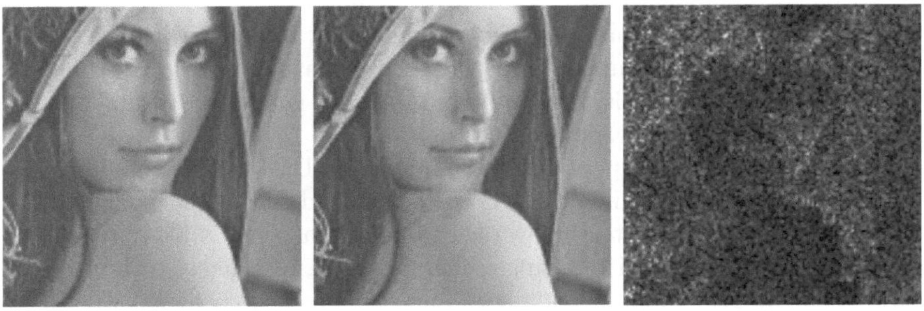

(a) Original image (b) Reconstructedimage (c) Error image

Fig. 2.9. Performance of DCT based image compression.

2.3 Motion Compensation Based Inter Frame Video Coding

Although the basic principles are the same, video can be compressed at a much higher ratio compared to still images, because in a sequence of video frames, little changes can be found between frames. Little change means a lot of redundant information which can be compressed effectively. Therefore video coding typically involve two stages, the Intra coding, which refers to the compression of a still image, as is described in the previous section, and the Inter coding, which reduces the temporal redundancy in between consecutive images in the video. The tools used to remove temporal redundancy is very similar to the predictive coding as is discussed in Section 2.2.1, with the difference that the basic unit for prediction is a macroblock (MB) which is of the size 16×16, and the prediction is based on the neighboring frames rather than inside the same frame.

2.3.1 Frame Difference and Motion Compensated Frame Difference

As is mentioned previously, video coding relies on removing redundancy from the source signal. We have introduced a number of schemes to remove the redundancy from individual images. In this section, we will show that higher compression ratios are only achievable by removing the redundancy that exists in successive images, i.e., to encode a new frame in the video sequence, only information which are different need to be coded and transmitted.

Although the difference between successive frames in a video sequence is small, it will become very large when the video contains fast motion scenes. Therefore to simply code the difference information is normally inefficient. Alternatively, motion estimation will help to locate the MB in the reference frame that is the best match of the current MB. This best matched MB in the reference frame can be used as a prediction of the current MB. The difference between the MB in the current frame and its best matched MB in reference frame is called the motion compensated difference, which forms a low-information-content prediction-error, and is sometimes called the difference along the motion axis. Therefore greater compression ratios are possible as we only need to send the motion vectors and the low-information-content prediction-error. Fig. 2.10 shows the comparison of the frame difference along the time axis and the motioned compensated difference between two consecutive frames in a video sequence "garden". Obviously the difference along the motion axis contains much less energy and can then be much easily compressed using the DCT based Intra coding method as described in previous section.

2.3.2 Block Matching Based Motion Estimation

Different techniques are used to estimate the motion vectors. One method is called block matching, in which a frame is divided into a number of non-overlapping macroblocks (MB) of size 16×16. The selected MB, called current MB, is moved around its position within a search area in the reference frame to find the best match in the reference frame, as shown in Fig. 2.11. The best match means the two MBs have the smallest matching error according to certain matching criteria. A motion vector is then issued, which is defined as the vector that pointing from the coordinate position of the current MB, to the position of its matched MB in the reference frame. The motion vector information forms part of the bit stream and is multiplexed with the motion compensated difference information, which has been Intra coded.

The motion vector is obtained by minimizing a cost function measuring the mismatch between the current MB and the MB in the reference frame. An often used searching criterion is called the mean absolute difference (MAD), which is defined as,

$$\mathrm{MAD} = \frac{1}{16 \times 16} \sum_{i=0}^{15} \sum_{j=0}^{15} \left| f(i,j) - r(i-d_x, j-d_y) \right|, \tag{2.8}$$

where, $-\frac{d_{\max}}{2} < d_x,\ d_y < \frac{d_{\max}}{2}$, $f(i,j)$ is the pixel in current frame, $r(i,j)$ is that in the reference frame, and $d_{\max}$ is the maximum searching displacement horizontally or vertically. For practical algorithms, it is often not necessary

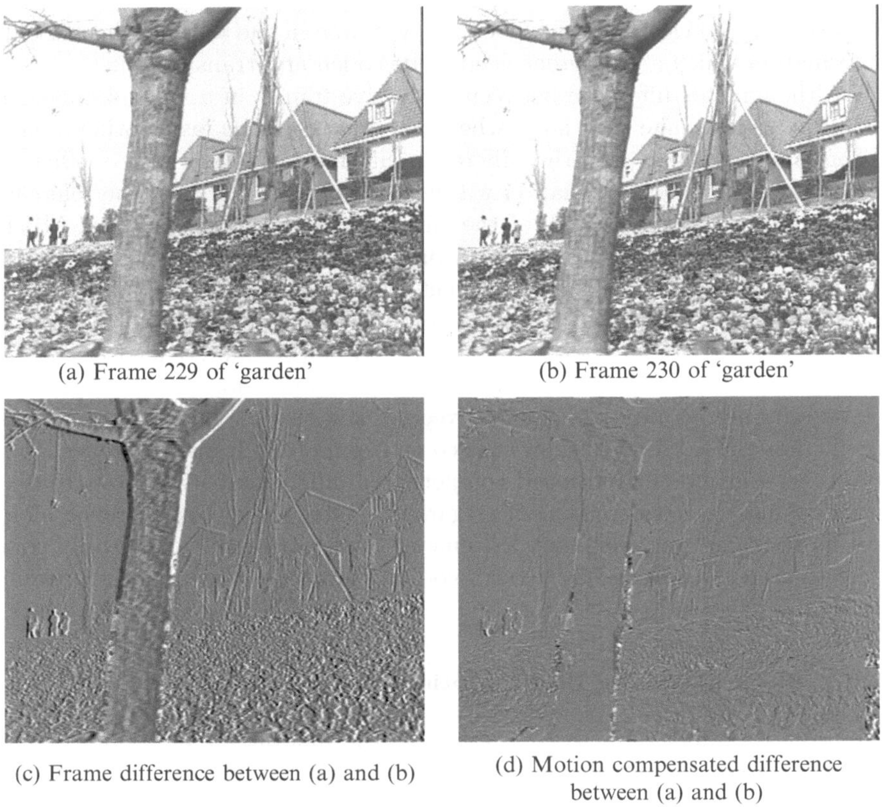

(a) Frame 229 of 'garden'

(b) Frame 230 of 'garden'

(c) Frame difference between (a) and (b)

(d) Motion compensated difference between (a) and (b)

Fig. 2.10. Frame difference and motion compensated frame difference.

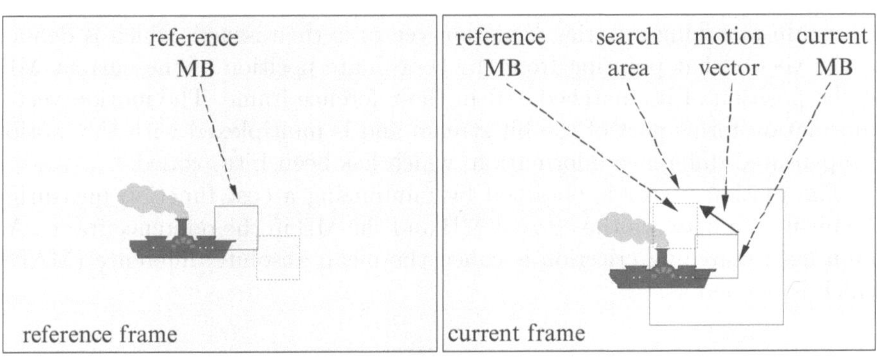

Fig. 2.11. Principle of motion estimation.

to compute the average difference as the block size is always fixed. Instead, we use sum of absolute difference (SAD), which is the same as Equation (2.8) without dividing 16×16.

The search area is defined around an MB in the current frame to cover any motion between successive frames. The full search motion estimation algorithm is the most straightforward block-matching algorithm, which can give the optimal estimation in terms of minimizing matching error by checking all candidates one by one. However, for a search area of 32×32 pixels, the total number of pixel to pixel comparison would be $(2 \times 8 + 1)^2 \times 16^2 = 73984$. For a 30 Hz SDTV format of video signal, we need to perform $704 \times 576 \times 25/16/16 = 39600$ block based motion estimations in a single second – this is equivalent to $73984 \times 39600 = 2.93$ billion pixel to pixel comparisons in one second. Therefore full search motion estimation is a very expensive process.

Numerous efforts have been made to find fast block-matching algorithms. Most of these methods assume that in the video sequence, objects move in translation in a plane parallel to camera plane, illumination is spatially and temporally uniform, and occlusion among objects are neglected. Fast motion estimation algorithms use different block-matching strategies and search patterns with various sizes and shapes, such as two dimensional logarithmic search [11], three-step search [12], four-step search [13], diamond search [14] and hexagon-based search [15], etc.

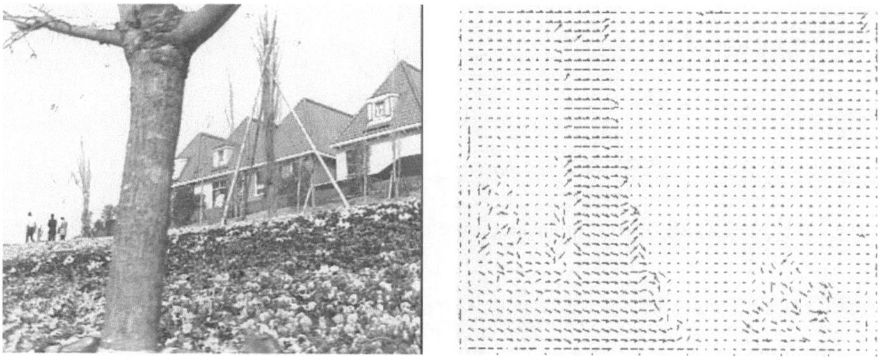

(a) Frame 229 of 'garden'   (b) Motion vectors for each MB

Fig. 2.12. Example of motion vectors.

Fig. 2.12 shows the 229th frame of sequence "garden" and its motion vectors. It can be seen from this figure that the motion vectors are usually very small, and are uniform in most of the area. Therefore it can be further compressed using DPCM coding following by entropy coding.

2.3.3 Motion Compensation

During the motion estimation, matched MB in the reference frame is used as a prediction of the current MB, and their difference forms a low-information-content prediction-error block. This prediction error will be compressed the same way as the DCT based Intra coding. Its corresponding motion vector is further compressed using DPCM coding. Both the motion vector and the prediction error are sent to the decoder, see Fig. 2.13(a). In the decoder, the motion vector is then used to decide the displacement in the reference frame, and the displaced MB in the reference frame will be extracted and used as the prediction for the current MB. In the meantime, the prediction error is Intra decoded, and added to the predicted MB to reconstruct the final MB. Fig. 2.13(b) shows the process of motion compensated decoding.

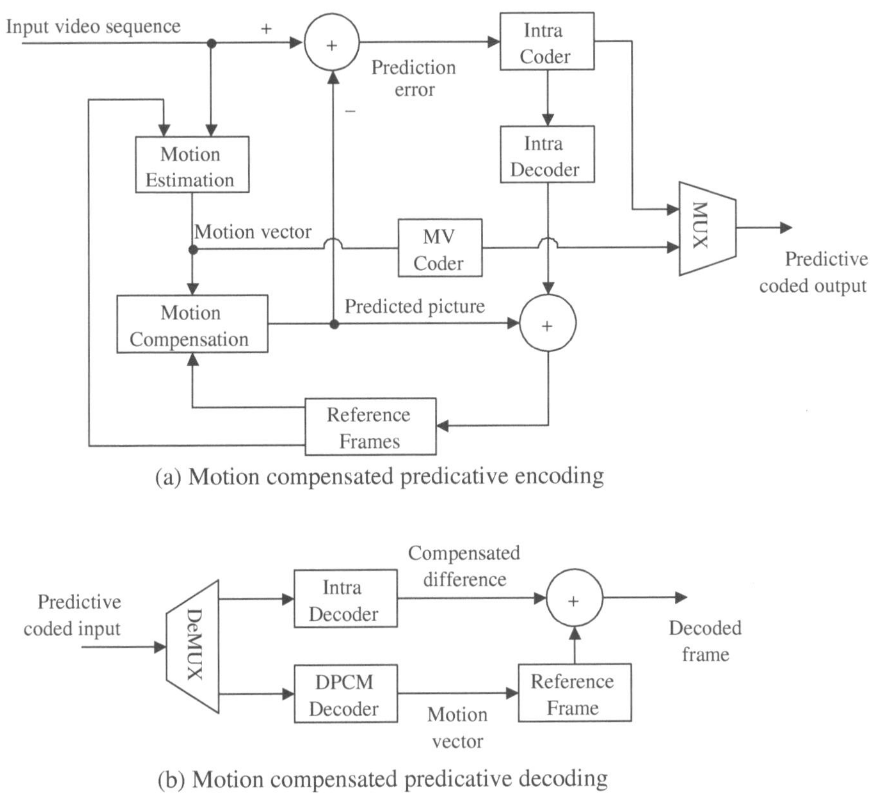

Fig. 2.13. Motion compensated predicative encoding and decoding.

2.3.4 Forward Prediction and Bi-Directional Prediction

Motion compensated prediction based on the past frame is basically unidirectional and is thus called forward prediction. Such predicted frames are designated as P-frames. Compared to Intra coded frames (I-frames), P-frames allow a higher data compression.

However, when an object moves, it conceals the background at its leading edge and reveals the background at its trailing edge. The newly revealed background will not have reference in previous frame. Similarly, when the camera pans, new areas come into view and nothing is known about them previously. Instead, we can find their reference in the frames after it, i.e., its future frames. This is possible if the frames are reordered and transmitted so that the future frames are received before the current frame. This type of prediction based on future and past frames is called bi-directional predictive coding.

Bi-directional predictive coding allows the current frame to be predicted from frames before and after the current frame, which are then interpolated to form the prediction for the current frame. The frame generated from bi-directional predictive coding is called the B-frame. B-frames can also be compressed through a prediction derived from a previous frame or a future frame alone. Similar to P-frames, the prediction error of the B-frame is further compressed by DCT based Intra coding. Fig. 2.14 shows the diagram of forward predictive coding (P-frame) and bi-directional predictive coding (B-frame).

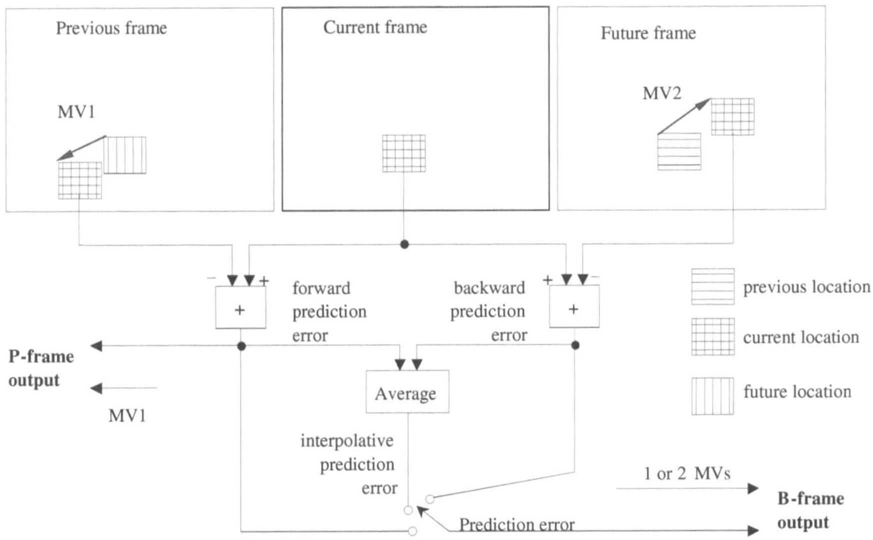

Fig. 2.14. Forward predictive coding and bi-directional predictive coding.

The advantages of bi-directional prediction are

- B-frames use much less data bits than P-frames.
- B-frames have less noise, which is the result of averaging between previous and future frames.
- Newly panned or uncovered area can be accurately predicted from the future reference frame.

2.4 Overview of Video Coding System

There are two main techniques used in all the video coding systems, i.e., the DCT based Intra frame data compression technique to remove the spatial redundancy in an image frame, as is described in Section 2.2, and the motion compensated prediction based Inter frame data compression to remove the temporal redundancy in between successive frames, as is described in Section 2.3. In this section we will introduce the architecture of the video coding system, and the coding and decoding process of various types of pictures.

2.4.1 Video Bitstream Hierarchy

The video coding standard is primarily a specification of bitstream semantics. The video bitstream is usually arranged in layers, each corresponds to a hierarchy, as is shown in Fig. 2.15. The functions of each of the hierarchy are very useful as are explained in the following:

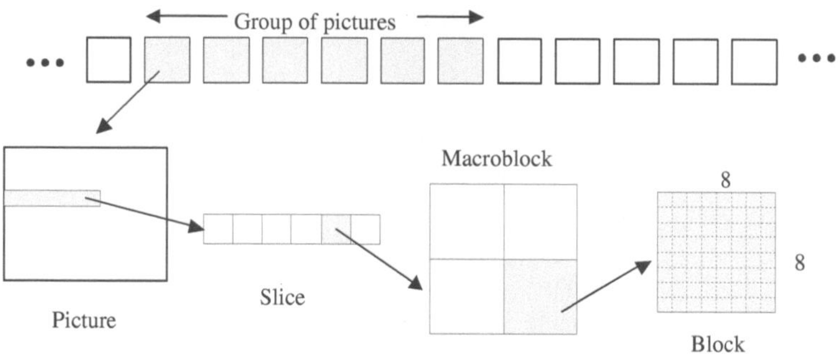

Fig. 2.15. Video bitstream hierarchy.

Video sequence: This is the highest layer which defines the context valid for the whole sequence. A video sequence consists of sequence header, the number of group of pictures (GOP), and end-of-sequence code. The sequence header initializes the state of the decoder. This allows a decoder to decode any sequence without being affected by past decoding history.

Group of pictures (GOP): A GOP consists of a series of one or more pictures intended to allow random access into the sequence. A GOP always starts with an I-picture.

Picture: The picture is the primary coding unit of the video sequence which consists of 3 rectangular matrices representing one luminance (Y) and two chrominance (C_b and C_r) components.

Slice: A slice is the layer for Intra frame addressing and (re)synchronization. It consists of one or more contiguous macroblocks. Slices should have the similar amount of data.

Macroblock (MB): A typical MB contains four Y blocks, one or two C_b and C_r blocks depending on whether it is 4:2:0 or 4:2:2 sub-sampled. MB is the basic unit for motion prediction and compensation.

blocks: A block is an 8×8 pixel section of luminance or chrominance components. It is the basic unit for DCT based Intra frame coding.

2.4.2 Picture Types

Most of video coding standards have three main picture types, and they are,

I-Picture: These are Intra coded picture, which means they are coded independent of any other pictures. All the MBs in an I-picture are Intra coded using DCT plus quantization plus zigzag scanning and run length coding followed by VLC coding.

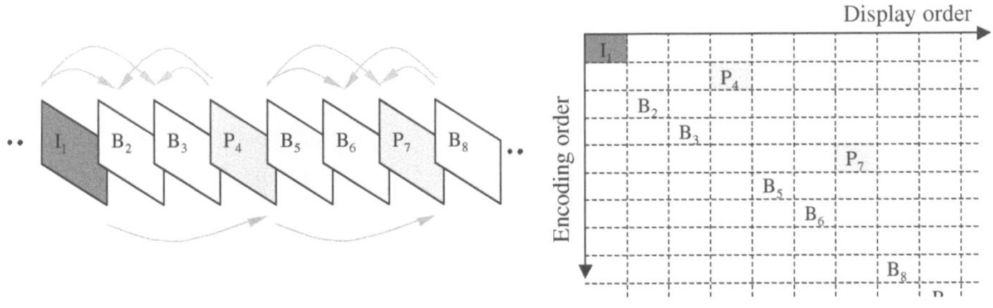

(a) MPEG picture structure (b) Encoding ord er and display order

Fig. 2.16. Picture types and their encoding/display order.

P-Picture: These are forward predicted pictures and are coded using motion compensation from previous I- or P-pictures. MBs in P-picture are mostly coded using forward predictive motion compensation. However if a good match can not be found in reference frame, it will be Intra coded.

B-Picture: These are the bi-directional predicted pictures, which are coded by interpolating between a previous and a future I- or P-picture. In a B-picture, there could be three different types of MBs, including B-block, P-block, and I-block. The default is B-block. If an MB can not find good reference in previous and future frames simultaneously, it will be coded using forward or backward predictive coding only. An Intra coding will be used if good match can not be found in either previous or future frames.

Fig. 2.16(a) shows the structure of the three picture types in an MPEG bitstream. Since B-pictures depend on the prediction based on the preceding and future I- or P-pictures, the future frame must be available before a current B-picture can be (de)coded. For this reason, the display order and coding order in an MPEG video sequence must be different, as is shown in Fig. 2.16(b). According to Fig. 2.16(b), the display order and coding order of a typical IBBPBB$\cdots$ coding can be listed in the following,

Display order: I_1, B_2, B_3, P_4, B_5, B_6, P_7, B_8, $\cdots$

Coding order: I_1, P_4, B_2, B_3, P_7, B_5, B_6, B_{10}, $\cdots$

2.4.3 Variable Data Rate and Rate Control

The number of bits produced for each frame vary with the type of pictures it is used. For example, I-frame requires most number of bits while B-frame requires the least. On the other hand, the complexity of the scene in the video signal can change dramatically over time, which results in significant changes in the resulting data bits. Therefore the bit rate of a video stream will not be constant but fluctuating. However, in some applications, such as broadcasting, the transmission bandwidth is fixed. Therefore it is necessary to control the output bit rate so that it will neither overflow nor underflow. Overflow means some of the data bits can not be transmitted, which results in data loss; On the other hand, underflow means that the resource (which is usually scarce in video coding) is not fully utilized.

In order to control the bit rate of the video stream, the encoded bitstream is buffered and the data are read out from the buffer at the required bit rate according to the channel requirement. The fullness of the buffer can used to control the quantization step in the encoder. For example, an increase in scene activity will result in the buffer filling up. In order to reduce the buffer fullness, we can increase the quantization step in the encoder, so as to reduce the output bit rate. On the other hand, if the buffer starts to empty, the quantization step should be reduced so that the output bit rate will increase. The compression ratio, as well as the coding quality, can vary considerably depending on the spatial complexity and the amount of motion in the video. A relatively simple and "static" scene leads to low compression ratio and high quality, and highly textured and "active" scene leads to high compression ratio and lower quality. If the quantization level is too coarse, it may result in significant coding artefact that is visually annoying [16].

In general, the quality of the frames used as references must be very good to prevent the errors from propagating to other frames in a GOP. For this reason, it is preferable to allocate more bits to I- and P-frames. Few bits are allocated to B-frames because they are not used as a reference frame and cannot spread errors to other frames. Furthermore, B-frames benefit from more extensive motion-compensation tactics and therefore naturally consume least amount of data bits.

Depending on the applications, rate control [10] can be implemented at frame level, slice level, MB level and even video object level. The lower level it goes, the more complicated the algorithm will be.

2.4.4 Video Encoder and Decoder

Fig. 2.17 shows the block diagram of a video encoder and video decoder. The encoding and decoding of the I-, P- and B-frames are explained as follows:

The first frame in the GOP will always be Intra coded. During Intra coding all the switches except K_2 are switched off, and each block of the I-frame is directly DCT transformed, quantized, zigzag scanned, run length coded and variable length coded as we described in Fig. 2.2. The Intra coded frame is also Intra decoded immediately, and is then stored as "previous frames" which will be used as the reference frame for predictive coding of P-frames and B-frames.

After the I-frame is coded, if there are B-frames, their encoding will be delayed until the following P-frame is coded as the encoding of B-frame depends on its future I- or P-frame. When encoding a P-frame, the switches are all switched on. An MB of the P-frame is motion estimated by searching on the reference frames (The previous I- or P-frame) to obtain motion vectors. The motion compensator then shift MB in the reference frame according to the motion vectors to get the predicted MB. This motion compensated MB is subtracted from the actual P-frame to produce the motion compensated error, which is also Intra coded. The motion vector for this MB is DPCM coded and variable length coded, which is eventually multiplexed with the prediction error information to form the bitstream of a P-block. As P-frame is also used as reference frame for predictive coding of other P-frames and B-frames, the P-frame will also be decoded and stored as "previous frames".

The encoder now starts encoding the B-frames that were skipped previously when the P-frame was coded. At this time K_2 and K_5 are switched off while the others are switched on as B-frame will not be used as reference frame. The motion estimator operates twice and calculates forward vectors from the previous I- or P-frame and backward vectors from the future I- or P-frame. These are used by the motion compensator to create three predicted frames: forward, backward, and interpolated. The input B-frame is subtracted from these predicted frames to form the prediction error, which will be Intra coded as before. The motion vector for this MB is, as in the P-block, also multiplexed with the error information to form the bitstream of the B-frame.

The output buffer is used as the data meter to monitor data flow out of the encoder. If the buffer is very full and is in danger of overflowing, the quantizer will increase its step size to reduce the data rate. If the buffer dries up, the quantizer will decrease its step size to increase the data rate. The quantization parameters will also be embedded into the output bitstream so the decoder knows which quantization parameters to choose.

To decode an I-frame, the switch K_6 and K_7 are both off. So an I-picture is simply variable length decoded, de-quantized and Inverse DCT transformed. This I-frame will need to be stored as the reference frames for decoding of following P- and B-frames.

To decode a P-frame, the switch K_6 is on but K_7 is off. The motion vector is de-multiplexed and used by the motion compensator to get motion compensated MB in the reference frame. The incoming prediction error is Intra decoded and added to the motion compensated MB to reconstruct the P-block. The P-frame also is stored as the reference for decoding of other P- and B-frames.

The decoding of the B-frame is very similar to that of P-frame. The motion vector is de-multiplexed and used to fetch the reference MB from the I- or P-frames to create the predicted MB. The prediction-error are decoded and added to the predicted MB to reconstruct the B-frame.

2.5 Overview of Video Coding Standards

Video communication is greatly dependent on good standards. The presence of standards allows for a larger volume of information exchange using a universal language that is understood by all parties, thereby benefiting the equipment

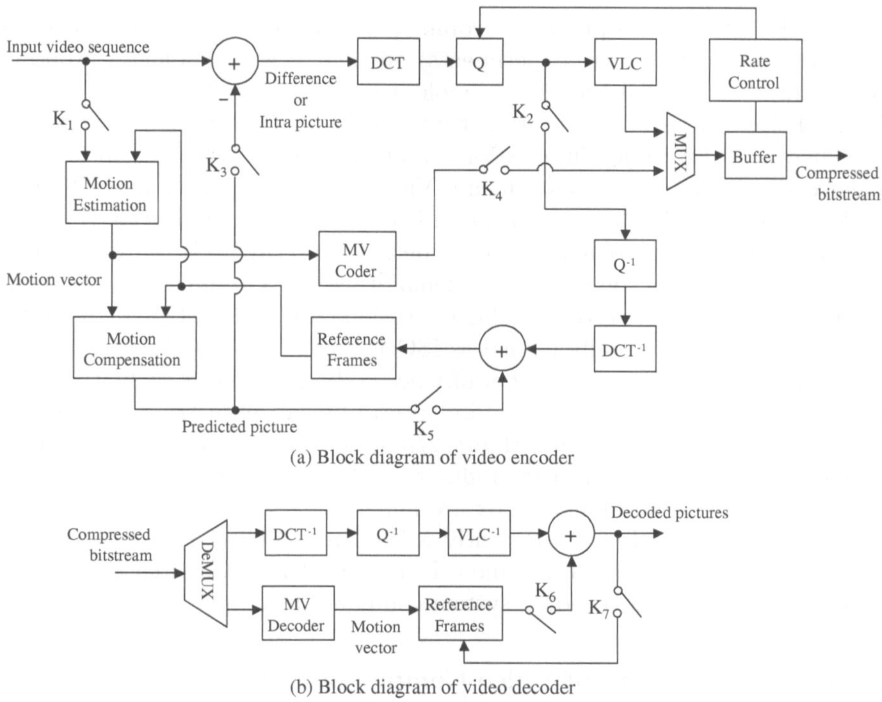

Fig. 2.17. Block diagram of the generic video encoder and decoder.

manufacturers, service providers and the customers. Standards are the universal language that the different parties can communicate with one another.

In general, a video coding standard have two separate parts, the normative parts and the non-normative parts. The normative parts must be implemented as directed. The non-normative parts are recommendations or suggestions outside of the standard, but are helpful in implementing the standard. In many video coding standards, only the bit stream syntax (semantics) is the normative part of the standard, which specifies the requirements related to the process of decoding a bit stream encoded by that standard. The encoding part is always non-normative and it doesn't address, therefore, the methods and techniques required for encoding a video sequence. A standard with normative decoding and informative encoding is usually called an open standard. The open standard has the advantage of allowing for continuous improvements in encoding techniques. It is possible that newly invented technologies can be used to encode the video signal with better coding quality or efficiency even after the standard has been finalized long ago.

Although the standard does not specify how an encoder or a decoder should be designed, it does provide the simulation software that consists of a software decoder and encoder. This software is usually called the verification model or test model. It aims to provide a common platform for different parties to conduct experiments (core experiments) on their new technologies proposed to the standard, so that the best technology can be adopted into the standard. It also helps interested parties to get quickly familiarized to the standards.

There are two major international standard bodies working on creating video coding standards. One of them is Video Coding Experts Group (VCEG) under International Telecommunication Union – Telecommunication (ITU-T), and the other is The Moving Picture Experts Group (MPEG), a group formed under the auspices of the the International Standards Organization (ISO) and the International Electro-technical Commission (IEC). The MPEG committee for video coding is formally named as ISO-IEC/JTC1/SC29/WG11.

MPEG has developed a number of video coding standards such as MPEG-1/2/4, with applications mainly in entertainment industry and Internet streaming. On the other hand, H.261/2/3 are developed by VCEG for applications mainly in communication industry such as video conferencing or video telephony. Strictly speaking, H.26x are not international standards but only recommendations of ITU-T. Recently MPEG and VCEG have been jointly developed a new video coding standard called H.264/AVC, witch is a simpler and much efficient video coding system compared to its predecessors.

2.5.1 A Brief History of Video Compression Standard

The history of video compression can trace back as early as 1940s when the analog television [17] was first designed, which used many elegant compression techniques to reduce the signal bandwidth. For example, the use of interlaced scanning has actually reduced half of the signal bandwidth compared to sequential scanning; the bandwidth of the color component is only one quarter of that of the luminance; the two color difference signals are modulated on two subcarrier which are of the same frequencies but orthogonal to each other; the modulated color subcarrier is frequency interleaved with the luminance signal so that it did not occupy extra bandwidth, etc.

The first digital video coding standards started in 1982 when the COST211 video codec, based on DPCM coding was standardized by CCITT (now called ITU-T), under the H.120 standard. The H.120 codec's target bit rate is 2 Mbit/s for PAL system and 1.544 Mbit/s for NTSC system. However, the video quality, although having very good spatial resolution, has a very poor temporal quality. It was soon realized that in order to improve the picture quality without exceeding the target bit rate, less than one bit should be used to code each pixel. This is only possible if a group of pixels are coded together, such that the bit per pixel is fractional. This led to the design of so-called block-based video coding, and one of the first block-based video coding standards is H.261.

2.5.2 H.261

During the late 1980s study period, of the 15 block based videoconferencing proposals submitted to the ITU-T, 14 were based on the Discrete Cosine Transform (DCT) and only one on Vector Quantization (VQ). In the late 1980s it was clear that the combination of Inter frame predictive coding and the Intra frame DCT based coding greatly improved picture quality over H.120. This effort led to the first practical digital video coding standard. The H.261 [18] design was a pioneering effort, laid the framework for all subsequent international video coding standards (MPEG-1/2/4, H.262/3/4). H.261 video coding standard was designed and optimized for low target bit rate applications suitable for transmission of color video over ISDN at $p \times 64$ kbits/s with low delay; here p specifies an integer with values between 1 and 30, This allows the transmission of H.261 video over more than one ISDN channel. H.261 uses DCT based Intra frame coding to removes the spatial redundancy, and motion compensation based Inter frame coding to remove the temporal redundancy. Other details of the standards are listed in the following.

- Frame formats are CCIR 601 CIF (352×288) and QCIF (176×144).
- A macroblock spans a 16×16 pixel area with 4 Y blocks and one C_r block and one C_b block., so the video is $4:1:1$ sub-sampled.
- I-frames use 8×8 DCT transform followed by entropy coding.
- P-frames use motion compensated predictive coding. The reference frame is always the previous I-frame.
- No bi-directional predictive coding
- A uniform quantization is used instead of using a quantization table.

From the above list we can see clearly that almost all the techniques used in H.261 can be found in late standards in one way or another. The continuous efforts in improving coding efficiency have resulted in significant improvements in coding efficiency, and a new standard, H.263, has been created. H.263 retains most of the functions the H.261 has, and is backward-compatible to it. This makes the H.261 essentially obsolete. H.261 is a major historical milestone in the development of video coding standards.

2.5.3 MPEG-1

The ISO/IEC Moving Picture Experts Group (MPEG) was formed in 1988. Its first video coding standard, MPEG-1 [19] was originally designed for typical applications using non-interlaced video PAL system and NTSC system for video quality comparable to that of Video Home System (VHS). The bit rate ranges from 1.2 to 1.5 Mbits/s, which was the maximum data rate of the CD-ROM at that time. Besides the multimedia CD-ROM applications, it is also a popular video format on the Internet in early days. In addition, MPEG-1 is the standard of the video coding in Video CD, which is the most popular video distribution format throughout Asia after VHS video cassette.

The work of MPEG-1 started in May 1988, and was adopted as the international standards in 1993. MPEG-1 consists of the following five parts,

- ISO/IEC 11172–1, System, defines how multiple video and audio streams can be multiplexed into one stream, and how synchronous playback can be realized.
- ISO/IEC 11172–2, Video, compression standard.
- ISO/IEC 11172–3, Audio, compression standard. Level 3 of MPEG-1 audio is the most popular standard for digital compression of audio known as MP3.
- ISO/IEC 11172–4, Conformance testing, defines procedures to test validity of bitstreams and compliance of decoders to the standard.
- ISO/IEC 11172–5, Software simulation, consists of a software decoder and an encoder, that helps interested parties to get quickly accustomed to MPEG Video and Audio.

Similar to H.261, MPEG-1 uses DCT based Intra frame coding to remove the spatial redundancy, and motion compensation based Inter frame coding to remove the temporal redundancy. It allows forward, backward, and interpolative predictions. The motion vectors will typically have the precision of half pixel.

Constraint Parameter Set

MPEG-1 has recommended a constraint parameter set that the MPEG-1 compatible decoder must be able to support. The main purpose of having this set of restrictions is to make sure that the decoder should be designed in a way that it is competitive in terms of cost, and will not be easily put out of the market. It should be noted that by no means the application of MPEG-1 is limited to this constraint parameter set.

Parameters	**CPS**	**PAL(SIF)**	**NTSC**
Horizontal size (pixel)	720	352, 176	352, 176
vertical Size (pixel)	576	288, 144	240, 120
total # of MBs/pic	396	396	330
total # of MBs/sec	9900	9900	9900
picture rate	30	25	30
bit rate (Mbps)	1.86	1.5	1.5
decoder buffer (bits)	376832	–	–

MPEG-1 for Video CD

One of the most successful applications of MPEG-1 is its use in Video CD, a requirement to shoehorn moving pictures into the data rate of a normal "White Book" Compact Disc player. In order to meet the desperately low bit rate allowed, MPEG-1 has not only to eliminate redundancy but also to eliminate a fair amount of information as well. The source entropy is reduced by sub-sampling in all three dimensions.

The following steps show an example of how an ITU R-601, 4:2:2 PAL component video input can be converted to a format that is suitable for storage in Video CD using MPEG-1 video coding,

- Discarding every other field. This results in a progressive scan system with a frame rate of 25 or 30 Hz. It also halves the data rate and neatly circumvents interlace handling. It halves the vertical resolution of the video frames.
- The horizontal resolution is halved by sub-sampling to 352 luminance pixels per line.
- The chroma signals are sub-sampled horizontally so that there are 176 pixels per line.
- The chroma signals are also sub-sampled vertically so that on alternate lines there are no chroma pixels. This is so-called 2:1:0 coding. This preprocessing produces what is known as the Source Input Format (SIF).

Beside reducing the resolution, discarding every other field damages the motion portrayal ability of the system and makes it the same as the motion picture film. Thus the common claim that MPEG-1 offers VHS quality is not really true.

2.5.4 MPEG-2

Following the success of MPEG-1, MPEG-2 [20] aims to provide a generic coding method for high quality moving pictures and associated audio. The target applications are CCIR 601 TV and HDTV. The MPEG-2 core algorithm is still a hybrid DCT/motion compensation scheme which is backward compatible to MPEG-1 and can be considered as the superset of MPEG-1. This is the first joint work between MPEG and VCEG. Therefore MPEG-2 can also be called as H.262. Similar to MPEG-1, MPEG-2 has achieved tremendous success in the application of digital versatile disk (DVD) and digital television broadcasting.

In order to support a diverse range of applications, MPEG-2 integrated many different algorithmic "tools" into the full standard. To implement all the features of the standard in all decoders is unnecessarily complex and costly, so a small number of subsets of the full standard, known as profiles and levels, have been defined. Besides the profiles and levels, MPEG-2 introduced a number of other extension compared to MPEG-1, those include interlaced coding, different zigzag scan patterns, and spatial, temporal and SNR scalability, etc.

MPEG-2 Profiles and Levels

MPEG-2 is designed to support a wide range of applications and services of varying bit rate, resolution, and quality. MPEG-2 standard defines 4 profiles and 4 levels for ensuring inter-operability of these applications. The profile defines the color space, resolution, and scalability of the bitstream. The levels define the range of frame resolution, luminance sample rate, the number of video and audio layers supported for scalable profiles, and the maximum bit rate per profile. The following table shows the MPEG-2 Profiles and Levels.

	Simple Profile	Main Profile	SNR Profile	Spatial Profile	High Profile
	no B pictures				spatial or SNR
High Level $1920 \times 1080 \times 30$ $1920 \times 1152 \times 25$		≤ 80			≤ 100 Mbps
High-1440 $1440 \times 1080 \times 30$ $1440 \times 1152 \times 25$		≤ 60		≤ 60	≤ 80 Mbps
Main $704 \times 480 \times 30$ $704 \times 576 \times 25$	≤ 15	≤ 15	≤ 15		≤ 20 Mbps
Low $352 \times 240 \times 30$ $352 \times 288 \times 25$	≤ 15	≤ 4	≤ 4		≤ 20 Mbps

MPEG-2 Scalability

Scalable video is only available on Main and higher profile. Currently there are four scalable modes, and these are,

Spatial Scalability: The spatial scalability codes a base layer at lower resolution, and the up-sampled reconstructed base layers are then used as prediction for the enhancement layers.

Data Partitioning: Data partitioning is a frequency domain method that breaks the block of 64 DCT quantized transform coefficients into two partitions. The first, higher priority partition forms the base layer, which contains the header information, motion vectors and more critical lower frequency coefficients. The lower priority partition is in the enhancement layer that carries higher frequency AC data.

SNR Scalability: SNR scalability is a spatial domain method where the base layer uses coarse quantization, and the prediction errors will be further quantized and VLC coded to form the enhancement layer. The enhancement layer is used to refine the base layer to construct a higher quality picture.

Temporal Scalability: The base layer codes video at a lower frame rate, and the intermediate frames can be coded in the enhancement layer using the base layer information as reference for prediction.

Theoretically there can be as many enhancement layers as possible, each refines the previous layer to achieve an improved video quality. However, multi-layer scalability results in heavy overheads and thus reduces the coding efficiency compared to non-scalable video. Therefore only two layers (base layer and enhancement layer) are usually used in MPEG-2 scalable video coding.

MPEG-2 Interlaced Coding

MPEG-2 supports both progressive scanning and interlaced scanning. Interlaced scanning is the scanning method used in the analogue television systems where odd lines of a frame are scanned first as one field (odd field), and even lines (field) are then scanned after the odd field.

An interlaced video coding can use two different picture structures: frame structure and field structure. In the frame structure, lines of two fields are coded together as a frame, the same way as in sequential scanning. One picture header is used for two fields. In the field structure, the two fields of a frame are coded independently, and the odd field is followed by the even field. However cross field predictive coding is possible as the two fields can be treated as two independent frames. The interlaced video sequence can switch between frame structure and field structure on a picture-by-pictures basics.

Alternate Zigzag Scanning

In interlaced scanning, adjacent scan lines come from different fields, and vertical resolution is reduced when there is motion in the scene. Therefore the frequency distribution of the DCT coefficients will have different pattern as is the case of non-interlaced video. A new zigzag scanning is designed to optimize the coding efficiency of the interlaced video, so as to make sure that the lower frequency coefficients will be scanned first.

Other Extensions of MPEG-2

MPEG-2 provides error concealment tools for the decoder in the case of packet loss during transmission. There are a number of ways to conceal errors due to packet loss, such as spatial neighborhood block averaging, temporal neighborhood block averaging, and temporal motion vectors averaging.

Another extension of MPEG-2 is the use of variable bit rate coding (VBR), which allows encoder to adjust the bit rate or quality level based on the spatial and temporal complexity of each video segment. More complicated video segments require more bits to code, and less complicated video segments can be coded using a lower bit rate. Variable bit rate coding is an important advancement in video/audio encoding technology, which has found good success in Super Video CD.

2.5.5 H.263

H.263 [21] was defined by ITU-T) as the next generation video coding for picture phones over analog subscriber lines. It has overtaken H.261 as dominant video-conferencing coding technique. The activities of H.263 started around November 1993, and the standard was adopted in March 1996. The main goal of this endeavor was to design a video coding standard suitable for applications with bit rates below 64 kbits/s (the so-called very-low bit-rate applications). During the development of H.263, it was identified that the near-term goal would be to enhance H.261 using the same framework, and the long-term goal would be to design a video coding standard that may be fundamentally different from H.261 in order to achieve further improvement in coding efficiency. As the standardization activities move along, a number of different versions of H.263 emerge, and they are named H.263+ (January 1998), and H.263++ or H.263 2000 (November 2000). H.263 is widely used as coding engine for Internet video streaming, and is also the coding core of the MPEG-4 standard.

The First Version of H.263

Based on H.261, MPEG-1 and MPEG-2, the first version of H.263 [21] has introduced many improvements, which makes it having a superior quality to H.261 at all bit rates and improved coding efficiency by a factor of two at very low bit rate. These improvements can be grouped into two categories, baseline algorithm features and enhanced modes which are optional. The baseline algorithm features include half-pixel motion compensation, 3-D variable length coding of DCT coefficients, median motion vector prediction, deleteable GOB header overhead etc. The enhanced modes include increased motion vector range with picture extrapolation, overlapped block motion compensation with picture extrapolation, bi-directional prediction and arithmetic entropy coding.

H.263+

The H.263+ [22] standard incorporates numerous enhancements and new features over the original H.263 design and is even better suited to low bit rate and Internet applications. Compared to H.263, H.263+ has the following improvements such as advanced Intra coding using spatial prediction, de-blocking filter, reference picture selection, customized and flexible video formats, scalability for resilience and multi-point and supplemental enhancement information, etc.

H.263++

H.263++ [23] project added a few more enhancements to H.263+ in late 2000. Those include error resilient data partitioning, 4×4 block size motion compensation, adaptive quantization, enhanced reference picture selection, inverse DCT mismatch reduction, de-blocking and de-ringing filters, as well as error concealment. Its Annex X also defines Profiles and Levels to group optional modes and parameters to improve inter-operability above the baseline capability.

2.5.6 MPEG-4

The MPEG-4 standard is fundamentally different in nature from its predecessors. It represents the scene as the composition of video objects, rather than just TV-like raster scan digital signal. In MPEG-4, the smallest entity in a picture is not a pixel, but an object with its associated shape, texture, and motion. Thus MPEG-4 is often referred as the second generation video coding standard, or the object based video coding standard.

The audio, video, graphics and other multimedia components of MPEG-4 are known as objects. These can exist independently, or a few of them can be grouped together. The result of grouping objects is an MPEG-4 scene. The strength of this object-oriented approach is that any of the components can be easily manipulated, optimally represented and interacted. Fig. 2.18 shows an example of how an MPEG-4 video scene can be segmented into a number of video objects and the background.

The advantages of the object based coding is its similarity to the HVS, easier to interact with objects in the picture and good potential for use in various applications. However it is very difficult to properly define, segment and track the video objects, and needs very complicated interface to conventional display. Fig. 2.19 shows how an MPEG-4 object can be decoded and composed to reconstruct the original video scene, and Fig. 2.20 shows the MPEG-4 scene graph structure of Fig. 2.19.

Besides the object based coding, MPEG-4 has provided a number of advanced tools for shape coding, motion estimation and compensation, texture coding, error resilience, sprite coding and scalability, such as,

- Shape coding: can be performed in binary mode or greyscale mode.
- Motion coding: 16×16 or 8×8 block based, variable object boundaries, overlapped block motion compensation, half-pixel resolution.
- Texture coding: based on 8×8 DCT, variable object boundaries, coefficient prediction.
- Wavelet transform based still texture coding.
- Sprite coding, which is an extended, panoramic image used for background pictures. This extended image is coded and transmitted in advance. On the receiver side, an image patch is extracted from the extended image and is used as a background picture of the decoded image.
- Model based coding.
- Face object coding.
- Mesh object coding.

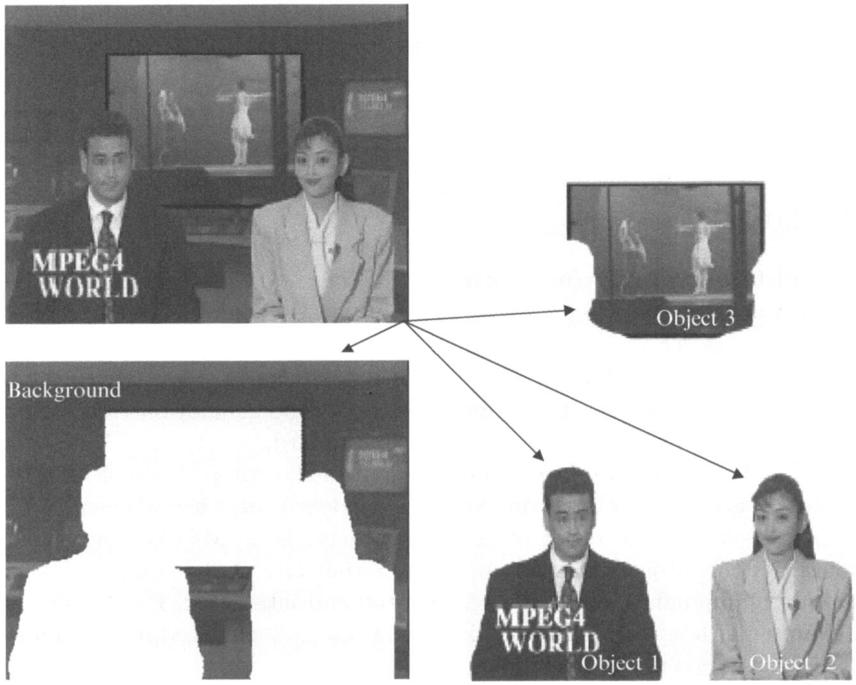

Fig. 2.18. MPEG-4 video objects.

- Object based scalable coding, both temporal and spatial.

Obviously, MPEG-4 provides the best possible choice for any multimedia application or service that needs to provide bandwidth efficiency, interactivity, adaptability, content based access, summarization, authoring and content re-purposing. However, the technical and computational complexity of the encoder lead to a substantial delay in developing the tools needed for a fully functional implementation of MPEG-4. The currently available tools only implement the basic specifications, which aim only for achieving better compression ratios, or adaptive bit rate or quality. Therefore, the advanced functionality of object manipulation is still not achievable. However, there is an intense research activity going on in the fields of video segmentation, object detection, modelling and recognition, and scene understanding. It is believed that many advanced techniques are likely to become available in near future.

2.5.7 H.264/AVC

H.264 Advanced Video Coding (H.264/AVC) [24, 25] is again the results of joint effort between MPEG and VCEG. It was developed in response to the growing need for higher compression of video signal for various applications

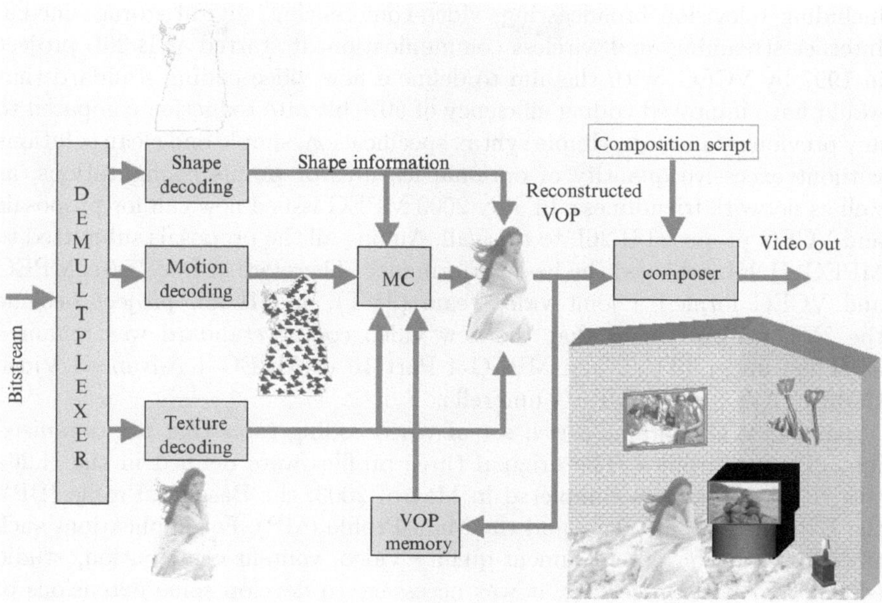

Fig. 2.19. Coding of MPEG-4 video objects.

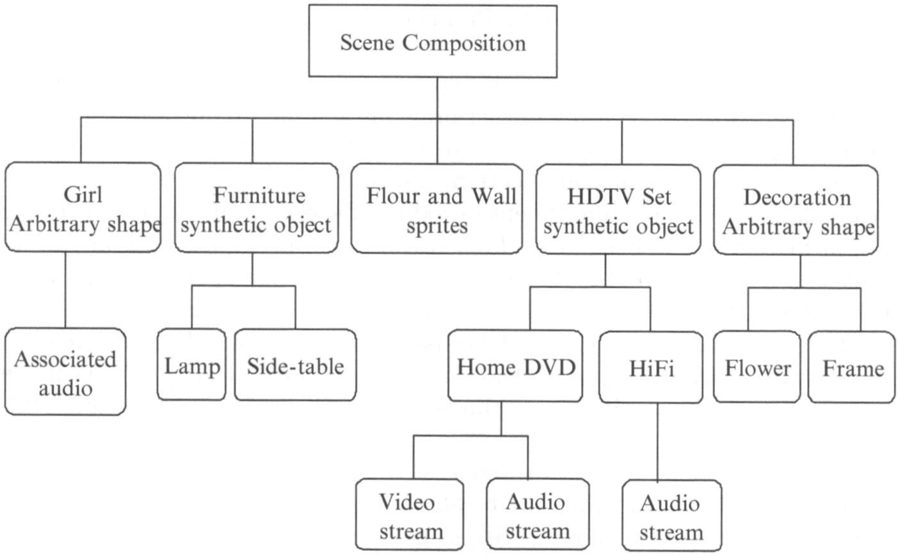

Fig. 2.20. Composition of MPEG-4 video objects.

including television broadcasting, video-conferencing, digital storage media, Internet streaming, and wireless communication. It started as H.26L project in 1997 by VCEG, with the aim to define a new video coding standard that would have improved coding efficiency of 50% bit rate reduction compared to any previous standards, simple syntax specification, simple and clean solutions without excessive quantity of optional features or profile configurations, as well as network friendliness. In July 2000 MPEG issued new call for proposals and VCEG proposed H.26L to this call. Among all the proposals submitted to MPEG, H.26L achieved the best performance. Therefore in Dec. 2001, MPEG and VCEG formed a joint video team (JVT), and H.26L project became the JVT project. After that the new video coding standard was renamed as H.264 under ITU-T and MPEG-4 Part 10 or MPEG-4 Advanced Video Coding (AVC) under MPEG umbrella.

H.264/AVC contains a rich set of video coding tools that are organized into different profiles. The original three profiles were defined in the H.264 specification that was completed in May of 2003: the Baseline Profile (BP), the Extended Profile (XP) and the Main Profile (MP). For applications such as high-resolution entertainment-quality video, content-contribution, studio editing and post-processing, it was necessary to develop some extensions of the tool set for professional video applications. This effort has resulted in a new set of extensions which are named the .fidelity range extensions (FRExt). These extensions include four new profiles: the High Profile (HP), the High 10 Profile (Hi10P), the High 4:2:2 Profile (H422P), and the High 4:4:4 Profile (H444P).

H.264/AVC represents a major step forward in the development of video coding standards. It typically outperforms prior standards by a factor of two or more, particularly in comparison to H.262/MPEG-2 and H.263++. This improvement enables new applications and business opportunities to be developed. However the improvement in coding efficiency is at the cost of coding complexity, which is believed to be 3–5 times more complex than any of its predecessors. However the phenomenon of Moore's Law makes this problem less important. Furthermore, H.264 is a collaboratively designed open standard with the aim of very small licensing cost. This will help to create a competitive market, keeping prices down and ensuring that products made by a wide variety of different manufacturers will be fully compatible with each other.

Compared to the previous standards, H.264/MPEG-4 AVC is not a fundamentally different method, but rather a significant refinement of well-established methods. Following list some new techniques that H.264/AVC has implemented,

- spatial prediction in Intra coding with two block size of 16×16 and 4×4
- adaptive block size motion compensation with variable block size of 4×4, 4×8, 8×4, 8×8, 8×16, 16×8 and 16×16
- 4×4 integer transformation

- multiple reference pictures (up to seven)
- content adaptive binary arithmetic coding (CABAC)

Fig. 2.21 shows the block diagram of the H.264/AVC encoder. In the diagram we have specified the new features related to various function blocks.

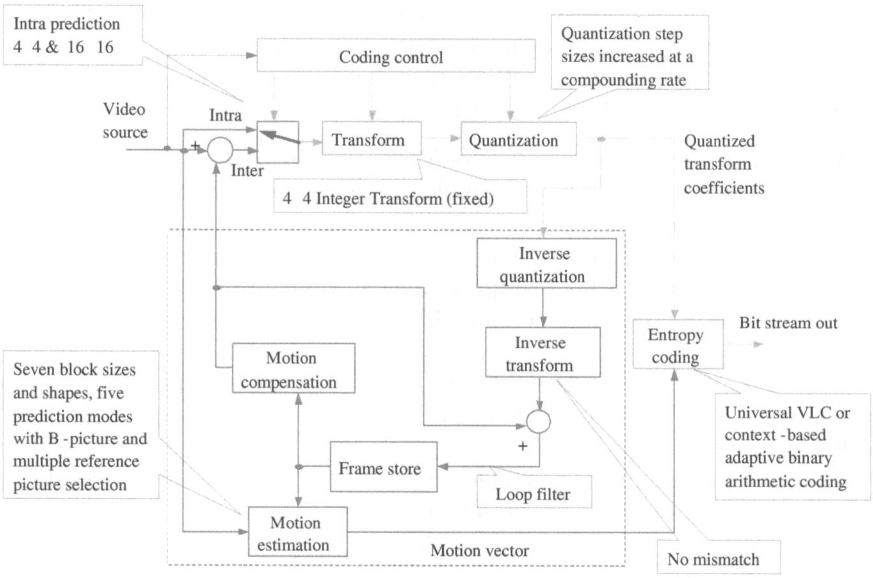

Fig. 2.21. H.264/AVC encoder block diagram.

The increased coding efficiency of the H.264/AVC has led to new application areas and business opportunities. There are strong interests of adopting it in various industries such as digital television broadcasting over cable, satellite, terrestrial, etc., as well as the high definition DVD. Another interesting business area is streaming TV signal over ADSL networks, as it is now possible to transmit video signals at about 1 Mbit/s with SDTV quality. In the field of mobile communication, H.264 will play an important role because the bandwidth will remain to be the bottleneck of multimedia services, even under the third-generation mobile (3GPP and 3GPP2) networks.

2.6 Summary

Video has always been the backbone of multimedia technology. In the last two decades, the field of digital video coding has been revolutionized by the advent of various standards like MPEG-1 to MPEG-4 and H.261 to H.263++, and

H.264. These techniques and standards have revolutionized the three main industries including broadcasting, communication and personal computers. This chapter provides a basic overview of the principle of video coding, with the focus on the core techniques and various standards. Due to the space limit, a lot of technical details have to be left out. We also refrain from introducing complex mathematics, only to the extent that it helps the reader to understand the techniques. However, we hope this chapter could serve as a good foundation for further study or research work.

Although it is always difficult to try guessing the future, it looks quite secure to identify a few basic trends for video coding, notably:

- The importance of new video coding tools will become less obvious as the existing standards have occupied or are occupying the existing and emerging markets.
- Comparing to the growth of bandwidth and storage capacity, the progress of video coding is much less impressive now and it will be even so in future.
- The existing generic video coding scheme has almost reached its theoretical limit.
- A change of paradigm is needed in order to achieve another 50% of bit savings – future coding schemes are believed to be more specialized and less generic.
- More intelligent image and video analysis tools are needed so that the coding is customized to nature of the video.

References

1. ITU-R Recommendation (1995): BT-500.7: Methodology for the subjective assessment of the quality of television pictures. ITU Geneva, Switzerland
2. VQEG (2000): Final report from the video quality expert group on the validation of objective models of video quality assessment. `http://www.vqeg.org/`
3. Rao, K.R. and Yip, P. (1990): Discrete cosine transform: algorithms, advantages, applications. Academic Press, Inc. London
4. Shi, Y.Q. and Sun, H. (2000): Image and video compression for multimedia engineering: fundamentals, algorithms, and standards. CRC Press
5. Elias P. (1955): Predictive coding, parts i and ii. IRE Trans. Information Theory, **IT-1**, 16
6. Huffman, D.A. (1952): A method for the construction of minimum redundancy codes. Proceedings of the Institute of Radio Engineers, **40**, 1098–1101
7. Rissanen J. (1976): Generalized Kraft inequality and arithmetic coding. IBM Journal of Research and Development, **20**, 198–203
8. Chen, W.H. and Pratt, W.K. (1984): Scene adaptive coder. IEEE Trans. on Communications, **32**, 225–232
9. Ahumada Jr., A.J. and Peterson, H. A. (1993) A visual detection model for DCT coefficient quantization. Computing in Aerospace, **9**, 314–318
10. Ribas-Corbera, J. and Lei, S. (1999): Rate control in DCT video coding for low-delay video communications. IEEE Trans. Circuits Syst. Video Technol., **9**, 172–185

11. Jain, J.R. and Jain, A.K. (1981) Displacement measurement and its application in interframe image coding. IEEE Trans. on Communications, **COM-29**, 1799–1808
12. Li, R., Zeng, B., and Liou, M.L. (1994) A new three-step search algorithm for block motion estimation. IEEE Trans. Circuits Syst. Video Technol., **4**, 438–443
13. Po, L.M. and Ma, W.C. (1996): A novel four-step search algorithm for fast block motion estimation. IEEE Trans. Circuits Syst. Video Technol., **6**, 313–317
14. Zhu, S. and Ma, K. K. (2000): A new diamond search algorithm for fast block-matching motion estimation. IEEE Trans. Image Processing, **9**, 287–290
15. Zhu, C., Lin, X., and Chau, L.P. (2002): Hexagon-based search pattern for fast block motion estimation. IEEE Trans. Circuits Syst. Video Technol., **12**, 349–355
16. Pan, F., Lin, X., Rahardja, S., Lin, W., Ong, E., Yao, S., Lu, Z., and Yang, X. (2004): A locally-adaptive algorithm for measuring blocking artifacts in images and videos. Image Communication: Signal Processing, **19**, 499–506
17. Grob, B. (1984): Basic television and video systems, 5th Ed., McGraw-Hill
18. ITU-T Recommendation H.261 (1990): Video codec for audiovisual services at p x 64 kbit/s, Geneva. Revised (1993) Helsinki
19. ISO/IEC 11172-2 (1993): Information technology — Coding of moving pictures and associated audio for digital storage media at up to about 1.5 Mbit/s – Video, Geneva
20. ISO/IEC 13818-2 (1995): Generic coding of moving pictures and associated audio information, Part 2: Video
21. ITU-T Recommendation H.263 (1996): Video coding for low bitrate communication
22. ITU-T Draft Recommendation H.263 Version 2 H.263+ (1997): Video coding for low bitrate communication
23. ITU-T Study Group 16: Video Coding Experts Group (Question 15) (1998): Doc. Q15F09. Report of the ad hoc committee H.263++ development, Seoul, Korea
24. ITU-T Rec. H.264 / ISO/IEC 11496-10 (2002): Advanced video coding. Final Committee Draft, Document JVTE022
25. Information Technology — Coding of audio-visual objects — Part 10: Advanced video coding. Final Draft International Standard, ISO/IEC FDIS 14496–10

3

Advances of MPEG Scalable Video Coding Standard

Wen-Hsiao Peng[1], Chia-Yang Tsai[1], Tihao Chiang[1], and Hsueh-Ming Hang[1]

National Chiao-Tung University
1001 Ta-Hsueh Rd., HsinChu 30010, Taiwan
pawn@mail.si2lab.org; cytsai.ee90g@nctu.edu.tw; tchiang@mail.nctu.edu.tw; hmhang@mail.nctu.edu.tw

Summary. To support clients with diverse capabilities, the MPEG committee is defining a novel Scalable Video Coding (SVC) framework that can simultaneously support multiple spatial, temporal and SNR resolutions under the constraints of low complexity and small delay. In order to fulfill these requirements, two main approaches have been considered as the potential technologies. One is the Wavelet-Based Scheme and the other is the Scalable Extension of MPEG-4 AVC/H.264. The latter has been finally chosen as the MPEG SVC standard to be finalized in 2007. This chapter gives a brief overview on the latest advances in these technologies with a focus on the MPEG standard activities.

3.1 Introduction

Scalable Video Coding (SVC) attracts wide attention due to the rapid growth of multimedia applications over the Internet and wireless channels. In these applications, the video may be transmitted over error-prone channels with fluctuating bandwidth. The clients, which consist of different devices, may have different processing power and spatial resolutions. Fig. 3.1 shows an example of Scalable Video Coding in a streaming environment, where a single bit-stream is broadcast to various clients through various heterogeneous networks. As shown, the challenge is how to generate such a bit-stream which matches the capabilities of the different devices.

To support clients with diverse capabilities in the areas of complexity, bandwidth, power and display resolution, the MPEG committee is in the process of defining a Scalable Video Coding (SVC) framework that can simultaneously support multiple spatial, temporal and SNR resolutions under the constraints of minimum complexity and small delay. More than 20 proposals were submitted during the request for proposal stage of the inquiry [1] in February 2004. These proposals can be roughly classified into the following two categories. One is the Wavelet-Based Scheme and the other the

W.-H. Peng et al.: *Advances of MPEG Scalable Video Coding Standard*, Studies in Computational Intelligence (SCI) **58**, 55–80 (2007)
www.springerlink.com

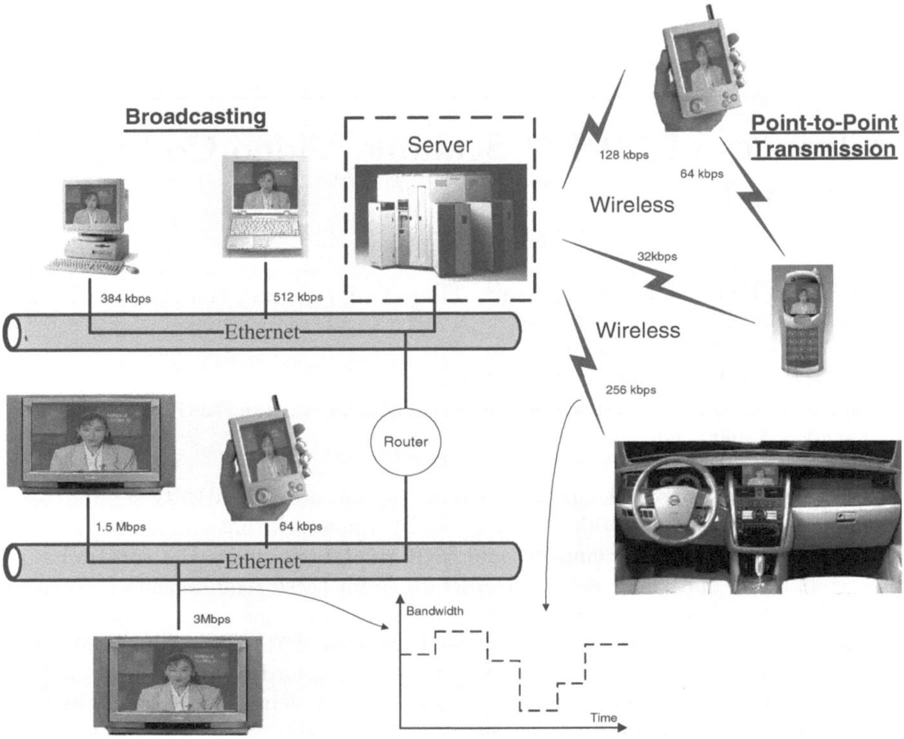

Fig. 3.1. Application framework for Scalable Video Coding.

AVC/H.264-based approach [2]. In addition, and depending on the transform order in the spatio-temporal domain, the wavelet-based scheme can be further divided into two variations. That is the "2D+t(+2D)" and "t+2D" structures [2]. In order to distinguish the differences, Fig. 3.2 gives a comparison of the architecture of these two variations.

To achieve temporal scalability, both the wavelet-based scheme and the AVC-based approach adopt the technique of Motion Compensated Temporal Filtering (MCTF). To achieve the SNR scalability with a fine granularity, the AVC-based scheme uses a context-adaptive bit-plane coding [3, 4]. The wavelet-based scheme employs an embedded quantizer with arithmetic coding [5, 6, 7] for the same purpose. For spatial scalability, the wavelet-based scheme uses the advantages of multi-resolution property of wavelet transform. The AVC-based scheme exploits the layered coding concept used in MPEG-2, H.263, and MPEG-4.

A test has been done comparing these technologies [8]. The AVC-based scheme has a better quality for several features and was adopted as the joint ITU and ISO MPEG SVC standard draft. The MPEG committee also established an ad-hoc group to further study wavelet-based technologies for possible

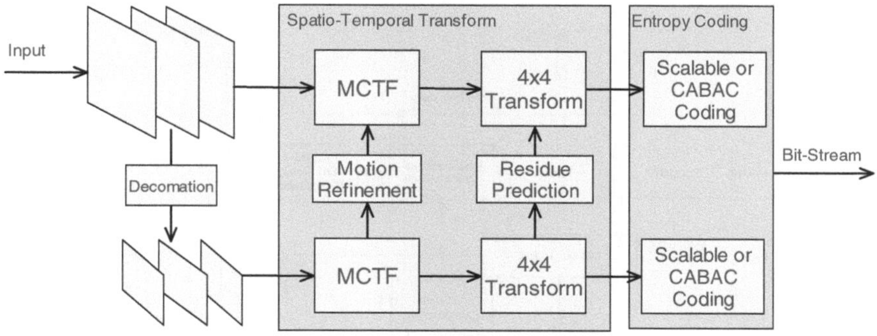

(a) An AVC/H.264-based approach (also DCT-based)

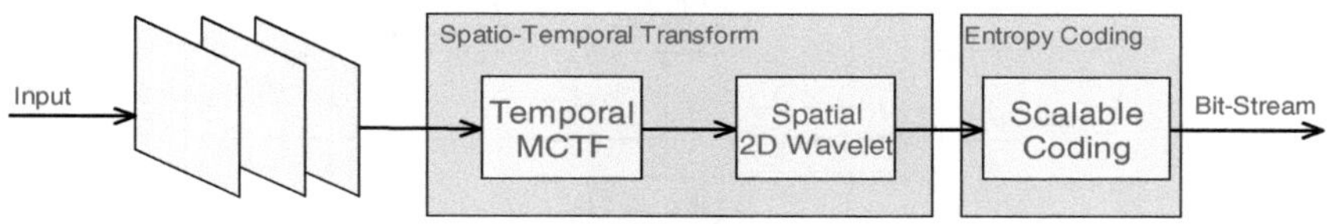

(b) A wavelet-based approach with "t+2" structure

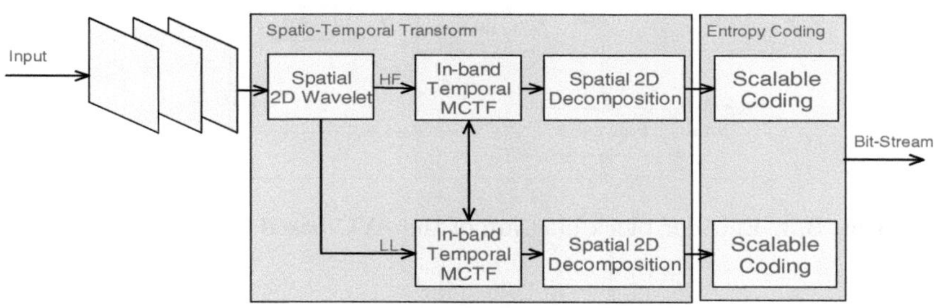

(c) A wavelet-based approach with "2D+t+2D" structure

Fig. 3.2. An architectural level comparison for various SVC algorithms [2].

future video coding applications. In this chapter, we give a brief overview of the latest advances in these technologies. The rest of this chapter is organized as follows. Section 3.2 elaborates the details for each dimension of scalability in the AVC-based approach and Section 3.3 describes the basis and variations of the wavelet-based scheme. It also compares this with the performance with that of the AVC-based scheme. The latest MPEG activities in SVC are summarized Section 3.4.

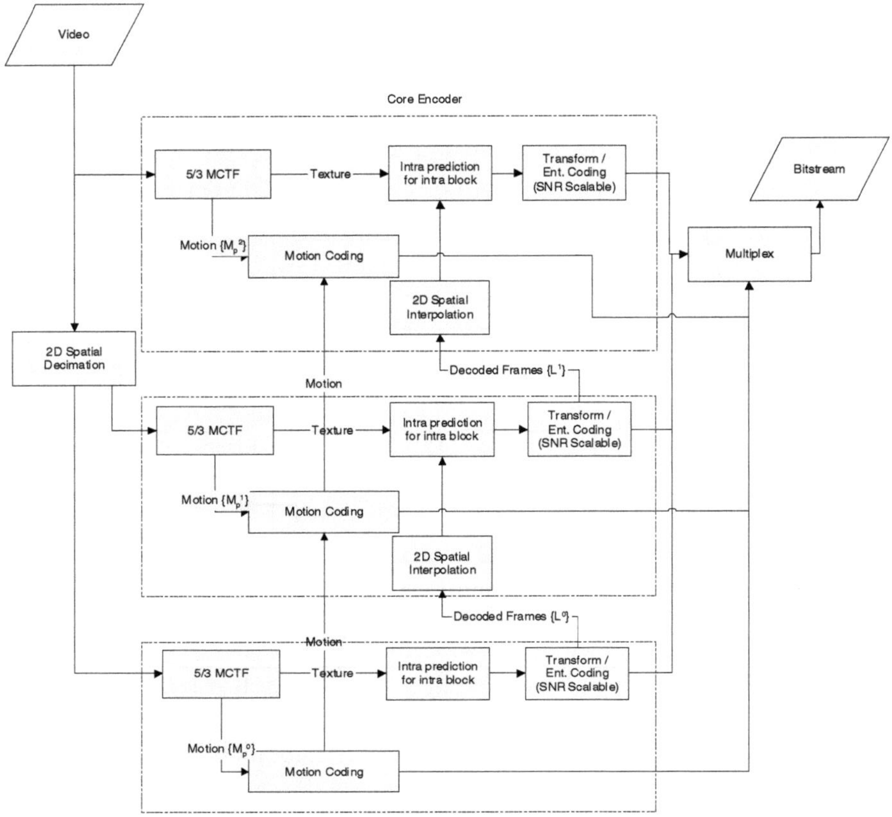

Fig. 3.3. Encoder block diagram of the AVC-based SVC scheme [3].

3.2 Scalable Extension of AVC/H.264

In order to simultaneously support spatial, temporal and SNR scalability, a scalable version of AVC/H.264 was proposed [3]. Fig. 3.3 shows the encoder structure of the AVC-based scheme. To facilitate the spatial scalability, the input video is decimated into spatial resolutions. The sequence in each spatial resolution is coded as a separated layer using AVC/H.264. Within each spatial layer, Motion Compensated Temporal Filtering (MCTF) is employed in every Group Of Pictures (GOPs) to provide the temporal scalability. In order, to remove redundancy existing among spatial layers, a considerable degree of inter-layer prediction is incorporated. The residual frames existing after the inter-layer prediction are then transformed and successively quantized for SNR scalability. In the following subsections, we elaborate the details for each dimension of scalability.

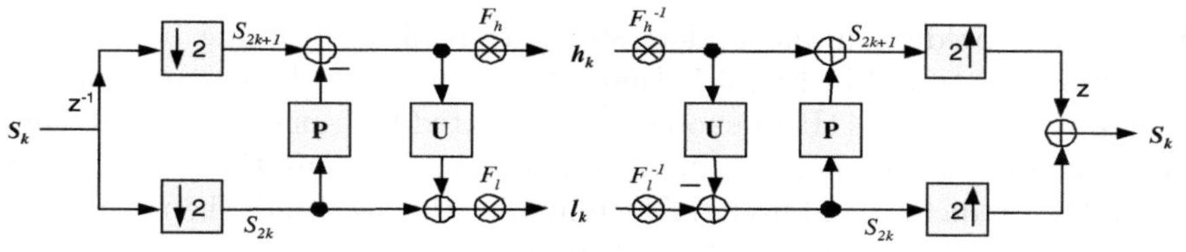

Fig. 3.4. Lifting scheme for the (5, 3) wavelet transform [3]. (a) Decomposition. (b) Reconstruction.

3.2.1 Temporal Scalability

Motion Compensated Temporal Filtering (MCTF)

The temporal scalability is achieved by Motion Compensated Temporal Filtering (MCTF), which is responsible for the wavelet decomposition/reconstruction along the motion trajectory. The MCTF is conducted independently in each spatial layer.

To reduce complexity and ensure perfect reconstruction, the MCTF is implemented by a Lifting Scheme. Particularly, in SVC [9], the MCTF is largely restricted to a special Lifting Scheme that has only one prediction or update step. Fig. 3.4 shows an example of such a scheme. Here S_k denotes the k-th input frame and S_{2k} represents an even-indexed frame. The term S_{2k+1} stands for an odd-indexed frame. As shown, the decomposition mainly consists of 3 operations, which are (1) Polyphase Decomposition, (2) Prediction, and (3) Update. To produce the high pass signal h_k, an odd-indexed frame is predicted from the output of the Prediction Filter (**P**), which uses the even-indexed frames as input. The residue then forms the high pass frame. Accordingly, in order to generate the low pass frame l_k, an even-indexed frame is updated using the output of the Update Filter (**U**), which takes the high-pass frames as input,

$$h_k \triangleq S_{2k+1} - P_{(5,3)}(S_{2k}) = S_{2k+1} - \frac{1}{2}\left(S_{2k} + S_{2k+2}\right), \tag{3.1}$$

$$l_k \triangleq S_{2k} + U_{(5,3)}(h_k) = S_{2k} + \frac{1}{4}\left(h_k + h_{k-1}\right). \tag{3.2}$$

For better understanding, we show the MCTF structure using the (5, 3) wavelet. Eq. (3.1) and (3.2) define the operations of prediction and update steps for the (5, 3) wavelet. According to Eq. (3.1), the high pass frame h_k is the residual frame after an odd-indexed frame is predicted from the adjacent even-indexed frames. Similarly, using Eq. (3.2), the low pass frame l_k is obtained by updating an even-indexed frame by means of the adjacent high pass frames. The prediction and update steps are realized by using bidirectional prediction illustrated in Fig. 3.5. Here $\{\mathbf{L}^n\}$ stands for the low-pass original frames at the level n. $\{\mathbf{H}^n\}$ denotes the associated high-pass frames. To effectively remove the temporal redundancy, motion compensation is conducted before the prediction and update. To minimize the overhead, the motion vectors for the update steps are derived from those used for the prediction. By using n decomposition stages, up to n levels of temporal scalability can be achieved. The video of lower frame rates can be obtained from the low-pass frames derived from higher levels,

$$h_k \triangleq S_{2k+1} - P_{(\text{Haar})}(S_{2k}) = S_{2k+1} - S_{2k}, \tag{3.3}$$

$$l_k \triangleq S_{2k} + U_{(\text{Haar})}(h_k) = S_{2k} + \frac{1}{2}h_k. \tag{3.4}$$

In addition to the $(5,3)$ wavelet, the Haar wavelet is also used in the current SVC algorithm. This is used particularly, to improve coding efficiency. The terms in $(5,3)$ and the Haar wavelets are adaptively switched at the macroblock level. Eq. (3.3) and (3.4) specify the corresponding operations of the prediction and the update steps for the Haar wavelet. Similarly to the $(5,3)$ wavelet, the filtering of Haar wavelet can be simplified to operate as an unidirectional prediction.

Hierarchical B Pictures

In SVC [9], the base layer must be compatible with the main profile of H.264/AVC [10]. The compatibility is achieved by using a representation of the hierarchical B pictures for the lowest spatial layer. With hierarchical B pictures, the temporal update step is omitted, and this leads to a purely predictive structure as shown in Fig. 3.6. Here A denotes the anchor frames and B^n represents the B pictures of the level n. In addition, the coding order in a GOP is specified by a series of numbers.

Similarly to the layers encoded with MCTF, the first picture is independently coded as an IDR picture, and all remaining pictures are coded in "B$\cdots$BP" or "B$\cdots$BI" groups of pictures using the concept of hierarchical B pictures. For the prediction of a B picture at the level l, the reference frames come from the set $\{\{A\} \cup \{B^n \mid n < l\}\}$. For instance, the B pictures of the level 1, (i.e., the pictures labelled as B^1 in Fig. 3.6,) use only the surrounding anchor frames $\{A\}$ for prediction. Similarly, the pictures B^l use the surrounding anchor frames $\{A\}$ as well as the $\{B^n \mid n < l\}$ for prediction. As shown, the same dependency structure as the MCTF without the update steps is used. Moreover, the structure of hierarchical B pictures can be supported by the syntax of H.264/AVC [10].

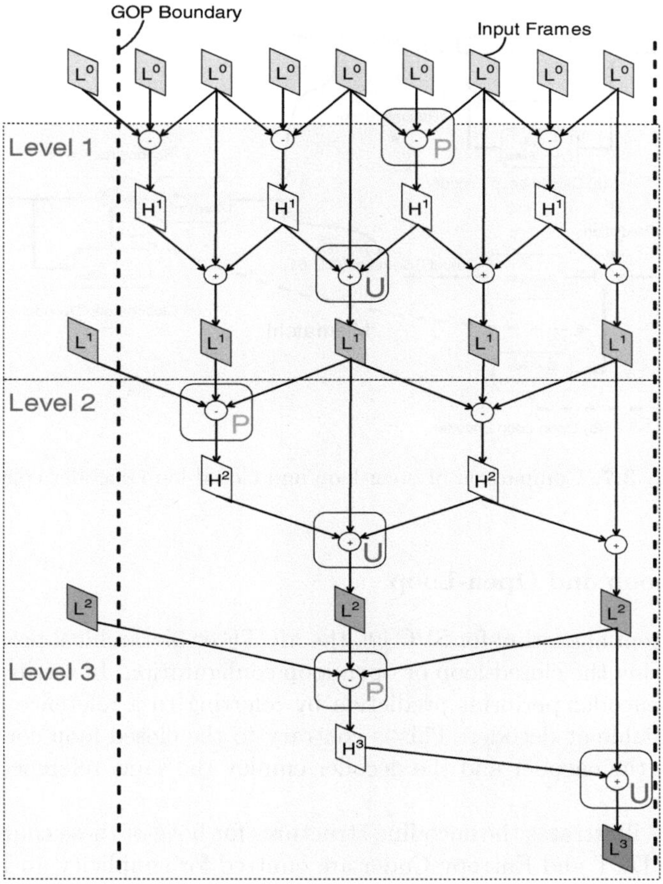

Fig. 3.5. MCTF structure for the (5, 3) wavelet.

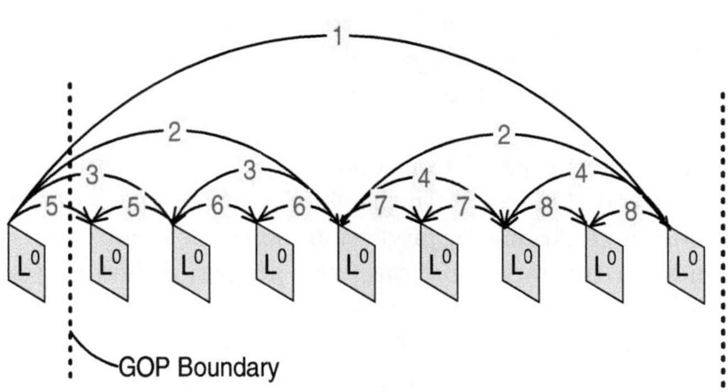

Fig. 3.6. Structure of hierarchical B pictures.

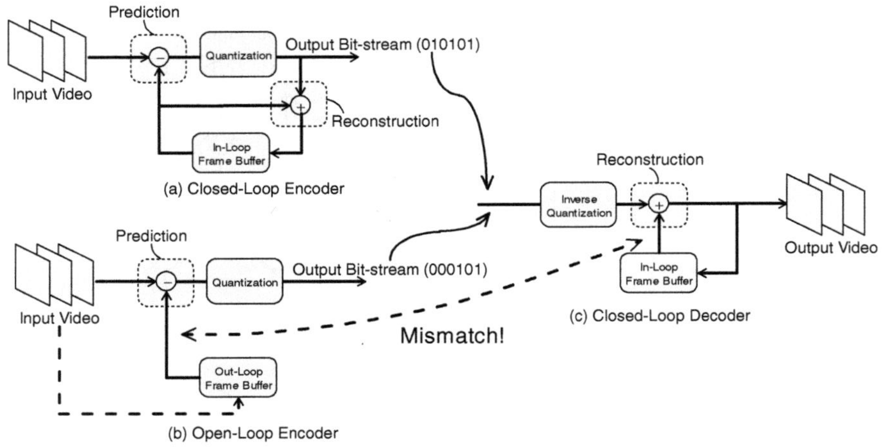

Fig. 3.7. Comparison of open-loop and closed-loop encoder control.

Closed-Loop and Open-Loop

In the current algorithm for SVC [9], the MCTF or hierarchical prediction can be done using the closed-loop or open-loop configuration. In setting the open-loop, the encoder performs prediction by referring to a reference frame that is not available at decoder. This is contrary to the closed-loop configuration. Here both the encoder and the decoder employ the same reference frame for prediction.

Fig. 3.7 illustrates the encoding structures for both of these configurations, where the DCT and Entropy Coder are omitted for simplicity. In Fig. 3.7(a), the in-loop frame buffer keeps identical content as the one at the decoder in Fig. 3.7(c). Particularly, the reference frame at encoder is produced by a Reconstruction Loop, which has the same structure as the decoder. For the open-loop configuration, the out-loop frame buffer in Fig. 3.7(b) may have different contents from the in-loop frame buffer at the decoder. In practice, the reference frame in the out-loop frame buffer can be arbitrarily generated by the encoder.

The configuration of prediction loop affects the prediction efficiency and the quality of decoded video. With the closed-loop configuration, the encoder uses the reconstructed frame for prediction. Since the quality of reconstructed frame depends on the target bit rate, the prediction becomes less efficient when the video is encoded at a very low bit rate. Poor prediction efficiency causes reduced coding efficiency and rate-distortion performance. On the other hand, one can freely refer to the original frame for better prediction in the open-loop configuration. However, mismatch errors are created because the original frame is only available at the encoder. At the decoder, the reference frame is a quantized version of the original one. Quantization errors cause the mismatch between the reference frames at encoder and decoder. Thus, even if the prediction residues are correctly received by decoder, the output video will still contain errors.

In summary, closed-loop prediction has reduced efficiency and thus produces more prediction residues, which degrade coding efficiency. On the contrary, open-loop prediction provides better efficiency but creates mismatch errors. Both prediction efficiency and mismatch errors influence the quality of the output video. Thus, the loop configuration is used as an encode option for the trade-off between prediction efficiency and mismatch error.

The Update Step

In MCTF, the update step performs low-pass filtering along the motion trajectory. It provides better coding efficiency by removing both temporal noise and aliasing. In addition, using the update step, the fluctuation of decoded quality between even frames and odd frames can be reduced in open-loop configuration [11].

However, the gain of coding efficiency and subjective quality comes at the cost of extra complexity. For the update step, the derivation of motion vector needs intensive branch instructions. Moreover, the motion compensation for adjacent high-pass frames demands extra memory bandwidth. In addition, the buffer management for reference frames becomes more complex.

In [11], the role of the update step in MCTF is investigated. The studies indicate that disabling the update step at decoder does not degrade the visual quality and the PSNR performance of the decoded video while comparing with the case of enabling the update step. Specifically, enabling the update step at encoder reduces the fluctuation in quality between even and odd frames. However, disabling the update step at decoder side does not show significant differences in terms of PSNR or of subjective quality. As a result, the update step is adopted as an encoder option in SVC. The MCTF at decoder becomes a purely predictive structure and reduces the complexity of decoder by 50%.

Comparison of MCTF and traditional GOP structure

In SVC [3], MCTF is a key technology for temporal scalability. In addition, it has been shown in [12] that MCTF also provides higher coding efficiency than the traditional GOP structure.

For a better understanding, Fig. 3.8 depicts the comparison of rate-distortion performance with different GOP structures. As shown, the MCTF with closed-loop configuration outperforms the traditional "IBBPBBP···" structure in all cases. Moreover, the closed-loop configuration provides better rate-distortion performance than the open-loop one. In particular, with open-loop configuration, the MCTF may have worse performance than traditional "IBBPBBP···" structure. An example is shown in Fig. 3.8(d).

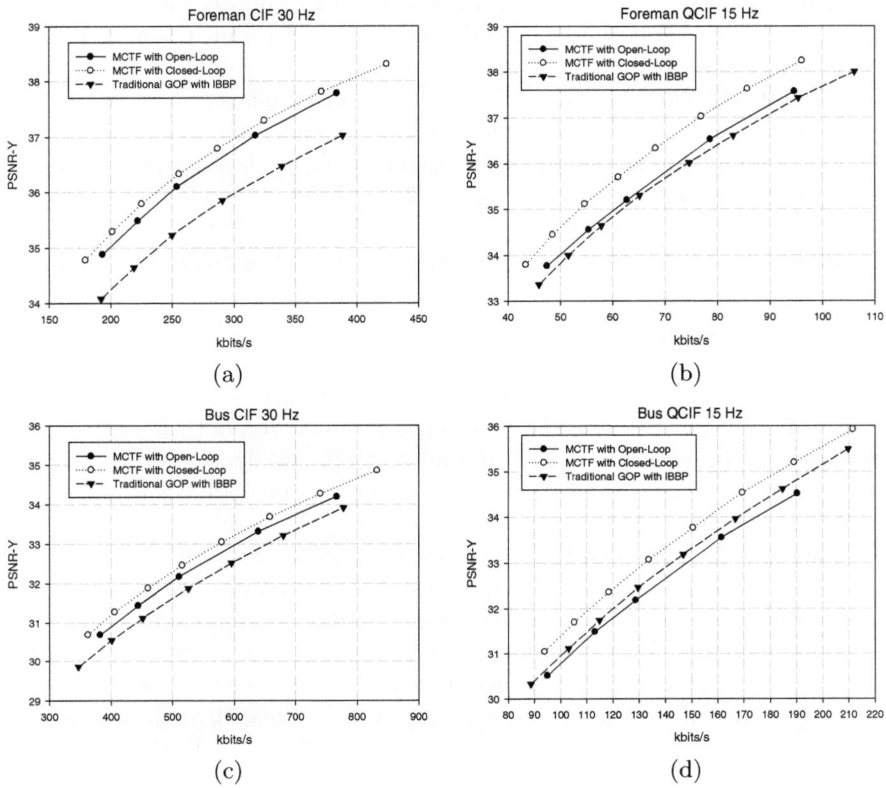

Fig. 3.8. Comparision of PSNR performance between the GOP structures of MCTF and IBBP. All schemes are coded with single layer configuration [12].

In summary, from the perspective of prediction efficiency, MCTF shows better performance than traditional GOP structure of "IBBPBBP· · · ." It is a tool for temporal scalability, and also for coding efficiency.

3.2.2 Spatial Scalability and Inter-Layer Prediction

The spatial scalability is achieved by the concepts used in MPEG-2, H.263, or MPEG-4. Sequences of different spatial resolutions are coded in separated layers. Conceptually, a pyramid of spatial resolutions is provided.

To remove the redundancy among different spatial layers, a large degree of inter-layer prediction is incorporated. Specifically, the residues and motion vectors of an enhancement-layer frame are predicted from the those in the subordinate layers. Fig. 3.9 presents an example of inter-layer prediction with 2 spatial layers. The spatial base layer is coded with the structure of hierarchical B pictures and the spatial enhancement-layers are coded by the MCTF.

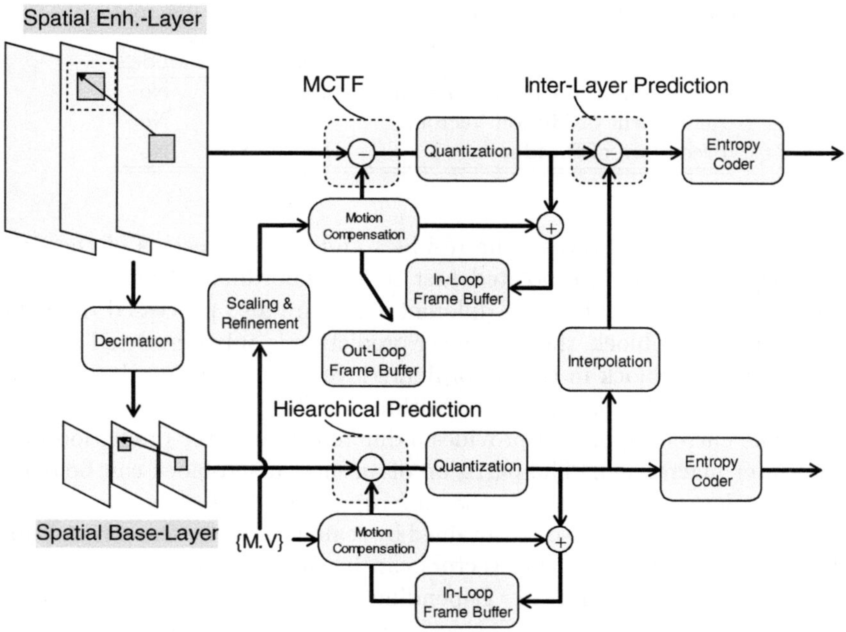

Fig. 3.9. Structure of inter-layer prediction.

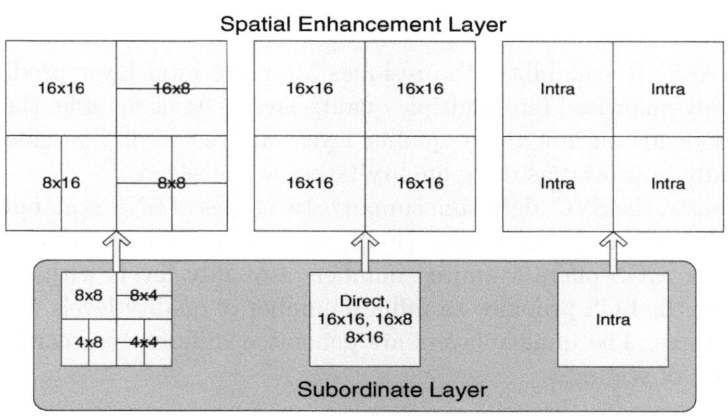

Fig. 3.10. Extension of prediction/partition information for the inter-layer prediction.

Table 3.1. Inter-layer prediction modes for an inter macroblock.

	Mode0	Mode1	Mode2
Extension of Macroblock Partition	Yes	Yes	No
Refinement of Motion Vector	No	Yes	No
Prediction of Residue	Yes	Yes	No

In the prediction process, the residues and motion vectors of the subordinate layers will be interpolated first if the subordinate layer has a lower resolution. The macroblocks of different types are also processed differently. For an intra macroblock, the inter-layer prediction is only permitted if the corresponding 8×8 block in the subordinate layer is further encoded within an intra-coded macroblock. Prediction within an inter macroblock is always enabled. The current approach provides 3 different inter-layer prediction modes for an inter macroblock. The partition of an inter macroblock can be derived from the relevant sub-blocks at the subordinate layer as shown in Fig. 3.10. The motion vectors can also be obtained by scaling those for the corresponding sub-blocks. The scaled motion vectors can be further refined in the quarter-pel range between -1 and $+1$. Depending on the macroblock partition and the refinement of motion field, Table 3.1 is used to summarize the inter-layer prediction modes for an inter macroblock.

3.2.3 SNR Scalability

To achieve SNR scalability, the residues after the inter-layer prediction are successively quantized into multiple quality layers. At client side, the decoded quality depends on how many quality layers are received. The video quality is gradually improved as more quality layers are received.

Currently, the SVC algorithm supports two types of SNR scalability, which are Fine Granularity Scalability (FGS) and Coarse Granularity Scalability (CGS). The CGS offers a limited number of quality levels with distinct bit rates while the FGS provides an infinite number of quality levels with continuous bit rates. The quality layers are generated differently according to the granularity of scaling.

Coarse Granularity Scalability

To achieve CGS, the stack structure shown in Fig. 3.9 is used. This is done in a different manner to spatial scalability. The CGS is achieved by encoding the video of the same spatial resolution in different spatial layers. Thus, each spatial layer is used as a quality enhancement-layer. Fig. 3.11 illustrates the prediction structure of CGS, where one base-layer and two quality enhancement-layers are generated where Qp0 > Qp1 > Qp2. Compared to the stack structure in Fig. 3.9, the interpolation of prediction residues and

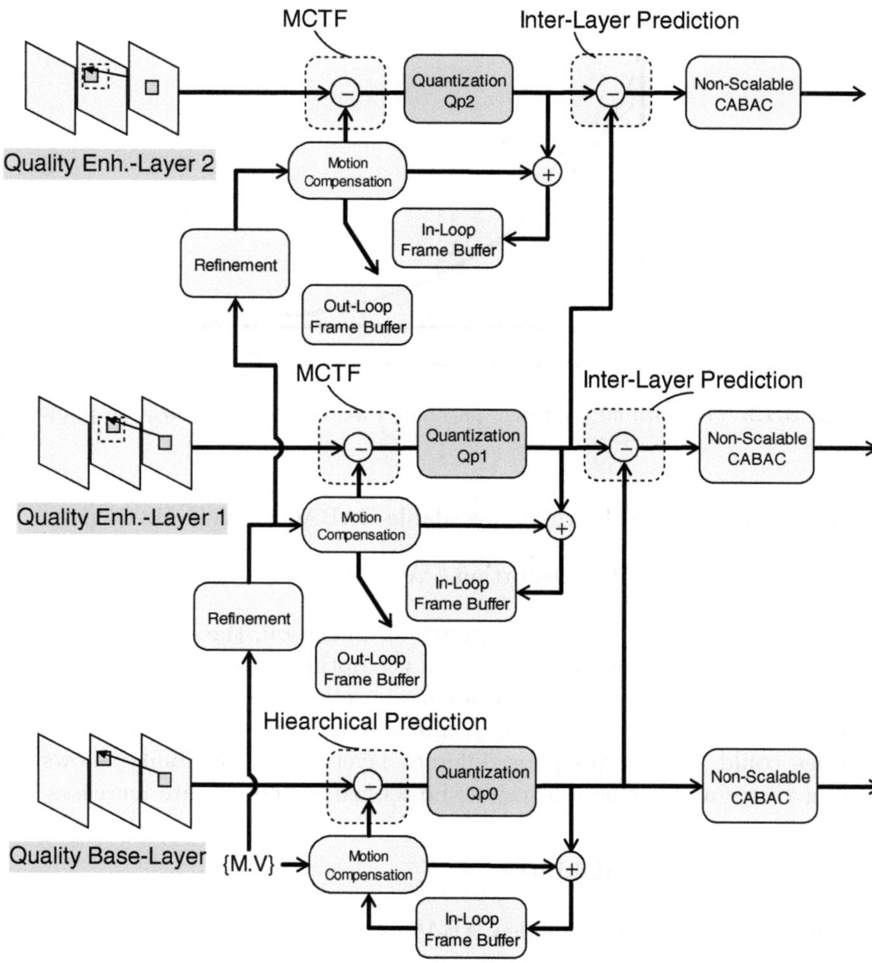

Fig. 3.11. Prediction structure of coarse granularity scalability.

the scaling of motion vectors are omitted since different quality layers have the same resolution.

Although the same resolution is used for each layer, different quality layers are optimized for different bit rates. For instance, if the base layer is coded and optimized for the bit rate $R1$, the first quality layer will be coded at a higher bit rate $R2$. In the same way, the next quality layer will be coded for the bit rate $R3$ with $R3 > R2 > R1$. To achieve the target bit rate for each layer, different quantization parameters are applied. In addition, the redundancy between quality layers is removed by using inter-layer prediction. Thus, each quality layer records the differences between the signals obtained with two different quantization parameters. The prediction residues at each

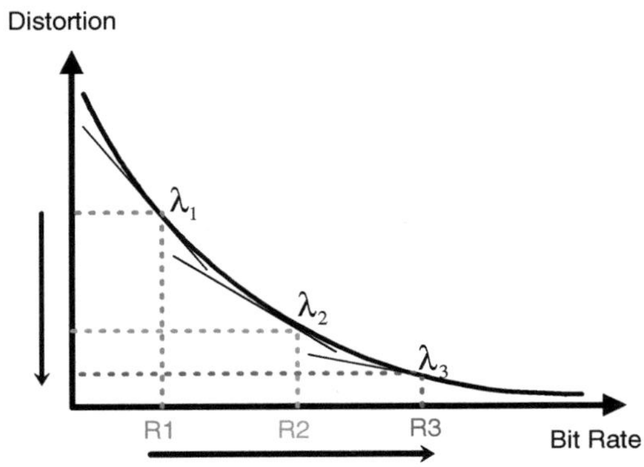

Fig. 3.12. The optimal Lagrange parameter at different optimization points.

quality layer are coded by the non-scalable CABAC in AVC/H.264 [10],

$$J = \text{Distortion} + \lambda \times (\text{BitRate})\,. \tag{3.5}$$

According to the theory of Lagrange optimization, the optimal Lagrange parameter (i.e., the λ factor) varies with the optimization point as illustrated in Fig. 3.12. Thus, if the criterion for mode selection is to minimize the Lagrange cost as defined in Eq. (3.5), different motion vectors and prediction residues could be generated for different layers. Such flexibility allows the motion vector and prediction residue be refined as the bit rate increases.

Fine Granularity Scalability

To achieve FGS, the non-scalable CABAC is replaced by an embedded cyclical block coding [13]. By using embedded coding, the bit-stream of a quality layer can be arbitrarily truncated for FGS.

In Cyclical Block Coding [13], each quality layer is coded using two passes. These are the Significant Pass and the Refinement Pass. The significant pass first encodes the insignificant coefficients that have zero values in the subordinate layers. The refinement pass then refines the remaining coefficients within range –1 to +1. During the significance pass, the transform blocks are coded in a cyclical and block-interleaved manner. By contrast, the refinement coefficients are coded in a subband by subband fashion [13].

Fig. 3.13 gives an example of cyclical block coding [13]. For simplicity, we assume all the coefficients are to be coded in the significant pass. As shown, each coding cycle in a block includes an EOB symbol, a Run index and a non-zero quantization level. The EOB symbol is coded first for indicating whether there are non-zero coefficients to be coded in a cycle. In addition, the Run index represented by several significance bits is used to locate the non-zero

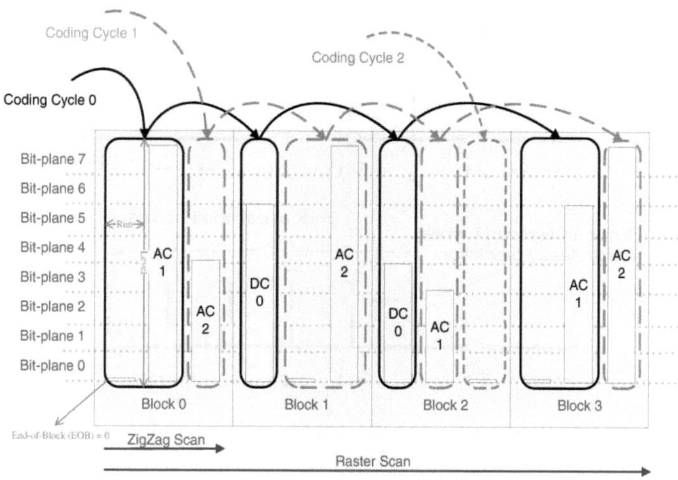

Fig. 3.13. Illustration of cyclical block coding.

Table 3.2. Comparison of fine granularity scalability and coarse granularity scalability.

	FGS	CGS
Quantization	Smaller step size	Larger step size
Motion Vector of Quality Layers	Shared	Independent
Prediction Mode of Quality Layers	Shared	Independent
Prediction of MCTF Residues	Yes	Adaptive
Entropy Coding of Quality Layers	Scalable	Non-Scalable

coefficient. To further reduce the bit rate, all the symbols are coded by a binary arithmetic coder.

In addition to using a Scalable Entropy Coding, Table 3.2 highlights other differences between FGS and CGS. In FGS, the quality layers are generated by successive quantization with each succeeding smaller step size. The quality layers of FGS use the same motion vector and prediction mode. The inter-layer prediction of MCTF residues is always enabled. Since the Motion Vector and Prediction Mode are not refined along with the increase of bit rate, the FGS is preferable for the applications with a smaller range of scalability. The flexibility of CGS is suitable for the requirement of larger scalable range. In recent studies [14], it has been proved that applying Adaptive Refinement of Motion Vector and Prediction Mode in FGS can further improve the PSNR by 1 dB. Thus, in the latest joint draft of SVC, the FGS maintains the same flexibility as CGS for better coding efficiency [14]. Multiple prediction loops may be created in the quality enhancement-layer.

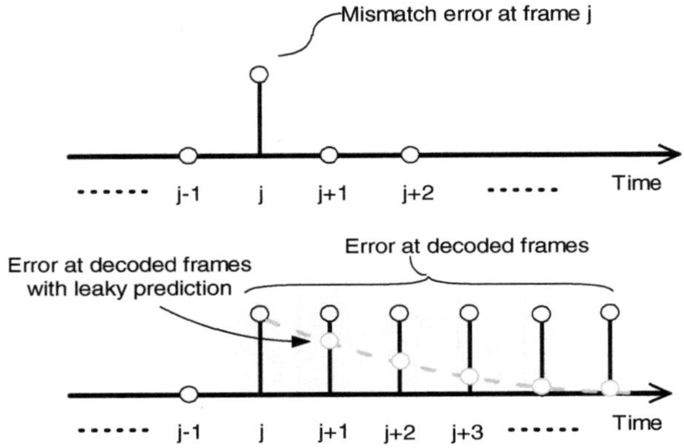

Fig. 3.14. Illustration of mismatch error and drifting behavior.

Fine Granularity Scalability in Low-Delay Applications

Applications with Real-Time or Interactive features normally have the constraint of Low-Delay. In these applications, the extra delay for MCTF or Hierarchical Prediction is not permissible. Thus, the traditional GOP structure of "IPPP⋯" is preferred for low-delay applications.

With the GOP structure of "IPPP⋯," it has been shown in [15, 16] that the mismatch error will cause further drifting error. In FGS, the quality enhancement-layer may not perform in the expected manner. Thus, a mismatch error could occur. Due to drift, the mismatch error of the frame j will propagate to later frames as illustrated by Fig. 3.14. Accordingly, mismatch errors at different instances of time are accumulated in the temporal direction, which significantly degrade the quality of the decoded video.

To reduce drifting errors, the concept of leaky prediction [15, 16] is adopted by the current SVC algorithm. The concept is to introduce an in-loop gain factor α at both encoder and decoder to cause the mismatch error to decay. For better understanding, Fig. 3.15 illustrates the configuration of prediction loop when the leaky prediction scheme is enabled. The transmission error is modelled by adding an error term $E(t)$ to the prediction residue of encoder, $R(t)$. The gain factor α is constrained in the interval of $[0, 1)$. The transmission error will decay in an exponential manner and the error is circulated in the reconstruction loop of decoder. The dashed line in Fig. 3.14 characterizes the effect of drifting behavior with leaky prediction.

3.2.4 Combined Scalability

In SVC [9], all of the scalability can be combined to simultaneously support a wide range of spatial, temporal, and SNR scalability. Fig. 3.16 illustrates the use of Combining Different Scalability. In this example, the Spatial Base

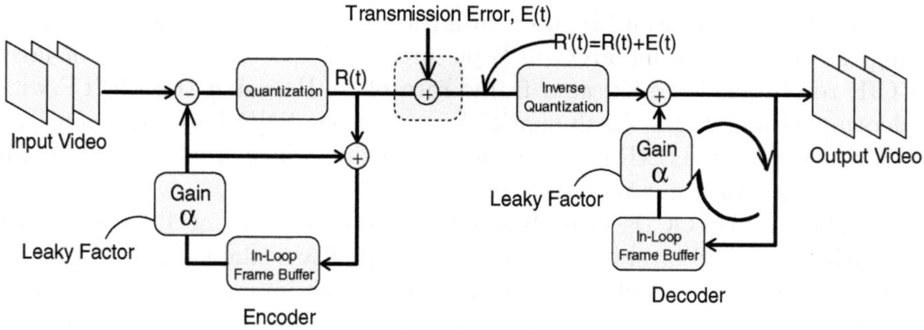

Fig. 3.15. Configuration of prediction loop for leaky prediction.

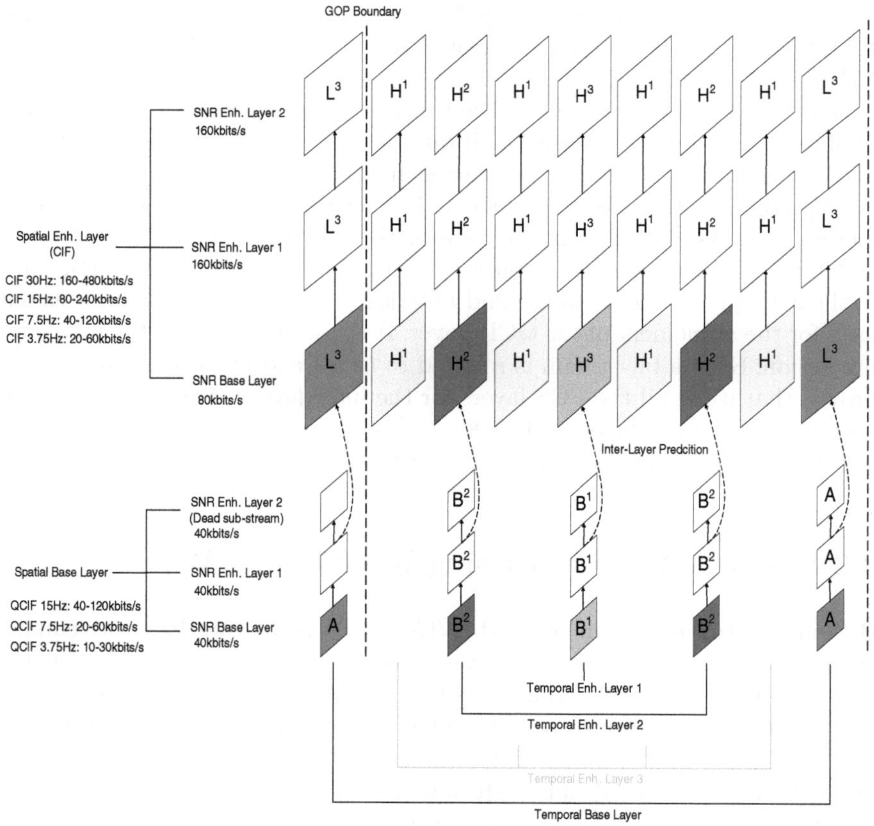

Fig. 3.16. Example of combining spatial, temporal, and SNR scalability.

Layer (in QCIF resolution) is coded at a frame rate of 15 Hz with H.264/AVC using the structure of hierarchical B pictures. The spatial enhancement layer in CIF resolution is coded at a frame rate of 30 Hz using the MCTF with 4 decomposition stages. Each spatial layer has one SNR base layer and two FGS layers. For each SNR layer, the left hand side of Fig. 3.16 specifies its bit rate at maximum frame rate.

As shown, the QCIF layer has a maximum bit rate of 120kbits/s. By truncating the FGS layers, one can obtain a quality scalable bit-stream with a bit rate ranging from 40kbits/s which implies a minimum guaranteed quality to 120kbits/s. Also, a bit-stream of reduced frame rate can be extracted by dropping the B pictures in a dyadic manner. For instance, one can obtain a QCIF sequence of 7.5 Hz by dropping the frames labeled as B^2. A frame rate of 3.75 Hz can be obtained by discarding all the B pictures. Together with the SNR scalability, we can have a QCIF bit-stream with bit rate ranging from 10kbits/s to 120kbits/s and associated frame rate starting from 3.75 Hz to 15 Hz.

For the combined scalability, the same techniques can be applied in order to obtain a CIF bit-stream with a bit rate ranging from 20kbits/s to 480kbits/s and corresponding frame rate starting from 3.75 Hz to 30 Hz. Due to the inter-layer prediction, the decoding of the CIF layer requires the bit-streams of the QCIF layer. As a result, the bit rate of the CIF layer at 30 Hz starts from 160kbits/s, which includes the bit rates of the QCIF bit-streams. Particularly, in the example of Fig. 3.16, the 2nd FGS layer of the QCIF resolution is only used for the refinement of the QCIF layer. It is not exploited for the inter-layer prediction. Such a bit-stream is referred to as a Dead-Substream. It has been proved that using all the FGS layers for the inter-layer prediction may not be optimal for coding efficiency [17, 18]. Dead-Substream provides the flexibility to select an optimal truncation point for the inter-layer prediction.

3.3 Scalable Approach Using Inter-Frame Wavelet

By contrast to the aforementioned AVC-based scheme that basically employs the hybrid coding structure, a wavelet-based scheme using (t+2D) structure was proposed in [5, 19]. Similar to the AVC-based approach, the wavelet-based scheme can produce a fully embedded bit-stream that simultaneously supports spatial, temporal, and SNR scalability. However, a major difference between the AVC-based approach and the Wavelet-Based approach is that all the predictions in the latter case are conducted in an open-loop manner. The open-loop prediction provides more flexibility for bit-stream extraction and is more robust with respect to transmission errors. A recent variation can include a closed-loop prediction structure but it is not yet popular.

Fig. 3.2(b) shows the basic structure of a wavelet-based scheme using the t+2D structure. Within each GOP, MCTF is used for temporal decomposition. Particularly, the temporal low-pass frames are recursively generated via motion compensated filtering to achieve the temporal scalability. Other possible structures will be discussed in Sec. 3.3.4. To achieve the spatial scalability, the 2-D wavelet decomposition is done for each frame after the MCTF. To further reduce the bit rate and generate a scalable bit-stream, the wavelet coefficients are coded using a scalable entropy coder such as zero-tree coder or other types of arithmetic coder. By means of proper extraction techniques a single bit-stream with scalable spatial, temporal and SNR parameters can be produced. Similar wavelet video coding schemes but with specific features have been suggested by several other researchers [20, 21].

Historically, the wavelet-based schemes fell short in video quality in the MPEG standard competition in 2004. An ad hoc group in MPEG with a coined name VidWav was formed and has continued to study the wavelet video coding technique for the past two years. Based on the software originally developed by Microsoft Research Asia, this group produced a common simulation platform for testing and improving wavelet video algorithms [22, 23]. Additional reports on the recent VidWav group activities are summarized in [24] and [25].

In the following subsections, we give a brief overview of the basic concepts of the wavelet video scheme. The MPEG VidWav evaluation software will often be used for illustration. Although there are a number of on-going research works outside MPEG, our description focuses only on the MPEG related wavelet video projects. An interesting phenomenon is that over the past 3 years, several tools such as MCTF originally proposed for the wavelet schemes are now included in the AVC-based SVC with an open-loop concept. These tools have been discussed in the previous sections and we will minimize the overlap here. Some AVC tools such as the AVC base-layer are tested under the wavelet structure and the Variable Block-Size Motion Compensation.

3.3.1 Temporal Scalability

To provide the temporal scalability, the wavelet-based scheme also adopts the MCTF as described in Section 3.2.1. The MCTF concept was first proposed for wavelet coding [5]. Typically, Haar or $(5, 3)$ wavelets are used.

To improve the accuracy of the motion field so as to improve coding performance, several techniques for better motion estimation have been proposed in [26, 27]. Particularly, in [27], a novel structure, known as Barbell-Lifting, is presented. The basic idea is to use a "barbell" function for generating the prediction/update values in the lifting structure. Specifically, for each pixel in the high-pass frame, the prediction value is obtained by using a set of pixels as the input to the barbell function. It has been shown that the prediction using the barbell function offers a superior performance when compared to the conventional scheme using a single-pixel. It often reduces the mismatch of motion in the prediction and update steps. However, in the conventional t+2D structure, the motion vectors are estimated at the highest spatial resolution. In reconstructing the spatial low-resolution images the temporal prediction

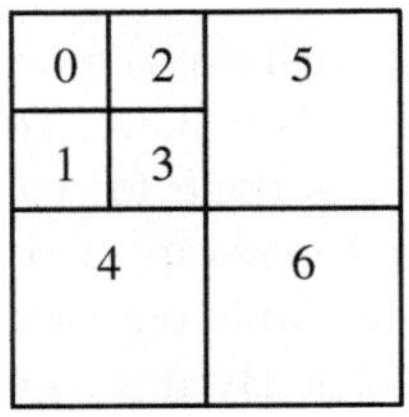

Fig. 3.17. Spatial sub-bands after a typical 2-level wavelet decomposition [22, 23].

uses a scaled down version of the motion vectors, which are inadequate from time to time. One solution to this problem is the 2D+t structure, which is also called in-band MCTF [20]. We will discuss the 2D+t(+2D) structure in Section 3.3.4.

3.3.2 Spatial and SNR Scalability

To achieve spatial scalability, a separable 2-D wavelet transform is applied to both the temporal low-pass and the high-pass frames. Similarly to JPEG2000, when only the low-resolution images are to be reconstructed, we decode the corresponding lower sub-band coefficients. A typical 2-level 2-D wavelet decomposition is shown in Fig. 3.17.

To provide the SNR scalability with fine granularity, an embedded zero-tree coding [6] can be used after the spatial decomposition. In addition to [6], other methods such as embedded zero-block coding (EZBC) [5] and embedded block coding with optimized truncation (EBCOT) [7] are also commonly used for coding the wavelet transform coefficients. This is done to reduce the temporal redundancy among successive frames. These coding techniques are used in the VidWav software and can be further extended to a 3-D structure such as 3-D EBCOT as proposed in [21].

3.3.3 Motion Scalability

The compressed bit-stream includes both the texture and the motion information. The bit-stream for the texture part can be almost arbitrarily truncated. However, the motion information can not be easily partitioned in the original wavelet video proposal, Motion Compensated Embedded Zero Block Coding (MC-EZBC) [5]. This is because the motion information can be large and can amount to consume a large percentage of the transmitted data in the low bit rate applications. This leads to few bits available for transmitting texture data. This results in poor subjective image quality. To solve this problem, motion information should also be represented in a scalable manner.

In [28], a scalable representation of motion information is proposed for the MC-EZBC scheme. Furthermore, in [29], the motion information is partitioned into multiple "motion layers". Each layer records the motion vectors with a specified accuracy. The lowest of these layers denotes only a rough representation of the motion vectors. The higher layers are used to refine the accuracy. Different layers are coded independently so that the motion information can be truncated at the layer boundary.

Due to the mismatch between the truncated motion information and the residual data, the schemes with scalable motion information have drifting errors. As a result, a linear model is proposed in [26] to provide a better trade-off between the scalable representation and the rate-distortion performance.

3.3.4 The (2D+t+2D) Structure

The 2D+t structure is suggested to reduce the drawbacks of the t+2D structure such as inaccurate motion vectors at lower spatial resolutions and drifting errors. Fig. 3.2 (c) shows a typical 2D+t+2D scheme. The 2D+t structure is also given where the second spatial decomposition is omitted. The first 2D spatial transform is usually a multi-level dyadic wavelet transform and is called the pre-spatial decomposition or transform. In this structure, MCTF is applied to each spatial sub-band generated by the pre-spatial transform. One drawback is that the motion estimation on the low-resolution images is not as good as the high resolution motion estimation. This is because only low-resolution references are used.

Based on the above observations, a second spatial wavelet decomposition, called post-spatial decomposition (or transform) is added as shown in Fig. 3.2(c) [22, 23]. The VidWav evaluation software is able to produce various combinations of pre- and post-spatial decompositions. Three examples are shown in Fig. 3.18. The first example, Fig. 3.18 (a), is a conventional t+2D scheme outputs with 3 temporal levels. The resulting four temporal sub-bands are t-LLL, t-LLH, t-LH, and t-H. A 2-level or 3-level post-spatial decomposition is then applied depending on the temporal sub-band. Since the t-H sub-band contains high-pass signals, it is reasonable to choose a smaller band split. Fig. 3.18 (b) shows a two-level pre-spatial decomposition. Only the lowest spatial band is further split by the post-spatial transforms. Fig. 3.18 (c) demonstrates a possible combination based on a similar concept when the pre-spatial transform has only two levels. This structure provides a lot of flexibility in trading the temporal with the spatial coding efficiency. For example, it enables the inter-layer prediction between the lower and higher spatial resolutions. This is an idea adopted by the AVC-based SVC. More sophisticated schemes in the 2D+t+2D category are also suggested as an addition to the VidWav software such as the Spatial-Temporal tool (STool). Here the inter-layer prediction is applied to the lower spatial band after MCTF [24, 25].

3.3.5 Enhanced Motion Compensated Filtering

Another problem in the conventional t+2D structure is that it produces image artifacts on low-pass temporal filtered images due to incorrect motion vectors.

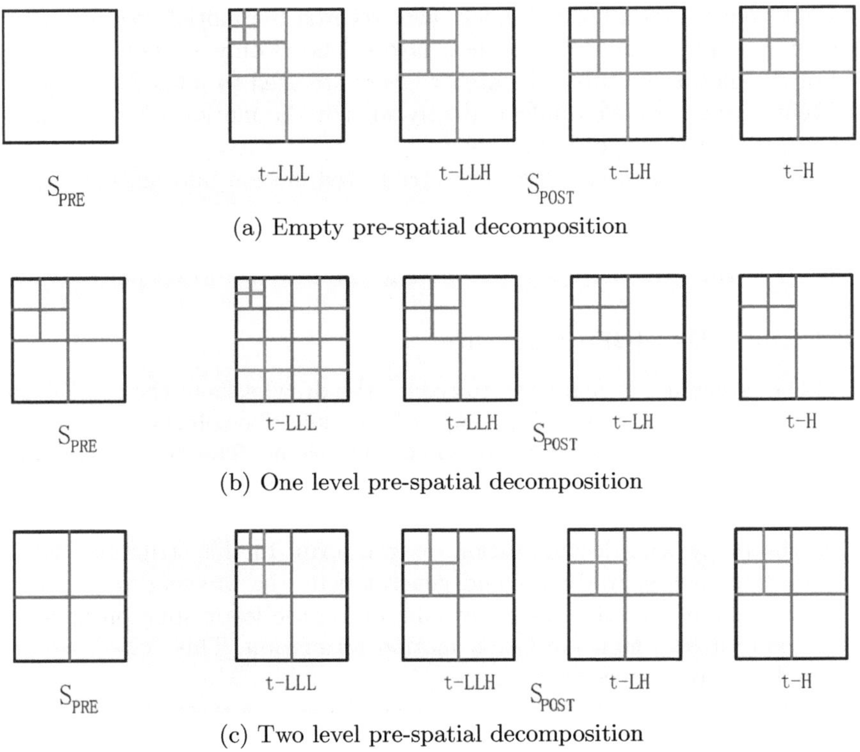

Fig. 3.18. Three examples of pre- and post-spatial decompositions [22, 23].

These artifacts are particularly visible after a few levels of temporal filtering. One remedy for this is by using the original frames as the low-pass frames. It essentially skips the update step in the lifting scheme. The disadvantage of this method is that it lowers the coding efficiency.

Another tool available in the VidWav software is leaky motion compensation. It is caused when high quality images are used for motion compensation, drift errors occur when the decoder does not receive all the high quality image information. The low quality image motion compensation suffers coding efficiency loss. The leaky motion compensation is an in between compromise and is typically used for low spatial sub-bands. When encoding these sub-bands, the difference between the high quality reference and the low quality interpolated reference is attenuated by a leaky factor. This leaky factor is adjustable.

Some other tools available in the VidWav software are the mode-based temporal filtering where each macroblock uses either the low quality reference or the high quality reference to make the prediction. Another tool is the AVC base-layer. When used, the wavelet scheme is applied only to the enhancement layer [22, 23].

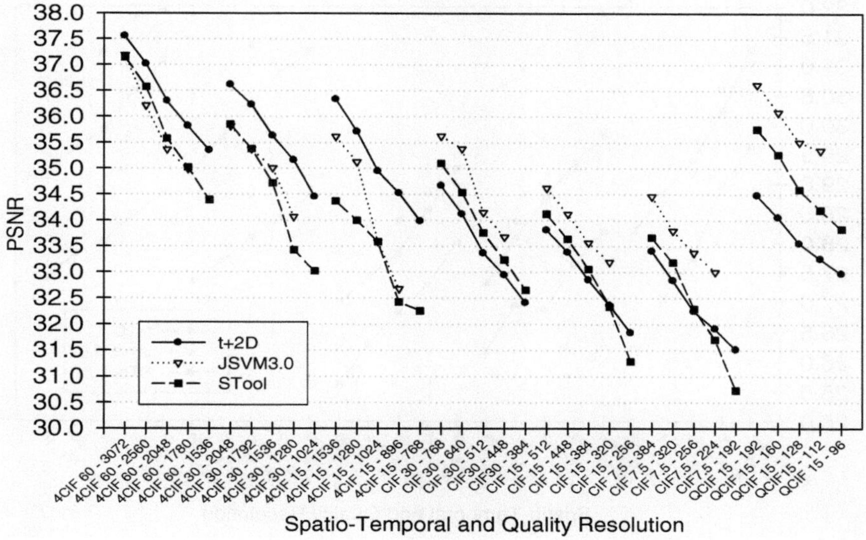

Fig. 3.19. Comparison of wavelet schemes with AVC-based SVC for the Harbour sequence [32].

3.3.6 Performance Comparison

The scalable extension of AVC/H.264 has been chosen to be the standard, the wavelet-based approach also has many promising features and open questions. In recent reports, the VidWave software can achieve comparable performance to the JSVM [24, 25, 30, 31, 32]. Figs. 3.19 and 3.20 show the performance comparison between the AVC-based scheme (denoted as JSVM) and the wavelet-based approach. They are extracted from the files in [32]. Fig. 3.19 is a case that favors the wavelet-based schemes. So far, the wavelet schemes show better results on high-resolution large motion pictures. The notion 4CIF is a picture format four times of the CIF size. This is about the size of the regular TV picture. Fig. 3.20 has nearly the worst performance of all wavelet schemes in [32].

Based on the comments and discussions in the VidWav group documents [24, 25, 30], the wavelet-based approach has its specific strengths but it also has weakness. Here is a brief summary. The advantages of the wavelet approach are as follows. The multi-resolution wavelets along both temporal and spatial axes provide a natural representation of image sequences. The wavelet video scheme provides a very large range of scalability. With the aid of embedded quantization and arithmetic coding, it offers an elegant, fine-grain SNR scalability. A typical wavelet video scheme has an open-loop structure, and it facilitates very flexible bit stream truncations. Another advantage of

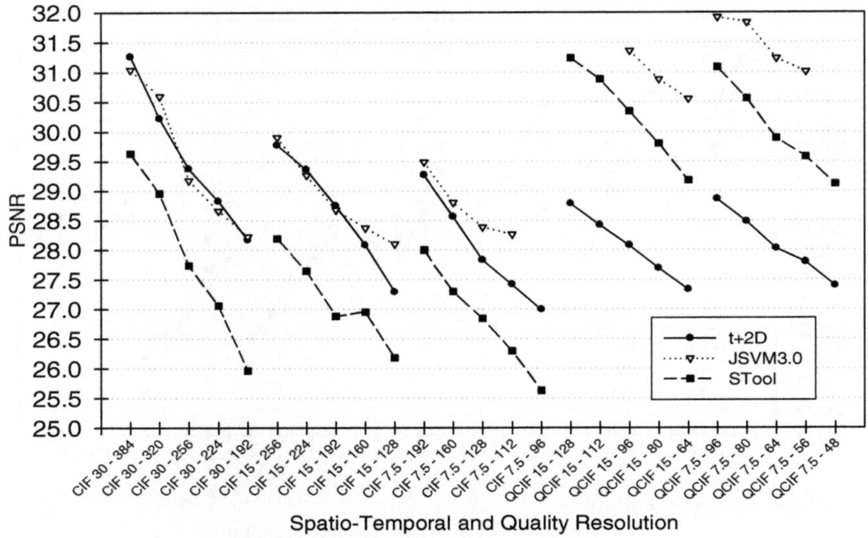

Fig. 3.20. Comparison of wavelet schemes with AVC-based SVC for the Mobile sequence [32].

the open-loop structure is that it eases the R-D optimization for selecting parameter values.

The current wavelet video schemes need improvement in some areas. The objective SNR is often good but the subjective image quality at lower bit rates is not as good as the images produced by AVC. This is often due to the low quality of the low pass temporal filtered pictures owing to incorrect motion vectors and/or down-sampling filters. High quality temporal references provide better coding efficiency but they induce drifting errors at low rates when high quality references are not available. A powerful tool, intra-prediction in AVC, is not well adopted by the wavelet scheme.

Overall, the wavelet video scheme is a relatively young structure in video coding. It seems to have a good potential in providing very good coding efficiency on the high-definition. That is in high rate, high resolution pictures. It offers also a high number of combined spatial-temporal scalable levels and extremely fine-grain SNR scalability. It may also do a better job for non-dyadic spatial scalability. With an open-loop structure, it can be more robust in coping with transmission errors. Finally, it can be made compatible with the JPEG2000 standard for single image compression [25].

3.4 Conclusions

In this chapter, we have reviewed the fundamentals of SVC and its latest development in the MPEG standard. Both the AVC-based approach and the wavelet-based scheme are capable of offering a fully scalable bit-stream. The AVC-based approach has been selected as the joint ITU and ISO MPEG SVC standard. The wavelet-based scheme still has the potential for use as a future video coding applications/standard. Research activities on the wavelet-based technology have been growing rapidly in the past a few years. The MPEG committee continuously keeps an ad-hoc group working on this subject. At the moment, a number of core experiments are in progress for the AVC-based SVC in MPEG. The target date of completing the MPEG SVC standard is 2007.

References

1. Ohm, J.R. (2004): registered responses to the call for proposals on scalable video coding. ISO/IEC JTC1/SC29/WG11, M10569
2. Reichel, J., Hanke, K., Popescu, B. (2004): Scalable video model v1.0. ISO/IEC JTC1/SC29/WG11, N6372
3. Reichel, J., Wien, M., Schwarz, H. (2004): Scalable video model 3. ISO/IEC JTC1/SC29/WG11, N6716
4. Ridge, J., Bao, Y., Karczewicz, M., Wang, X. (2005): Cyclical block coding for FGS. ISO/IEC JTC1/SC29/WG11, M11509
5. Hsiang, S.T., Woods, J.W. (2001): Embedded video coding using invertible motion compensated 3-D subband/wavelet filter band. Signal Processing: Image Communication, **16**, 704–724
6. Sharipo, J. (1993): Embedded image coding using zerotrees of wavelet coefficients. IEEE Trans. on Signal Processing, **41**, 3445–3462
7. Taubman, D. (2000): High performance scalable image compression with EBCOT. IEEE Transactions on Image Processing, **9**, 1158–1170
8. MPEG (2004): MPEG testing group: Subjective test results for the CfP on scalable video coding technology. ISO/IEC JTC1/SC29/WG11, N6383
9. Reichel, J., Schwarz, H., Wien, M. (2005): Scalable video coding working draft 2. ISO/IEC JTC1/SC29/WG11 and ITU-T SG16 Q.6, JVT-O201
10. Weigand, T. (2003): Draft ITU-T recommendation and final draft international standard of joint video specification (ITU-T Rec. H.264 — ISO/IEC 14496-10 AVC). ISO/IEC JTC1/SC29/WG11 and ITU-T SG16 Q.6, JVT-G050
11. Tabatabai, A., Visharam, Z., Suzuki, T. (2005): Study of effect of update step in MCTF. ISO/IEC JTC1/SC29/WG11 and ITU-T SG16 Q.6, JVT-Q026
12. Schwarz, H., Marpe, D., Wiegand, T. (2005): Comparison of MCTF and closed-loop hierarchical B pictures. ISO/IEC JTC1/SC29/WG11 and ITU-T SG16 Q.6, JVT-P059
13. Ridge, J., Bao, Y., Karczewicz, M., Wang, X. (2005): Cyclical block coding for FGS. ISO/IEC JTC1/SC29/WG11, M11509

14. Winken, M., Schwarz, H., Marpe, D., Wiegand, T. (2006): CE7: Adaptive motion refinement for FGS. ISO/IEC JTC1/SC29/WG11 and ITU-T SG16 Q.6, JVT-R022
15. Huang, H.C., Wang, C.N., Chiang, T. (2002): A robust fine granularity scalability using trellis based predictive leak. IEEE Trans. on Circuits Syst. for Video Technol., **12**, 372–385
16. Peng, W.H., Chen, Y.K. (2003): Enhanced mode-adaptive fine granularity scalability. Int'l Journal of Imaging Systems and Technology, **13**, 308–321
17. Amonou, I., Cammas, N., Kervadec, S., Pateux, S. (2005): Coding rate coverage extension with dead substreams in the SVM. ISO/IEC JTC1/SC29/WG11, M11703
18. Amonou, I., Cammas, N., Kervadec, S., Pateux, S. (2005): Response to CE 5: Quality layers. ISO/IEC JTC1/SC29/WG11 and ITU-T SG16 Q.6, JVT-O044
19. Ohm, J.R. (1994): Three-dimensional subband coding with motion compensation. IEEE Trans. on Image Processing, **3**, 559–571
20. Andreopoulos, Y., Munteanu, A., Barbarien, J., der Schaar, M.V., Cornelis, J., Schelkens, P. (2004): In-band motion compensated temporal filtering. Signal Processing: Image Communication, **19**, 653–673
21. Taubman, D., Mehrseresht, N., Leung, R. (2004): SVC technical contribution: Overview of recent technology developments at UNSW. ISO/IEC JTC1/SC29/WG11, M10868
22. Xiong, R., Ji, X., Zhang, D., Xu, J., Pau, G., Trocan, M., Bottreau, V. (2005): Vidwav wavelet video coding specifications. ISO/IEC JTC1/SC29/WG11, M12339
23. MPEG (2005): MPEG video group: Wavelet codec reference document and software manual. ISO/IEC JTC1/SC29/WG11, N7334
24. Brangoulo, S., Leonardi, R., Mrak, M., Pesquet, B.P., Xu, J. (2005): Draft status report on wavelet video coding exploration. ISO/IEC JTC1/SC29/WG11, N7571
25. Leonardi, R., Brangoulo, S., Signoroni, A. (2006): Status report version 1 on wavelet video coding exploration. ISO/IEC JTC1/SC29/WG11, N7822
26. Secker, A., Taubman, D. (2004): Highly scalable video compression with scalable motion coding. IEEE Trans. Circuits Syst. Video Technol., **13**, 1029–1041
27. Xu, J., Xiong, R., Feng, B., Sullivan, G., Lee, M.C., Wu, F., Li, S. (2004): 3D sub-band video coding using barbell lifting. ISO/IEC JTC1/SC29/WG11, M10569
28. Hang, H.M., Tsai, S.S., Chiang, T. (2003): Motion information scalability for MC-EZBC. ISO/IEC JTC1/SC29/WG11, M9756
29. Tsai, C.Y., Hsu, H.K., Hang, H.M., Chiang, T. (2004): Response to Cfp on scalable video coding technology: Proposal S08 – A scalable video coding scheme based on interframe wavelet technique. ISO/IEC JTC1/SC29/WG11, M9756
30. Xiong, R., Xu, J., Wu, F. (2005): Coding perfromance comparison between MSRA wavelet video coding and JSVM. ISO/IEC JTC1/SC29/WG11, M11975
31. Leonardi, R., Brescianini, M., Khalil, H., Xu, J.Z., Brangoulo, S. (2006): Report on testing in wavelet video Coding. ISO/IEC JTC1/SC29/WG11, M13294
32. Adami, N., Brescianini, M., Leonardi, R., Signoroni, A. (2005): Performance evaluation of the current wavelet video coding reference software. ISO/IEC JTC1/SC29/WG11, M12643

Part III

Various Data Hiding Techniques

4

A Bit-Level Visual Secret Sharing Scheme for Multi-Secret Images Using Rotation and Reversion Operations

Chin-Chen Chang[1,2], Tzu-Chuen Lu[2], and Yi-Hsuan Fan[3]

[1] Feng Chia University, Taichung, Taiwan, 40724, R.O.C.,
ccc@cs.ccu.edu.tw,
WWW home page: http://www.cs.ccu.edu.tw/~ccc
[2] Chaoyang University of Technology, Taiwan, 413, R.O.C.
tclu@cyut.edu.tw
[3] National Chung Cheng University, Chiayi, Taiwan, 621, R.O.C.

Summary. In 1995, Naor and Shamir proposed a visual secret sharing scheme to share a secret image with several participants. In this chapter, we extend the concept of visual secret sharing to gray-scale image visual secret sharing. This chapter applies the rotation and reversion operations to increase the security of the secret images and the utilization of the shared shadows. The experimental results show that the scheme can completely reconstruct the original gray-scale image, and the shadows can be used to hide more secret images. In addition, the proposed scheme can be extended to the application that some specific participants are only allowed to restore a certain amount of secret information.

4.1 Introduction

Secret sharing is a very interesting and important issue for variance applications, such as secure key management, secret data protection, and so on. In order to protect a secret file or text, we use a secret key to encrypt it. However, if unauthorized people or even our members use the secret key to decrypt the file, then the secret file is very likely to be stolen. Therefore, we need a secret key management to protect the secret key. The secret sharing system is a strategy formed to protect the secret key [1, 2].

Blakley [3] and Naor and Shamir [4] proposed their schemes for secret sharing. In Naor and Shamir's scheme, a key, which can be used to access many important files, is divided into several pieces, called shadows or shares. Then, those shadows are distributed to different participants. Each participant cannot retrieve any information from the shadow. When we need the key to access a file, a subset of participants can collect their shadows and reconstruct the key. A general secret sharing problem is t-out-of-n secret sharing. It is

C.-C. Chang et al.: *A Bit-Level Visual Secret Sharing Scheme for Multi-Secret Images Using Rotation and Reversion Operations*, Studies in Computational Intelligence (SCI) **58**, 83–101 (2007)
www.springerlink.com

also called $(t,\ n)$-secret sharing. The total number of participants sharing the secret key is n, and we need to have at least t of the shadows to reconstruct the secret key [5].

In 1995, Naor and Shamir introduced a new application, Visual Secret Sharing (VSS), for secret sharing. The basic problem with VSS is to share a secret image with several participants. For a general $(t,\ n)$-VSS scheme, the secret image is divided into n shadows, and each shadow is dispatched to different participants. The participant cannot find out any information from the shadow; because each shadow has only part of the secret information, and t or more shadows are needed to recover the secret image. They only become visible by stacking t shadows together. It is not necessary to use any complicated computation and other advanced cryptographic mechanisms to reveal the image.

Naor and Shamir's scheme is only suitable for a binary image composed of black and white pixels, but not for gray-scale or color images. Hence, the practical application of the scheme is limited. Some researchers converted the gray-scale image into halftone images as the secret data needed to replace the binary image. For example, Lin and Tsai [6] used dithering techniques to convert a gray-scale image into a binary image. Firstly, they divided a gray-scale image into several blocks. Secondly, they used a space-filling curve dither array to mix the order of the pixels in each block. Thirdly, they computed the score for each pixel in the block. If the score of the pixel is smaller than a dithering threshold, then the pixel is represented by a black bit. Otherwise, the pixel is represented by a white bit. After being converted, the binary image is obtained as the secret image. Then, they applied the general VSS scheme on the secret image to generate some shadows for the latter use.

Nevertheless, the quality of the recovered image is low when using this scheme on the binary images. From the human visual systems, we see that the revealed image is not clear when compared to the original. Therefore, many researchers reconsidered the physical properties of contrast, resolution, and color, of the image to improve the performance of VSS schemes [7, 8, 9].

In 2005, Lukac and Plataniotis [10] proposed a bit-level based VSS scheme operated directly on the bit planes of the secret image. That is, they decomposed the secret image into several bit planes and took each bit plane as a binary image. Their scheme could completely recover the original secret image. In this scheme, n participants could share one secret image.

However, for a company which owns a large number of secret images, each participant needs to maintain many secret shadows to recover the secret images as each shadow only can be used to recover one secret image. In order to broaden the utility of the shadow, Droste [11] introduced a new method for the VSS scheme. In Droste's VSS scheme, a shadow can contain several secret messages. That is, any t participants can recover a different secret image by using Droste's VSS scheme. Nevertheless, Droste's scheme is inefficient.

This chapter proposes an efficient VSS scheme that adopts Lukac and Plataniotis' bit-level concept to represent the secret image. The recovered image is the same as the original one. The scheme can also be used to share other secret messages among the participants.

4.2 Related Works

In Naor and Shamir's (t, n)-VSS scheme, the secret image is divided into n shadows for the different participants. Each pixel in the image is then expanded into sub-pixels for each shadow according to the encryption function and two codebooks, C_0 and C_1. Each codebook includes a number of pattern sets, and is used to generate the shadows for the participants. For a white pixel, the VSS scheme randomly chooses one pattern set from C_0. While for a black pixel, the scheme randomly chooses one pattern set from C_1.

Fig. 4.1 gives a (2, 2)-VSS example that is encrypted by using Naor and Shamir's VSS scheme. In Fig. 4.1, a secret image I is divided into two secret shadows, S^1 and S^2. Assume that the codebooks used in this example are C_0 and C_1 as shown in Fig. 4.2. Each codebook consists of six pattern sets. Each pattern set includes two patterns used to generate the shadows for S^1 and S^2.

The VSS scheme splits each pixel into two patterns, which are chosen from the codebooks C_0 and C_1, and then pastes the patterns in the shadows. For example, the i-th pixel of I in Fig. 4.1 is a black pixel. Hence, the scheme randomly chooses the fourth pattern set from C_1 and respectively pastes the patterns to S^1 and S^2. After encryption, the secret image is divided into two binary shadows, each of which is 2×2 times larger than the secret image. When we need to decrypt the secret image, the VSS scheme stacks a certain number of shadows to reveal the image. Following the same procedure, the reconstructed image I' is shown in Fig. 4.1.

Let us consider a real image with size 128×64 as the secret image. Fig. 4.3 demonstrates the (2, 2)-VSS scheme, where Fig. 4.3(a) is the input image and Fig. 4.3(b) and Fig. 4.3(c) are two generated shadows. Fig. 4.3(d) is the output which is four times larger than the original input.

In the decryption process, the VSS scheme stacks the shadows by using the decryption function $f_{\mathrm{d\_NS}}$ to reconstruct the secret image. The function $f_{\mathrm{d\_NS}}$ maps a certain number of blocks in each shadow into a binary pixel. This function is defined as follows:

$$f_{\mathrm{d\_NS}}(S_{\mathrm{i}}^1, S_{\mathrm{i}}^2) = \begin{cases} 1, & \text{if } S_{\mathrm{i}}^1 = 1 \cup S_{\mathrm{i}}^2 = 1, \\ 0, & \text{otherwise,} \end{cases} \tag{4.1}$$

where S_{i}^1 and S_{i}^2 are the i-th bit of S_1 and S_2, respectively. In Eq. (4.1), if both values of S_{i}^1 and S_{i}^2 are 1, it means that the color of the bit is black. And then, the color of the reconstructed bit is black.

The Naor and Shamir's scheme is simple and intuitive. However, the visual quality of the reconstructed image using the scheme is poor. In addition, the scheme cannot provide a perfect reconstruction of the pixel intensity aspect.

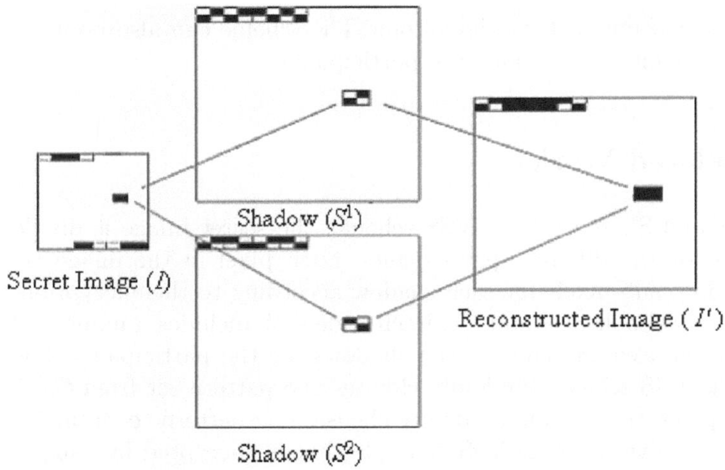

Fig. 4.1. The basic (2, 2)-VSS scheme.

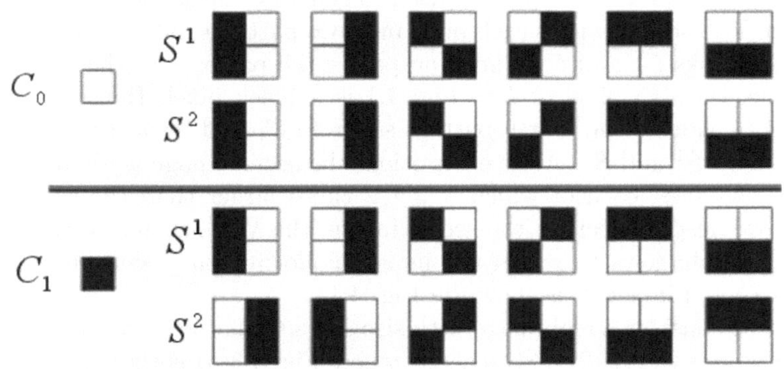

Fig. 4.2. Two codebooks for Naor and Shamir's (2, 2)-VSS scheme.

In order to improve the weaknesses of Naor and Shamir's scheme, Lukac and Plataniotis proposed a bit-level secret sharing scheme. In Lukac and Plataniotis's scheme, the gray-scale image is represented by eight bit planes. The example binary planes are shown in Fig. 4.4.

Lukac and Plataniotis regarded each plane as a secret image and used Naor and Shamir's VSS encryption process to generate the sub-shadows. The resultant sub-shadows of j-th plane are represented by α^{j} and β^{j}. Hence, the final shadows are composed according to

$$S_{\mathrm{i}}^1 = \alpha_{\mathrm{i}}^1 \times 2^7 + \alpha_{\mathrm{i}}^2 \times 2^6 + \cdots + \alpha_{\mathrm{i}}^7 \times 2^1 + \alpha_{\mathrm{i}}^8, \quad \text{and} \tag{4.2}$$

$$S_{\mathrm{i}}^2 = \beta_{\mathrm{i}}^1 \times 2^7 + \beta_{\mathrm{i}}^2 \times 2^6 + \cdots + \beta_{\mathrm{i}}^7 \times 2^1 + \beta_{\mathrm{i}}^8, \tag{4.3}$$

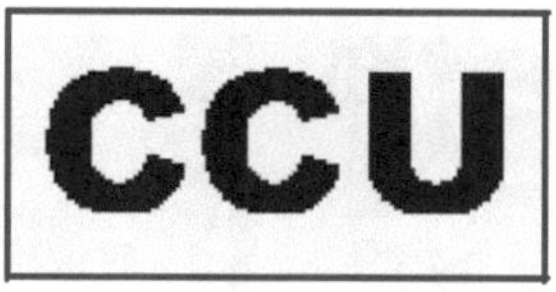

(a) the secret image of size 128 × 64

(b) the first shadow S^1

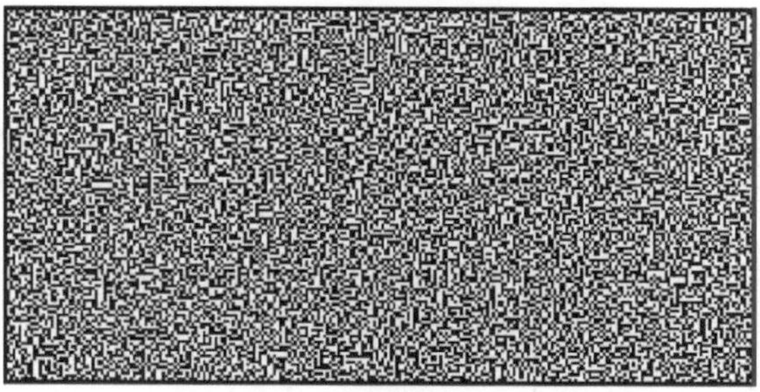

(c) the second shadow S^2

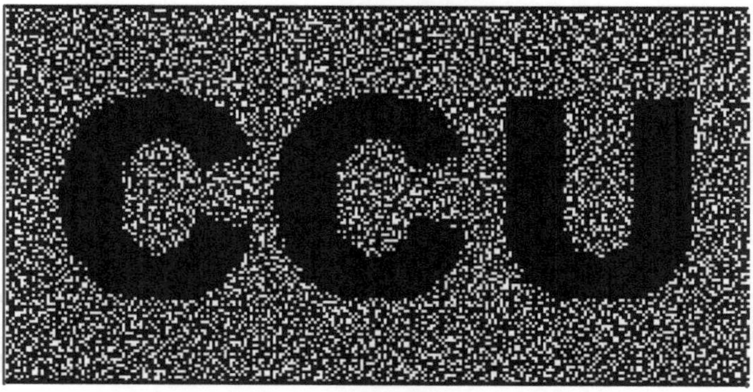

(d) the recovered image of size 256 × 128

Fig. 4.3. An example of (2, 2)-VSS scheme.

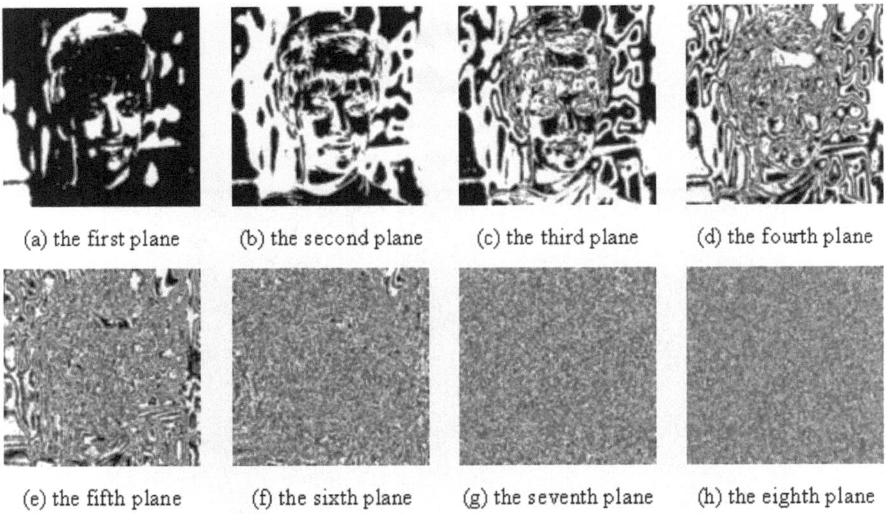

Fig. 4.4. The eight binary planes of the gray-scale image.

where α_i^j and β_i^j are i-th bits of α^j and β^j, respectively.

In the decryption process, the scheme stacks the shadows, S^1 and S^2, by using the decryption function f_{d_LP} to reconstruct the secret image. The function f_{d_LP} is defined as follows:

$$f_{d\_LP}(S_i^1, S_i^2) = \begin{cases} 1, & \text{if } \alpha_i \in C_1 \cap \beta_i \in C_1; \\ 0, & \text{otherwise.} \end{cases} \tag{4.4}$$

Lukac and Plataniotis' scheme can completely reconstruct the original secret image. In their scheme, several shadows can only be used to reserve one secret image. The utilization of the shadows is low. In this chapter, we shall adopt Lukac and Plataniotis' scheme to represent the secret image with bit-level. Furthermore, by our method each shadow can be used to carry more secret information.

4.3 The Proposed (2, 2)-VSS Scheme

In this section, we propose a bit-level based (2, 2)-VSS scheme to encrypt and decrypt gray-scale images. The diagram of the proposed scheme is shown in Fig. 4.5. Fig. 4.5(a) is the encryption process, while Fig. 4.5(b) is the decryption process.

4.3.1 The Encryption Process

The first step of the encryption process is to divide a gray-scale image into several sub-regions having a triangular shape. Each sub-region can be used to hide a secret image. Let $T = \{T_1, T_2, \cdots, T_{2^k}\}$ be the set of 2^k sub-regions, where T_i is the i-th sub-region. The total number of sub-regions in the gray-scale image is 2^k which means we have 2^k secret images in the gray-scale image.

In the second step, the gray-scale image is represented by eight bit planes. Let $P = \{P^1, P^2, \cdots, P^8\}$ be a set of eight bit planes of the image. Here $P^j = \{T_1^j, T_2^j, \cdots, T_{2^k}^j\}$ is the j-th plane, which consists of several sub-regions.

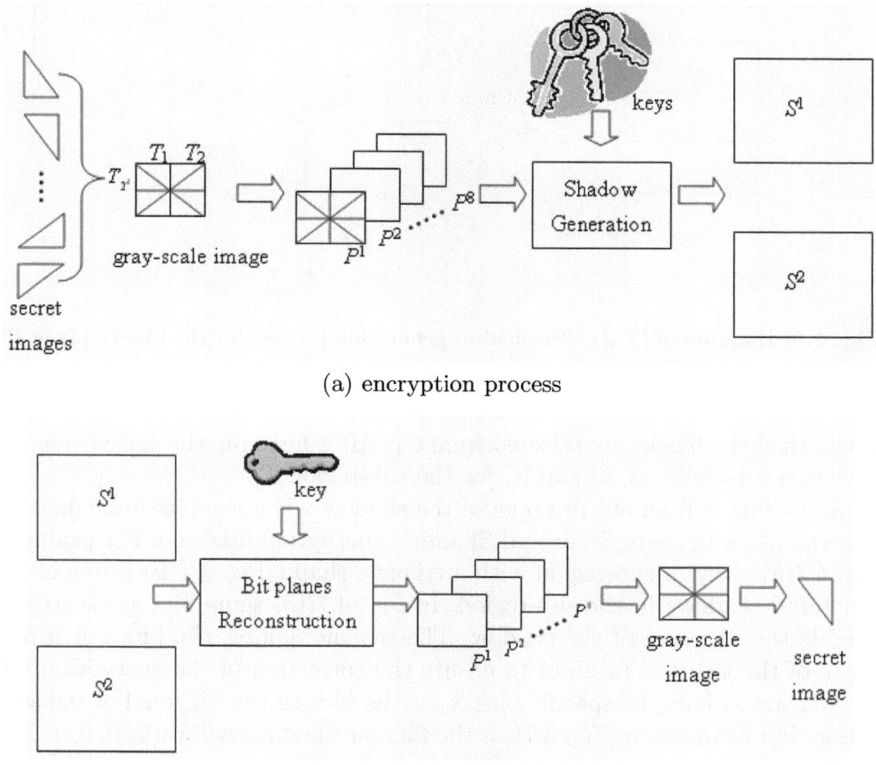

(a) encryption process

(b) decryption process

Fig. 4.5. Diagram of the proposed scheme.

The third step is to generate shadows for each binary plane P^j. The shadow generation process for P^j is shown in Fig. 4.6. The scheme splits each bit of the sub-region into several blocks by using Naor and Shamir's encryption function.

The encryption function maps each bit of T_i^j into a block of size 2×2 from C_0 or C_1 to different shadows. If the color of the input bit is white, then the blocks are randomly chosen from C_0. Otherwise, the color of the input bit is

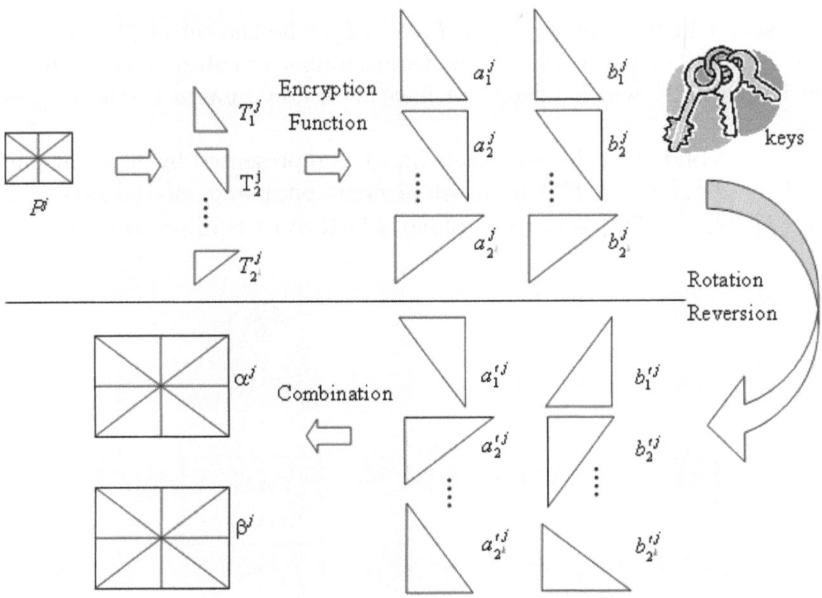

Fig. 4.6. Diagram of (2, 2)-VSS shadow generation process for the binary plane P^j.

black, then the blocks are selected from C_1. After finishing the encryption, we have two sub-shadows, a_i^j and b_i^j, for the sub-region T_i^j.

Some bits will be out of range of the shadow when the bits are expended into the block by using Naor and Shamir's encryption function. For example, Fig. 4.7(a) shows a sub-region with a triangle shape. Fig. 4.7(b) is one of the generated shadows in the sub-region. In Fig. 4.7(b), some bits are scattered outside the diagonal of the shadow. The scheme ignores the bits not in the range of the shadow. In order to ensure the correction of the decryption bit, the scheme assigns the specific blocks for the bits on the diagonal of the sub-region. For example, in Fig. 4.7(a), the bits on the diagonal are 0, 0, 0, 1, and 0. For the bit with value 0, the scheme assigns the blocks $\begin{bmatrix} 0\,0 \\ 1\,1 \end{bmatrix}$ and $\begin{bmatrix} 0\,0 \\ 1\,1 \end{bmatrix}$ for the first sub-shadow a_i^j and the second sub-shadow b_i^j, respectively. For the bit with value 1, the scheme assigns the blocks $\begin{bmatrix} 1\,0 \\ 1\,0 \end{bmatrix}$ and $\begin{bmatrix} 0\,1 \\ 0\,1 \end{bmatrix}$ for a_i^j and b_i^j, respectively.

In order to increase the complexity and enhance the security of the proposed scheme, the sub-shadows are placed in different locations of the plane by using a secret key. The scheme generates two random sequences, $RA^j = (ra_1\ ra_2\ \cdots\ ra_{2^k})$ and $RB^j = (rb_1\ rb_2\ \cdots\ rb_{2^k})$ for the j-th plane P^j by using the secret key, which is only known to the participants. Then, the scheme moves the i-th sub-shadow a_i^j to the ra_i-th location of the newly con-

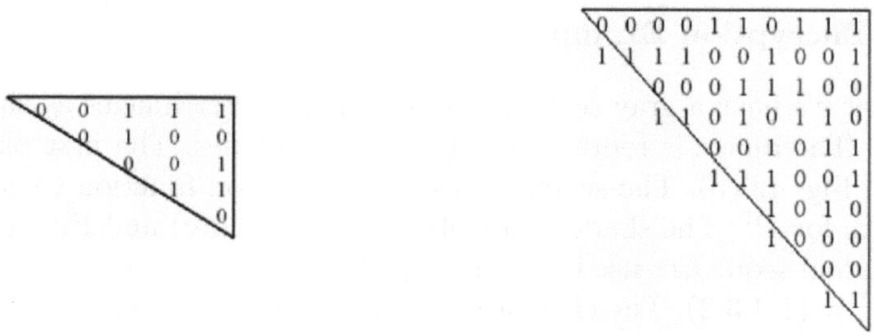

(a) the orignal binary sub-region (b) one of the shadows of the sub-region

Fig. 4.7. An example of a binary sub-region and ont of its generated shadows.

structed shadow α^j, and moves the i-th sub-shadow b^j_i to the rb_i-th location of the newly constructed shadow β^j.

However, the shape of the sub-shadow may not fit in with that of the new location. Hence, the scheme uses right-rotation, left-rotation, horizontal-reversion, and vertical-reversion operations to change the shape of the sub-shadow. A sub-region example after four operations is shown in Fig. 4.8. Let $\hat{a}^j_1, \hat{a}^j_2, \cdots$, and $\hat{a}^j_{2k}$, and $\hat{b}^j_1, \hat{b}^j_2, \cdots$, and $\hat{b}^j_{2k}$ be the new generated sub-shadows. Next, the scheme respectively combines the sub-shadows, $\hat{a}^j_1, \hat{a}^j_2, \cdots$, and $\hat{a}^j_{2k}$, and $\hat{b}^j_1, \hat{b}^j_2, \cdots$, and $\hat{b}^j_{2k}$ to form the shadows α^j and β^j, for the plane P^j.

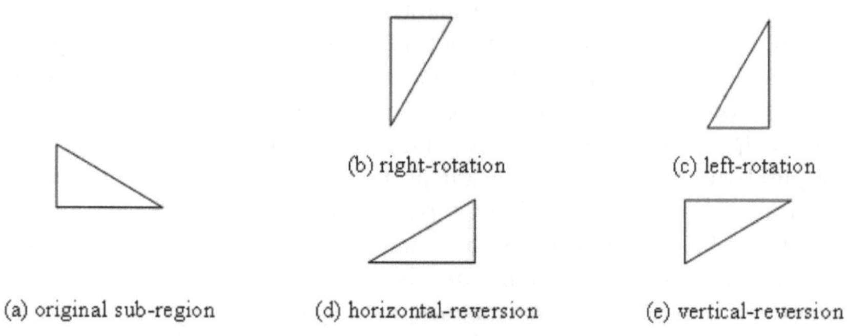

Fig. 4.8. An example sub-region after four operations.

Finally, the scheme collects the sub-shadows generated for each plane in order to compose the final shadows, which are expressed as

$$S^1 = \alpha^1 \times 2^7 + \alpha^2 \times 2^6 + \cdots + \alpha^7 \times 2^1 + \alpha^8, \quad \text{and} \tag{4.5}$$

$$S^2 = \beta^1 \times 2^7 + \beta^2 \times 2^6 + \cdots + \beta^7 \times 2^1 + \beta^8. \tag{4.6}$$

4.3.2 An Encryption Example

Assume that we have a gray-scale image with four secret images as shown in Fig. 4.9(a). The image is represented by eight bit planes. The first plane P^1 is shown in Fig. 4.9(b). The scheme uses the encryption function to generate two shadows for P^1. The shadows are shown in Fig. 4.9(c) and Fig. 4.9(d).

The random sequences used to rearrange the sub-shadows be $RA^1 = (3\ 2\ 1\ 4)$ and $RB^1 = (1\ 4\ 3\ 2)$. The element $ra_1 = 3$ means a_1^1 should be rearranged to the third location of the plane. The shape of a_1^1 is an inverted triangle. However, the shape of the third location of the plane is an equiangular triangle. In order to match the shape of a_1^1 with that of a_3^1, we use the vertical-reversion operation to reverse a_1^1. In addition, the element $rb_2 = 4$ means that b_2^1 should be put in the fourth location of the plane. For b_2^1, we use the horizontal-reversion operation to reverse b_2^1. The shadows α^1 and β^1 of P^1 are shown in Fig. 4.9(e) and Fig. 4.9(f), respectively. Following the same encryption process, we can obtain the final shadows S^1 and S^2 shown in Fig. 4.9(g) and Fig. 4.9(h), respectively.

4.3.3 The Decryption Process

Before starting the decryption process, the scheme decomposes each shadow into eight planes. For example, the first shadow S^1 is decomposed into eight bit planes, $\alpha^1, \alpha^2, \cdots, \alpha^8$. Next, the scheme performs the bit plane reconstruction process to reconstruct the original binary plane P^{j}. The diagram of the reconstruction process for P^{j} is shown in Fig. 4.10.

The first step of the reconstruction process is to separate the sub-region from the shadows α^{j} and β^{j}. The second step is to move the sub-shadows, $\hat{a}_{\mathrm{i}}^{\mathrm{j}}$ and $\hat{b}_{\mathrm{i}}^{\mathrm{j}}$, back to their original locations, $a_{\mathrm{i}}^{\mathrm{j}}$ and $b_{\mathrm{i}}^{\mathrm{j}}$. The scheme uses the random sequences, $RA^{\mathrm{j}} = (ra_1\ ra_2\ \cdots\ ra_{2^{\mathrm{k}}})$ and $RB^{\mathrm{j}} = (rb_1\ rb_2\ \cdots\ rb_{2^{\mathrm{k}}})$, to restore the original sub-shadows. Only legal participants own the secret keys used to generate the sequences RA^{j} and RB^{j} to rearrange the locations of the sub-shadows. In this step, right-rotation, left-rotation, horizontal-reversion, and vertical-reversion operations are also used to change the shape of the sub-shadows so as to fit in with the original locations.

In the third step, the decryption function is used to decrypt the secret information in the restored $a_{\mathrm{i}}^{\mathrm{j}}$ and $b_{\mathrm{i}}^{\mathrm{j}}$. The scheme stacks the sub-shadows, $a_{\mathrm{i}}^{\mathrm{j}}$ and $b_{\mathrm{i}}^{\mathrm{j}}$, using the decryption function $f_{\mathrm{d\_CLF}}$ to reconstruct the original sub-region $T_{\mathrm{i}}^{\mathrm{j}}$, which is defined as follows,

$$f_{\mathrm{d\_CLF}}(a_{\mathrm{i}}^{\mathrm{j}}, b_{\mathrm{i}}^{\mathrm{j}}) = \begin{cases} 1, & \text{if } a_{\mathrm{i}\gamma}^{\mathrm{j}} \in C_1 \cap b_{\mathrm{i}\gamma}^{\mathrm{j}} \in C_1; \\ 0, & \text{otherwise}, \end{cases} \tag{4.7}$$

where $a_{\mathrm{i}\gamma}^{\mathrm{j}}$ is the γ-th block of $a_{\mathrm{i}}^{\mathrm{j}}$, and $b_{\mathrm{i}\gamma}^{\mathrm{j}}$ is the γ-th block of $b_{\mathrm{i}}^{\mathrm{j}}$. Let $T_{\mathrm{i}\gamma}^{\mathrm{j}} = f_{\mathrm{d\_CLF}}(a_{\mathrm{i}}^{\mathrm{j}}, b_{\mathrm{i}}^{\mathrm{j}})$, where $T_{\mathrm{i}\gamma}^{\mathrm{j}}$ is the γ-th bit of $T_{\mathrm{i}}^{\mathrm{j}}$.

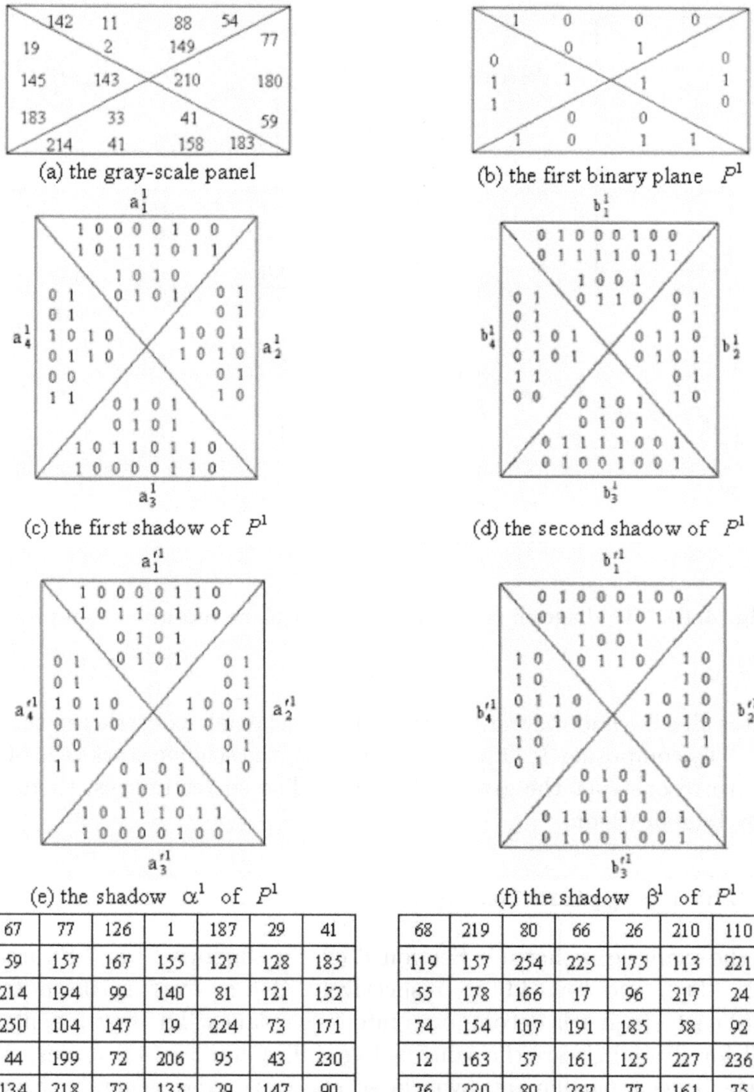

(a) the gray-scale panel
(b) the first binary plane P^1
(c) the first shadow of P^1
(d) the second shadow of P^1
(e) the shadow α^1 of P^1
(f) the shadow β^1 of P^1

238	67	77	126	1	187	29	41
180	59	157	167	155	127	128	185
102	214	194	99	140	81	121	152
10	250	104	147	19	224	73	171
133	44	199	72	206	95	43	230
58	134	218	72	135	29	147	90
83	125	5	147	88	224	124	235
245	159	70	170	55	162	129	61

(g) the first shadow S^1

68	219	80	66	26	210	110	104
119	157	254	225	175	113	221	211
55	178	166	17	96	217	24	188
74	154	107	191	185	58	92	213
12	163	57	161	125	227	236	123
76	220	80	237	77	161	75	222
163	190	74	146	48	230	120	212
106	104	95	210	92	225	202	117

(h) the second shadow S^2

Fig. 4.9. An encryption example employing the proposed scheme.

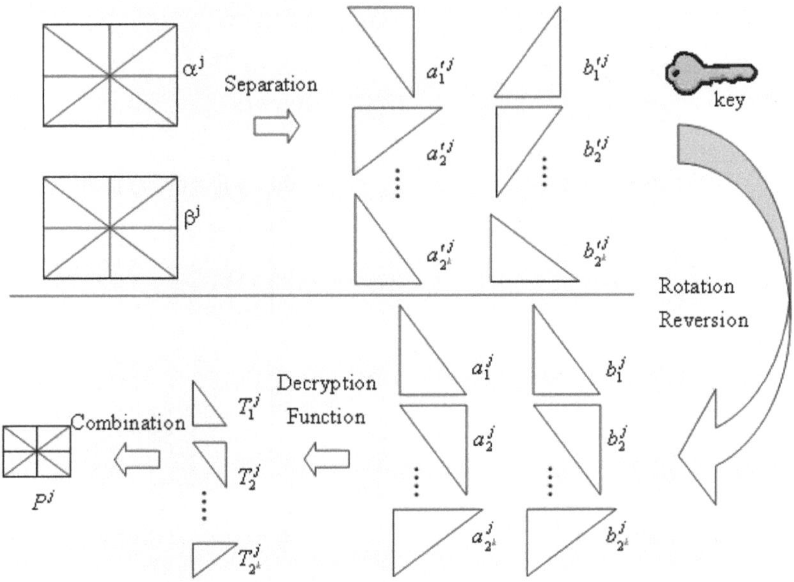

Fig. 4.10. The diagram of the (2,2)-VSS bit plane reconstruction process.

After all sub-shadows were decrypted, the scheme reconstructed the binary plane P^j by composing $T_1^j, T_2^j, \cdots, T_{2^k}^j$. Finally, the scheme stacks the obtained planes to reconstruct the gray-scale image. The secret images, then, can be seen by human vision.

4.3.4 The Decryption Example

Using the example as shown in Section 4.3.2, the shadows S^1 and S^2 are shown in Fig. 4.9(g) and Fig. 4.9(h), respectively. Before starting the decryption process, each shadow is decomposed into eight planes. The first two planes α^1 and β^1 for S^1 and S^2 are the same as Fig. 4.9(e) and Fig. 4.9(f), respectively. Because the legal participants own the secret keys used to generate the original random sequences, $RA^1 = (3\ 2\ 1\ 4)$ and $RB^1 = (1\ 4\ 3\ 2)$, the scheme can restore the sub-shadows of α^1 and β^1 into their original locations. The first element of RA^1 is 3, which means the first sub-shadow a_1^1 is reversed to become a_3^1. Therefore, we change the sub-shadow $\hat{a}_3^1$ into its original location 1. The second element of RB^1 is 4, which means the second sub-shadow b_2^1 is reversed to b_4^1. We change the sub-shadow $\hat{b}_4^1$ into its original location 2. The restored shadows are the same as those in Fig. 4.9(c) and Fig. 4.9(d).

The scheme next uses the decryption function to reconstruct the original binary plane. The first blocks of a_1^1 and b_1^1 are $\begin{bmatrix} 1\,0 \\ 1\,0 \end{bmatrix}$ and $\begin{bmatrix} 0\,1 \\ 0\,1 \end{bmatrix}$, both of which are selected from C_1. Hence, the first bit of T_1^1 is 1. The second blocks of a_1^1 and b_1^1 are $\begin{bmatrix} 0 & 0 \\ 1 & 1 \end{bmatrix}$ and $\begin{bmatrix} 0 & 0 \\ 1 & 1 \end{bmatrix}$, respectively, which are selected from C_0. Hence, the second bit of T_1^1 is 0. The final reconstructed plane is the same as the plane demonstrated in Fig. 4.9(b).

4.3.5 The Proposed Scheme Extension

The scheme places the sub-shadows in different locations using rotation and reversion operations on all planes to enhance the security. The legal participants can restore all of the information from the reconstructed image, since they own the secret keys to generate the random sequences to rearrange the rotated and reversed sub-shadows.

If a sender only wants to reveal part of the secret images to some specific participants, he can arrange part of the sub-shadows, which is available for the participants, in the fixed locations and randomly disperse the other sub-shadows to the remaining locations to increase the complexity of the decryption process. The participants are thereby unable to restore the complete secret images.

4.4 The Proposed (t, n)-VSS Scheme

In this section, the proposed (2, 2)-VSS scheme is extended into a (t, n)-VSS scheme. Here the gray-scale image is split into n shadows. In addition, any t legal participants can see the secret images by stacking their shadows together.

4.4.1 The Proposed Scheme Extension

Let $T = \{T_1, T_2, \cdots, T_{2^k}\}$ be the set of sub-regions, and each sub-region is used to paste a secret image. The scheme represents the image by eight bit planes. Let $P = \{P^1, P^2, \cdots, P^8\}$ be a set of eight planes. For each sub-region T_i^j, the scheme generates n sub-shadows for the sub-region using the encryption process. The shadow generation process is shown in Fig. 4.11.

The scheme maps each bit of T_i^j into a block from the codebooks C_0' or C_1' using different shadows. C_0' consists of several block patterns of the shadows generating for the white input bit, and C_1' consists several block patterns of the shadows generating for the black input bit. The probabilities of 0 and 1 appeared in the block are like.

The scheme next rearranges each sub-shadow in different locations on the plane. The scheme generates n random sequences for P^j by using the secret key to relocate the position of the sub-shadow. The right-rotation, left-rotation, horizontal-reversion, and vertical-reversion operations are used to change the shape of the sub-shadows so as to be suitable in the new location. The scheme

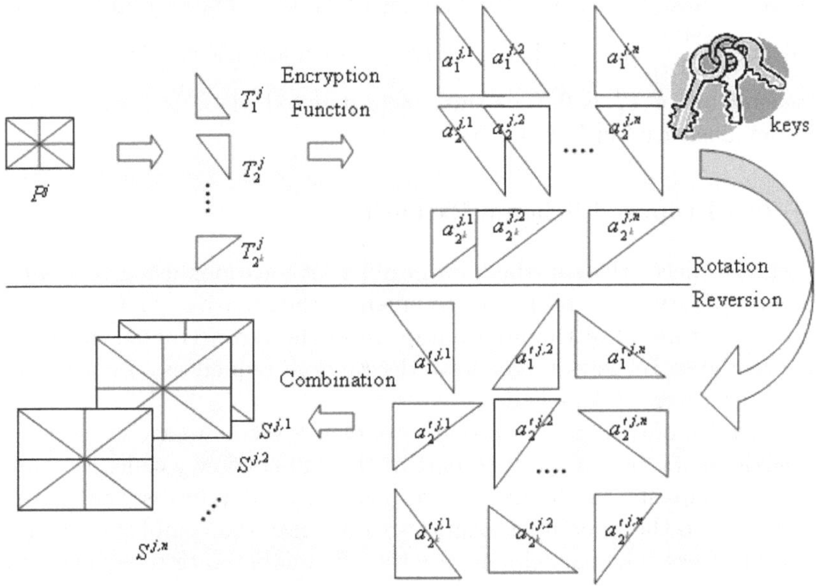

Fig. 4.11. Diagram of (t, n)-VSS shadow generation process for the binary plane P^{j}.

then combines the sub-shadows to form the shadows, $S^{\mathrm{j},1}, S^{\mathrm{j},2}, \cdots, S^{\mathrm{j},\mathrm{n}}$, for the plane P^{j}. The final shadows of the gray-scale image are expressed as

$$\begin{aligned}
S^1 &= S^{1,1} \times 2^7 + S^{2,1} \times 2^6 + \cdots + S^{7,1} \times 2^1 + S^{8,1}, \\
S^2 &= S^{1,2} \times 2^7 + S^{2,2} \times 2^6 + \cdots + S^{7,2} \times 2^1 + S^{8,2}, \\
&\vdots \\
S^{\mathrm{n}} &= S^{1,\mathrm{n}} \times 2^7 + S^{2,\mathrm{n}} \times 2^6 + \cdots + S^{7,\mathrm{n}} \times 2^1 + S^{8,\mathrm{n}}.
\end{aligned}$$

4.4.2 The Decryption Process for the $(t,\ n)$-VSS Scheme

The scheme decomposes each shadow into eight planes. The reconstruction process is then performed on those planes to reconstruct the original plane P^{j}, shown in Fig. 4.12.

In Fig. 4.12, each shadow is separated into 2^{k} sub-shadows. The scheme restores the sub-shadows, $\hat{a}_1^{\mathrm{j},\chi}, \hat{a}_2^{\mathrm{j},\chi}, \cdots$, and $\hat{a}_{2^{\mathrm{k}}}^{\mathrm{j},\chi}$, to their original locations, $a_1^{\mathrm{j},\chi}$, $a_2^{\mathrm{j},\chi}$, $\cdots$, and $a_{2^{\mathrm{k}}}^{\mathrm{j},\chi}$, where $1 \leq \chi \leq n$. The scheme uses the generated n random sequences to restore the original sub-region. Only legal participants who own the secret keys can generate the sequences needed to rearrange the locations of the sub-shadows.

The decryption function for the (t, n)-VSS scheme is next used to decrypt the secret information. The scheme stacks the sub-shadows, $a_1^{\mathrm{j},\chi}$, $a_2^{\mathrm{j},\chi}$, $\cdots$, and

$a_{2^k}^{j,\chi}$, by using the decryption function $f_{\mathrm{d\_CLF\_TN}}$ to reconstruct the original sub-region T_i^j. The function $f_{\mathrm{d\_CLF\_TN}}$ is defined as follows

$$f_{\mathrm{d\_CLF\_TN}}(a_i^{j,1}, a_i^{j,2}, \cdots, a_i^{j,n}) = \begin{cases} 1, & \text{if } a_{i\gamma}^{j,1} \in C_1' \cap a_{i\gamma}^{j,2} \in C_1' \cap \cdots \cap a_{i\gamma}^{j,n} \in C_1'; \\ 0, & \text{otherwise,} \end{cases} \tag{4.8}$$

where $a_{i\gamma}^{j,\chi}$ is the γ-th block of $a_i^{j,\chi}$. Let $T_{i\gamma}^j = f_{\mathrm{d\_CLF\_TN}}(a_i^{j,1}, a_i^{j,2}, \cdots, a_i^{j,n})$ where $T_{i\gamma}^j$ is the γ-th bit of T_i^j.

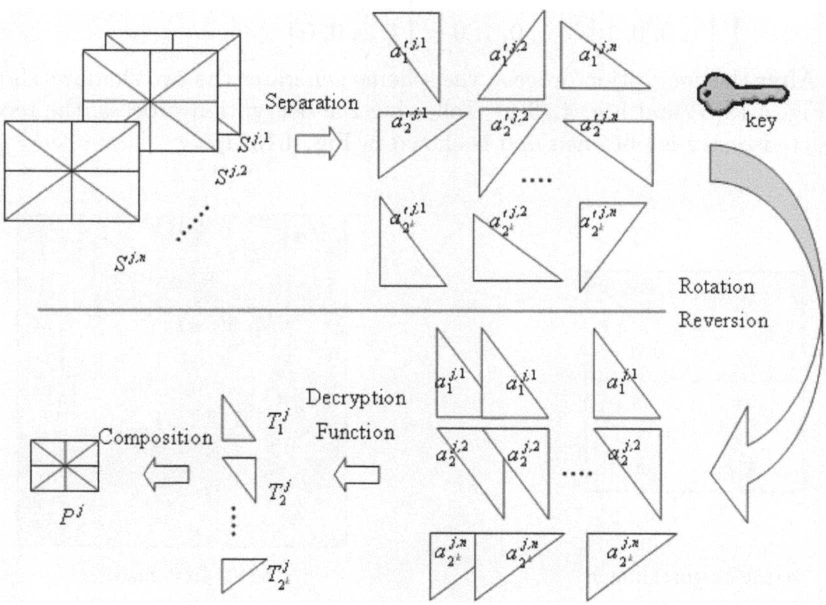

Fig. 4.12. Diagram of $(t,\ n)$-VSS bit plane reconstruction process for the binary plane P^j.

The scheme finally reconstructs the binary plane P^j and stacks the planes obtained to reconstruct the gray-scale image. The secret images can then be displayed by the human visual system.

4.5 Experiments and Results

In this section, the results obtained using our encrypted and decrypted schemes for information secret sharing are presented respectively and discussed in different applications to illustrate the efficiency and effectiveness.

In the first experiment, the proposed (2, 2)-VSS scheme is implemented and tested on an input image of size 512×512, which is shown in Fig. 4.13(a). The image consists of eight secret images. The codebooks C_0 and C_1 used in the experiment are

$$C_0 = \left\{ \begin{bmatrix} 0,0,1,1 \\ 1,1,0,0 \end{bmatrix}, \begin{bmatrix} 0,1,0,1 \\ 1,0,1,0 \end{bmatrix}, \begin{bmatrix} 0,1,1,0 \\ 1,0,0,1 \end{bmatrix} \atop \begin{bmatrix} 1,0,0,1 \\ 0,1,1,0 \end{bmatrix}, \begin{bmatrix} 1,0,1,0 \\ 0,1,0,1 \end{bmatrix}, \begin{bmatrix} 1,1,0,0 \\ 0,0,1,1 \end{bmatrix} \right\} \text{ and}$$

$$C_1 = \left\{ \begin{bmatrix} 0,0,1,1 \\ 0,0,1,1 \end{bmatrix}, \begin{bmatrix} 0,1,0,1 \\ 0,1,0,1 \end{bmatrix}, \begin{bmatrix} 0,1,1,0 \\ 0,1,1,0 \end{bmatrix} \atop \begin{bmatrix} 1,0,0,1 \\ 1,0,0,1 \end{bmatrix}, \begin{bmatrix} 1,0,1,0 \\ 1,0,1,0 \end{bmatrix}, \begin{bmatrix} 1,1,0,0 \\ 1,1,0,0 \end{bmatrix} \right\}.$$

After the encryption process, the scheme generates the two shadows shown in Fig. 4.13(b) and Fig. 4.13(c). Following the decryption process, the reconstructed image is obtained and is shown in Fig. 4.13(d).

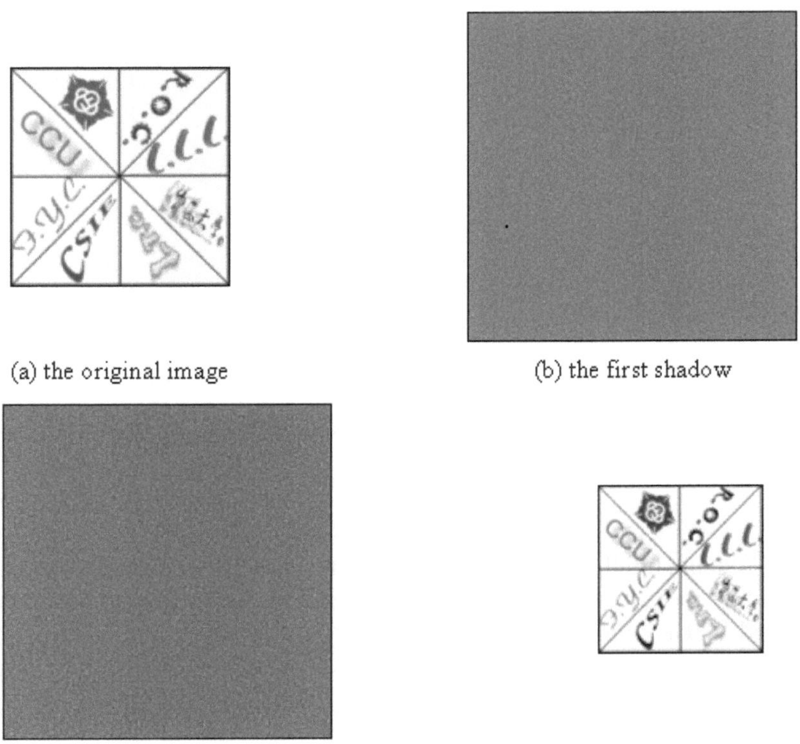

(a) the original image (b) the first shadow

(c) the second shadow (d) the decrypted image

Fig. 4.13. The (2, 2)-VSS scheme on the input image of size 512×512.

In this experiment, the participants can decrypt and recover all the shared secret information in all parts of the sub-shadows without being blocked. In the next experiment, we assume that the participants can only reveal the first secret image of the reconstructed image. The scheme arranges the sub-shadows of the first secret image in the fixed locations according to the generated random sequences, and randomly disperses the other sub-shadows on all planes. The final two shadows are shown in Fig. 4.14(a) and Fig. 4.14(b), respectively. The scheme, then, performs the decryption process to decrypt the shadows and reconstruct the secret image. The reconstructed image is shown in Fig. 4.14(c).

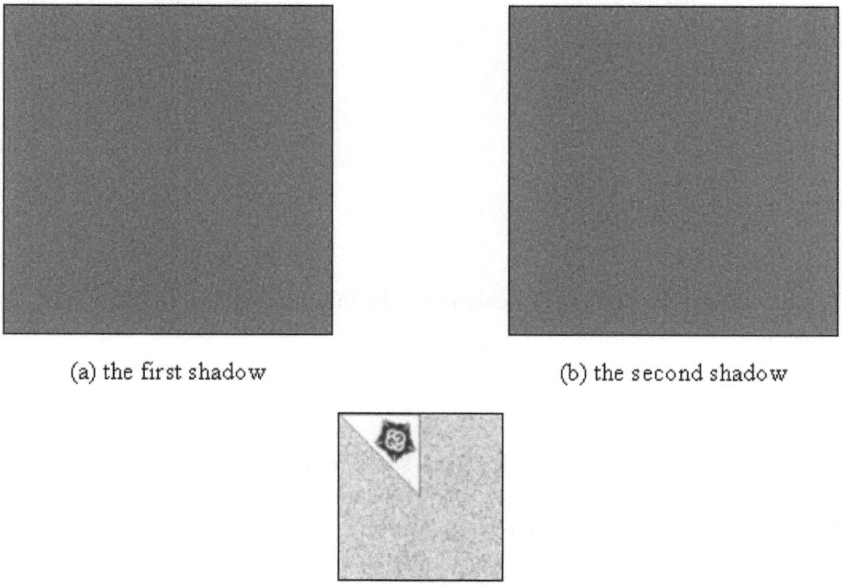

(a) the first shadow

(b) the second shadow

(c) the reconstructed image

Fig. 4.14. The (2, 2)-VSS scheme on the input image.

In Fig. 4.14(c), only the information in the first sub-region can be obtained. This constraint can increase the complexity and enhance the security of the secret information. The sub-shadows in each plane can also be randomly arranged in different position, so that the participants can obtain different parts of information in certain sub-regions by adopting the rotation and the reversion operations.

In the third experiment, we assume that the participants can reveal three secret images of the reconstructed image. The five shadows required are shown in Figures 4.15(a)–(e). The reconstructed image is shown in Fig. 4.15(f).

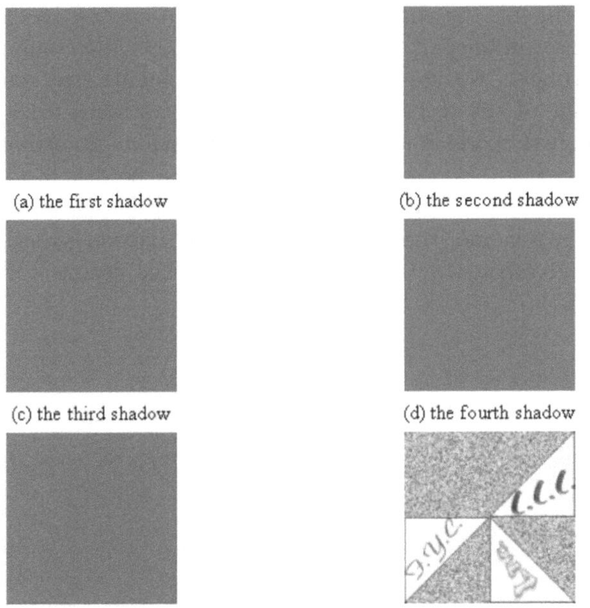

(a) the first shadow (b) the second shadow (c) the third shadow (d) the fourth shadow (e) the fifth shadow (f) the reconstructed image

Fig. 4.15. The (2, 5)-VSS scheme on the input image of size 512 × 512.

4.6 Conclusion

A visual secret sharing scheme for gray-scale images is proposed in this chapter. The image is divided into several sectors, and each sector can be used to hide a secret image. In order to completely recover the original image, the scheme represents the image by eight planes. The encryption process is then used to generate shadows for each plane. The scheme then uses the rotation and reversion operations to rearrange the sectors of each shadow.

In the decryption stage, only the legal participants who own the secret key needed to generate the random sequences for rearranging the sectors of the shadows can restore the original image and reveal the secret information. In addition, if the secret image owner only wants to share only a part of information with the participants, he can follow the same encryption process to generate the shadows, and then disperse the sectors, which do not belong to the participants. In this way, the participants can only retrieve their own part of the secret information but not the others'.

References

1. Chang, C.C. and Chuang, J.C. (2002): An image intellectual property protection scheme for gray-level images using visual secret sharing strategy. Pattern

Recognition Letters, **23**, 931–941
2. Hwang, K.F. and Chang, C.C. (2004): Recent development of visual cryptography. Intelligent Watermarking Techniques, World Scientific Publishing Company, Chapter 16, 459–480
3. Blakley, G.R. (1979), Safeguarding cryptographic keys. Proceedings of the National Computer Conference, New York, **48**, 313–317
4. Naor, N. and Shamir, A. (1995): Visual cryptography. Advances in Cryptology-Eurocrypt'94, Lecture Notes in Computer Science, Springer-Verlag, **950**, 1–12
5. Wu, H.C. and Chang, C.C. (2005): Sharing visual multi-secrets using circle shares. Computer Standards & Interfaces, **28**, 123–135
6. Lin, C.C. and Tsai, W.H. (2003): Visual cryptography for gray-level images by dithering techniques. Pattern Recognition Letters, **24**, 349–358
7. Blundo, C., Bonis, A.D. and Santis, A.D. (2001): Improved schemes for visual cryptography. Designs, Codes, and Cryptography, **24**, 255–278
8. Viet, D.Q. and Kurosawa, K. (2004): Almost ideal contrast visual cryptography with reversing. Visual Cryptography II: Improving the Contrast Via the Cover Base, Lecture Notes in Computer Science, Springer-Verlag, **2964**, 353–365
9. Verheul, E.R. and Tilborg, H.C.A. (1997): Constructions and properties of k out of n visual secret sharing schemes. Designs, Codes, and Cryptography, **11**, 179–196
10. Lukac, R. and Plataniotis, K.N. (2005): Bit-level based Secret sharing for image encryption. Pattern Recognition, **38**, 767–772
11. Droste, S. (1996): New Results on visual cryptography. Advances in Cryptology-Eurocrypt'96, Lecture Notes in Computer Science, Springer-Verlag, **1109**, 401–415

5

Adaptive Data Hiding Scheme for Palette Images

Chin-Chen Chang[1,2], Yu-Zheng Wang[2], and Yu-Chen Hu[3]

[1] Feng Chia University, Taichung, Taiwan, 40724, R.O.C.,
ccc@cs.ccu.edu.tw,
WWW home page: http://www.cs.ccu.edu.tw/~ccc
[2] Institute of Information Science, Academia Sinica, Taipei, 115, Taiwan, R.O.C.,
wyc@iis.sinica.edu.tw
[3] Providence University, Taichung, Taiwan, R.O.C.

Summary. In this chapter, we propose a new data hiding scheme for palette image applications that offer a high embedding capacity and good image quality. The clustering technique is adopted to obtain the goal of high embedding capacity and two embedding mechanisms. The first is the Cluster Ordering-and-Mapping Technique and the second is the combination technique. These are used to do embedding according to the size of the cluster. The former scheme embeds one bit in the image data with a cluster size of one, and the latter scheme makes more bits to be embedded in the image data. A larger cluster size is made possible by combining the elements of the cluster. According to our experimental results, the proposed method contains a perfect balance between embedding capacity and image quality.

5.1 Introduction

In recent years, data hiding techniques [1, 2] have formed a widely investigated field of research. The techniques are used to hide secret data, such as texts, audio, and digital images into cover medium. The traditional encryption techniques that encrypt the secret data by using a key leave clear marks on the encrypted data for attackers to trace down. Consequently there is an urgent need for better data hiding techniques. Data hiding techniques can camouflage the secret data so that attackers cannot easily detect the existence of the secret data. Image hiding techniques shown in Fig. 5.1 basically work by embedding secret information into a given image called the cover image or the host image. This done by seamlessly modifying the bits without creating noticeable artifacts [3, 4]. After embedding the secret data into the cover image, the resultant image is called the Stego-Image. As the Stego-Image conceals the existence of the secret data, only the receiver knows the data can then be correctly extracted. This technique can be used in many applications, such as Steganography, Secret Communication, Data Authentication, Annotation

C.-C. Chang et al.: *Adaptive Data Hiding Scheme for Palette Images*, Studies in Computational Intelligence (SCI) **58**, 103–122 (2007)
www.springerlink.com

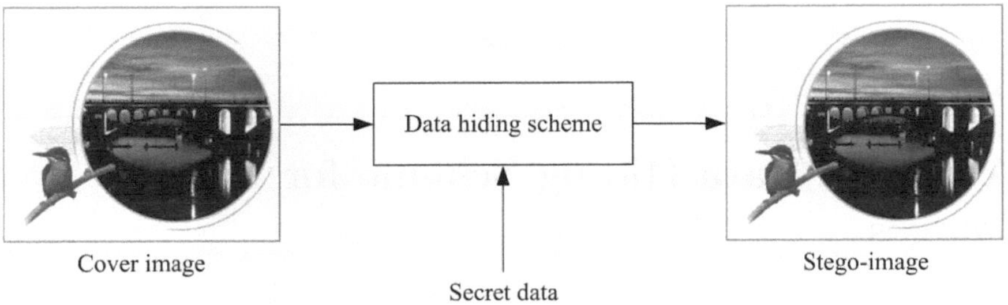

Fig. 5.1. Flowchart of data-hiding scheme.

Association, for example [5]. Several image hiding techniques have been developed for gray-scale as well as color images [6, 7, 8, 9], but less attention was paid to applications for Palette Images.

Palette-based images, or simply called Palette Images, are ubiquitous in modern computer systems. For example, GIF and 8-bit BMP files are some palette images widely used in multimedia applications. Each palette image consists of two components: a fixed lookup table called the Color Palette and a series of color indices called Image Data. Since image data in a palette image are not color values but rather indices of the color palette, it means that hiding data in a palette image is more challenging than in the pixel values of an image. We have two possibilities: the secret information can be embedded either in the color palette itself or in the image data. In the literature concerned, not much information can be found on palette image data hiding. In 1998, Kwan [10] proposed a program called "Gifshuffle" to embed data in GIF images. The idea is that the secret data used to permute the colors on the palette of an image in some specific order. For the 256 entries of a color palette, there are 256! possible permutations. So, at most $\log_2(256!)$ bits can be embedded into a GIF image. The advantage of this method is that the visual content of the cover image is not affected. However, security is weak because when the image is reloaded or saved, the image-processing software, whatever it may be, will usually rearrange the order of the colors on the palette according to some factors such as luminance, frequency of occurrence, for example. In 1999, Fridrich and Du proposed a method [11] to embed data into the parity bits of closest colors. The method first assigns a specific parity bit (0 or 1) to each color on the palette, and then modulates the index values to make the parities of the new index values replaced by the closest color equal to the bits of the embedded data. This adaptive method can embed an appropriate amount of data by modification of the pixel values. In 2004, Chang, Tsai and Lin proposed a method [12] to hide secret data based on the Color Clustering Technique. The colors in the palette are grouped into sub-clusters according to the relationship between the colors. For each image data, the hiding capacity is determined by the size of the sub-cluster of which it is a member. This method embeds a considerable quantity of data and has a good image quality. In 2004, Tzeng, Yang and Tsai proposed a method [13] based on a color-ordering relationship and a color-mapping function. The first is used to rearrange the order of the color according to the luminance of the color, and the second is used to embed data by the ordering of the color. The proposed method also considers the necessity of reducing local image content changes to achieve a good compromise between data-hiding capacity and image quality. Du and Hsu proposed an adaptive data hiding scheme [14] that embeds the secret data in the compressed codes of Vector Quantization (VQ) [15, 16]. This method uses a combination number to embed secret data. It offers a high embedding capacity, but it does not fit palette images. The modified color is easily detectable by human eyes. In this chapter, we propose a new scheme that offers a high embedding capacity and good image quality. The clustering technique is adopted in our proposed scheme for high embedding capacity. In addition, we use two embedding schemes, the Cluster Ordering-and-Mapping Technique and combination technique. The remainder of this chapter is organized as follows. In Section 5.2, we give a brief review of Tzeng et al.'s method. Our proposed method follows in Section 5.3. The experimental results are shown in Section 5.4. The conclusions are in Section 5.5.

5.2 Related Works

We briefly review some data-hiding schemes. In Subsection 5.2.1, we shall introduce codeword grouping scheme by Chang et al. [12], and review the color ordering and mapping developed by Tzeng et al. [13] in Subsection 5.2.2.

5.2.1 The Codeword Grouping Scheme

Chang et al. proposed an Adaptive Steganography for index-based images using a codeword grouping scheme that supports Adaptive Hiding Capacity. The palette-based image is one kind of Index-Based Images. The Codeword Grouping Scheme will group the colors of the palette into many sub-clusters according to the distance between colors that is less than the grouping threshold. Since the number of sub-cluster members determines the hiding capacity, the sub-clusters with larger members will be grouped first. Here, the number of sub-cluster members is restricted to the power of 2. From that, the colors of the palette are grouped into many sub-clusters with difference members according to difference grouping thresholds. For example, a palette with 256 colors will be grouped into 4-member, 2-member and 1-member sub-clusters according to grouping thresholds T_{M4}, T_{M2}. If the colors belong to the 4-member sub-cluster, the distance in between of them is less than T_{M4}. If the colors belong to the same 2-member sub-cluster, the distance between them is less than T_{M2}. The remaining colors are grouped individually as 1-member sub-clusters. In the embedding procedure, the number of sub-cluster members indicates how many secret bits can be embedded. If the number of sub-cluster members is n, then $\log_2 n$ secret bits can be embedded. The order of members in the sub-cluster is related to the embedded secret message. Therefore, the member whose order matches the embedded secret message is adopted to replace the original color index. For example, when there is a 4-member sub-cluster consisting of four members, ordered as 0, 1, 2, and 3, respectively. The color indices of these four members are 90, 80, 100 and 110. Since the number of this 4-member sub-cluster is 4, then 2 secret bits can be embedded. If the original index is 80, which is ordered as 1 in the sub-cluster, the 2-bit secret message to be embedded is valued as 3 (11 in binary), an index value of 110, of ordered as 3 in the sub-cluster, will be adopted to replace an original index 80.

5.2.2 The Color Ordering and Mapping Scheme

The goal of the color ordering and mapping scheme is to improve the performance of the scheme [11] proposed by Fridrich and Du in 1999. This embeds the secret data into the parity bits of closest colors. The flowchart of Tzeng et al.'s data-hiding scheme by color ordering and mapping is shown in Fig. 5.2.

To embed the secret data $A = \{a_1\ a_2\ \cdots\ a_w\}$ into the input color image I of $h \times w$ pixels, the image I is first compressed into the palette image with the color palette $C = \{c_i \mid 1 \leq i \leq n\}$ of n colors to generate the image data X, where $X = \{X(i,j) \mid 0 \leq i \leq h, 0 \leq j \leq w\}$. Before the embedding procedure is performed, the color palette is first sorted by the color-ordering relationship. Given two colors $c_1 = (r_1,\ g_1,\ b_1)$ and $c_2 = (r_2,\ g_2,\ b_2)$, the color-ordering relationship $R_{\text{color-order}}$ is defined as follows:

$$R_{\text{color-order}}: \begin{cases} c_1 > c_2, & \text{if } (l_1 > l_2) \text{ or } (l_1 = l_2 \text{ and } r_1 > r_2) \\ & \text{or } (l_1 = l_2 \text{ and } r_1 = r_2 \text{ and } g_1 > g_2); \\ c_1 = c_2, & \text{if } (l_1 = l_2 \text{ and } r_1 = r_2 \text{ and } g_1 = g_2); \\ c_1 < c_2, & \text{otherwise.} \end{cases} \tag{5.1}$$

The luminance values are calculated by Eq. (5.2) of the colors.

$$l = 0.3 \times r + 0.59 \times g + 0.11 \times b. \tag{5.2}$$

According to the color-ordering relationship $R_{\text{color-order}}$, the sorting result for all colors in the palette can be obtained. To embed the secret data into the image I, each pixel with image data $X(i,j)$ is processed in a raster-scanning manner. In this scheme, the four neighboring pixels are used to determine whether what the current pixel is embeddable. The four precedent neighbors of the current pixel are shown in Fig. 5.3.

A pixel is an embeddable pixel if it satisfies the following conditions:

1. The number of distinct colors of $X(i,j)$'s four precedent neighbors is larger than the threshold value T_α.
2. The maximum color difference between $X(i,j)$ and its four precedent neighbors is smaller than the threshold value T_β.

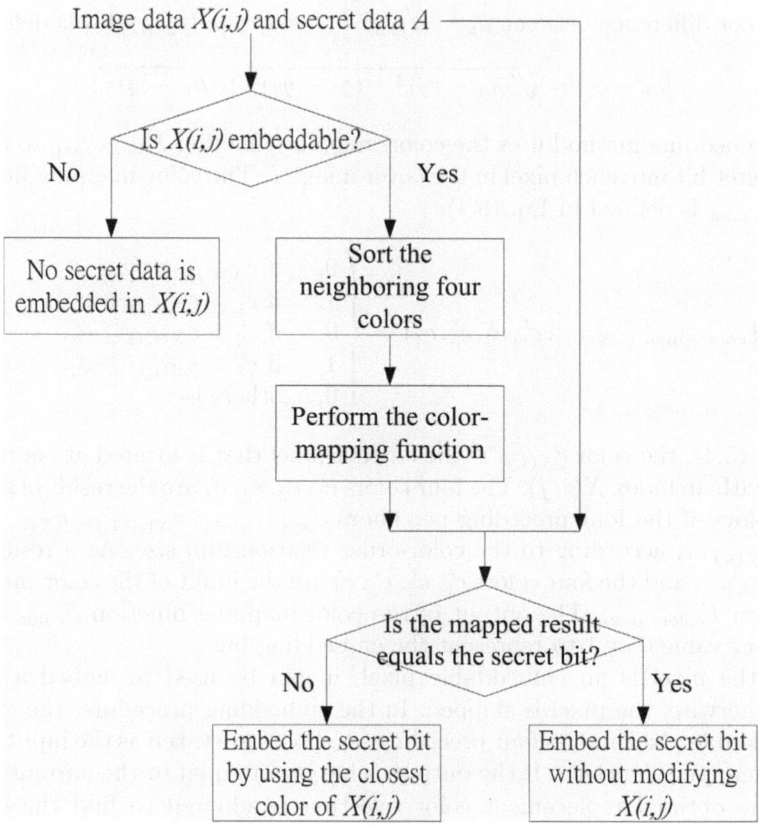

Fig. 5.2. Flowchart of Tzeng et al.'s data-hiding scheme.

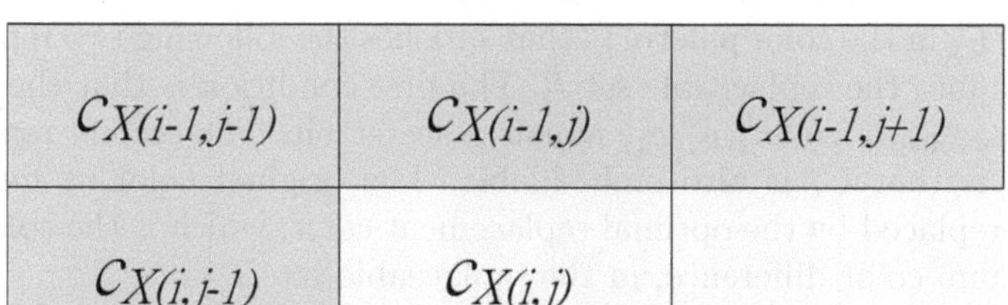

Fig. 5.3. The positions of four precedent neighbors of the current pixel indexed $X(i,j)$.

3. There exists a substitute color with the inverse mapping value of $X(i,j)$'s original color according to the color mapping function. And the maximum color difference between the substitute color of $X(i,j)$ and its four precedent neighbors is still smaller than the threshold value T_β.

The color difference between $c_1 = (r_1, g_1, b_1)$ and $c_2 = (r_2, g_2, b_2)$ is defined as

$$|c_1 - c_2| = \sqrt{[(r_1 - r_2)^2 + (g_1 - g_2)^2 + (b_1 - b_2)^2]}. \tag{5.3}$$

The embedding method uses the color-mapping function $F_{\text{color-map}}$ to embed one secret bit into each pixel in the cover image I. The color-mapping function $F_{\text{color-map}}$ is defined in Eq. (5.4).

$$F_{\text{color-map}}\left(c_{X(i,j)}, c_1', c_2', c_3', c_4'\right) = \begin{cases} 0, & \text{if } c_{X(i,j)} \geq c_1', \\ 1, & \text{if } c_1' > c_{X(i,j)} \geq c_2', \\ 0, & \text{if } c_2' > c_{X(i,j)} \geq c_3', \\ 1, & \text{if } c_3' > c_{X(i,j)} \geq c_4', \\ 0, & \text{otherwise.} \end{cases} \tag{5.4}$$

In Eq. (5.4), the color $c_{X(i,j)}$ is the current pixel that is located at coordinate (i, j) with an index $X(i, j)$. The four colors c_1', c_2', c_3', c_4' are the result of sorting the colors of the four preceding neighbors $c_{X(i-1,j-1)}$, $c_{X(i-1,j)}$, $c_{X(i-1,j+1)}$, and $c_{X(i,j-1)}$ according to the color-order relationship, size. As a result, the color $c_{X(i,j)}$ and the four colors c_1', c_2', c_3', c_4' are the input of the color-mapping function $F_{\text{color-map}}$. The output of the color-mapping function $F_{\text{color-map}}$ is a binary value 0 or 1 to represent the embedding bit.

If the pixel is an embeddable pixel, it can be used to embed a secret bit; otherwise, the pixel is skipped. In the embedding procedure, the current embeddable pixel and its four preceding neighbors are taken as the input to the color-mapping function. If the output value is not equal to the current secret bit, the optimal replacement color selection is adopted to find the closest color to replace it. Otherwise, the secret bit is embedded into the current embeddable pixel without modification.

The optimal replacement color selection uses the following steps: First, add each color C_i in the color palette C that satisfies the following two replacement conditions into the replaceable set R. The first condition is that the mapping value $F_{\text{color-map}}(c_i, c_1', c_2', c_3', c_4')$ equals a secret bit. The second replacement condition is that C_i is also embeddable. The original color of image data $X(i, j)$ is replaced by the optimal replacement color, which is the color having the minimum color difference, in the replaceable set R.

5.3 The Proposed Method

The goal of this data-hiding method is the ability to hide as many secret bits with the best image quality possible. To achieve the goal, the following techniques are employed. The cluster ordering-and-mapping technique, the combination technique are all employed. The proposed method consists of the following two main procedures, which are: the Embedding Procedure and the Extraction Procedure.

5.3.1 The Embedding Procedure

The cover image I has $h \times w$ pixels, and it is first quantized with the color palette P of n colors to generate the image data X. Before the secret A is embedded into the image data X, the colors in the palette are clustered by the proposed clustering technique. The flowchart of the clustering technique is depicted in Fig. 5.4.

To group the colors in the palette, the frequency of the color in the image data is counted for each color in the palette P. Initially, all clusters can be represented by $S = S_1, S_2, \cdots, S_m$, where $S_i = c_i$, $1 \leq i \leq n$, with n representing the number of the colors in the palette P. Each cluster satisfies $S_i \cap S_j = \emptyset$, for $i \neq j$. Therefore, each cluster S_i has one color c_i, and the number of the clusters m is equal to n.

The i-th maximum occurrence frequency of the colors in the palette P is then selected, beginning with $i = 1$, $1 \leq i \leq n$. This is included in the cluster S_i. To find the closest color of the i-th maximum color occurrence frequency, the cluster that the closest color belongs to is denoted as S_{nearest}. If the maximum color difference between each color in cluster and each color in cluster S_{nearest} is smaller than the threshold T_γ, S_i then S_{nearest} can be merged into the one cluster.

Whether the clusters are merged or not, i is augmented by one for next round of clustering steps. If two clusters are merged into one cluster the number of clusters m is decreased by one. The clustering step is terminated when the number of clusters m reaches the required value, or when i is larger than the number of colors in the palette n. Fig. 5.5 shows an example of the clustering scheme. Given a fixed threshold value T_γ, the clustering result of Fig. 5.5(a) can be obtained as shown in Fig. 5.5(b).

After the clustering technique is executed, the n colors in the palette are grouped into m clusters. In the proposed scheme, the cluster ordering-and-mapping technique and the combination technique are sequentially executed in order to embed the secret data A into the image data X.

In each technique, we first check the whether the image data $X(i, j)$ of one color pixel is embeddable. Only embeddable pixels are used in the embedding procedure. To determine whether one pixel is embeddable, two threshold values T_α and T_β are adopted. One pixel is embeddable if it satisfies the following requirements.

1. The number of distinct clusters in the four neighboring pixels is larger than T_α.
2. The maximum cluster difference is less than T_β. The Cluster Difference is the difference between the center of a cluster and that of another cluster.
3. When the size of a cluster is equal to one, if the replaced cluster of $X(i, j)$ is embeddable, then the pixel is an embeddable pixel.

On the first round, we embed a secret bit into $X(i, j)$, where the size of the cluster is one using the Cluster Ordering-and-Mapping Technique.

The flowchart of the Cluster Ordering-and-Mapping Technique is shown in Fig. 5.6. The Cluster Ordering-and-Mapping Technique is similar to the Color Ordering-and-Mapping Technique proposed by Tzeng et al. [13]. The major difference between the Cluster Ordering-and-Mapping Technique and the Color Ordering-and-Mapping Technique is that the first is based on the center of the cluster while the latter is based on the color.

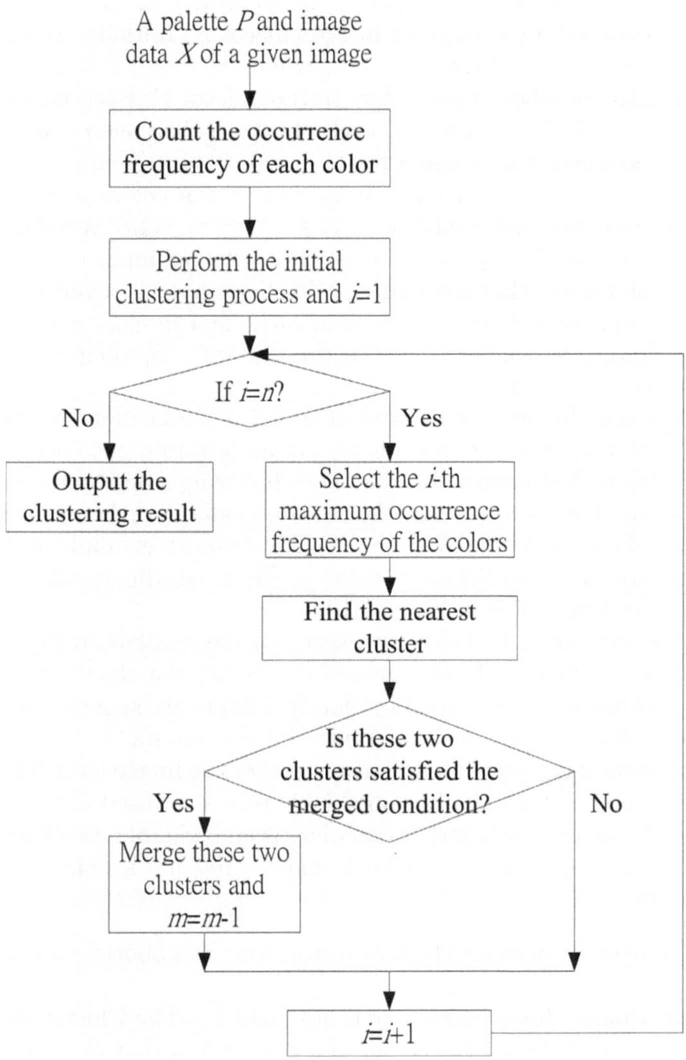

Fig. 5.4. Flowchart of the clustering technique.

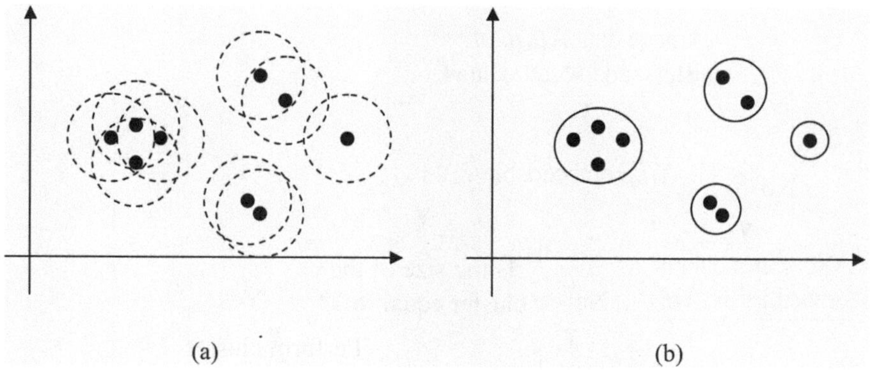

Fig. 5.5. Example of the clustering technique.

Assume that there are two clusters S_1 and S_2 where the centers are at $z_1 = (\overline{r_1}, \overline{g_1}, \overline{b_1},)$ and $z_2 = (\overline{r_2}, \overline{g_2}, \overline{b_2},)$. The cluster-ordering relationship between z_1 and z_2 may be defined as follows,

$$R_{\text{cluster-order}}: \begin{cases} z_1 > z_2, & \text{if } (\overline{l_1} > \overline{l_2}) \text{ or } (\overline{l_1} = \overline{l_2} \text{ and } \overline{r_1} > \overline{r_2}) \\ & \text{or } (\overline{l_1} = \overline{l_2} \text{ and } \overline{r_1} = \overline{r_2} \text{ and } \overline{g_1} > \overline{g_2}), \\ z_1 = z_2, & \text{if } (\overline{l_1} = \overline{l_2} \text{ and } \overline{r_1} = \overline{r_2} \text{ and } \overline{g_1} = \overline{g_2}), \\ z_1 < z_2, & \text{otherwise.} \end{cases} \tag{5.5}$$

Here, $\overline{l_1}$ and $\overline{l_2}$ are computed using the formula for the luminance shown in Eq. (5.2). To embed 1-bit secret data into the image data $X_{i,j}$ belonging to i-th cluster S_t, the cluster-mapping function $F_{\text{cluster-map}}$ defined by the following is used.

$$F_{\text{cluster-map}}(z_t, z_1', z_2', z_3', z_4') = \begin{cases} 0, & \text{if } z_t \geq z_1', \\ 1, & \text{if } z_1' > z_t \geq z_2', \\ 0, & \text{if } z_2' > z_t \geq z_3', \\ 1, & \text{if } z_3' > z_t \geq z_4', \\ 0, & \text{otherwise.} \end{cases} \tag{5.6}$$

Here z_1', z_2', z_3', form the sorting result, z_1' is the largest. The output of the cluster-mapping function $F_{\text{cluster-map}}$ is the bit to be embedded. We need to modify image data $X(i,j)$ if the output of the cluster-mapping function $F_{\text{cluster-map}}$ is not equal to the embedding bit. Let RID denote the image data that is selected to replace $X(i,j)$. The color c_{RID} has to satisfy the three conditions:

1. The size of the cluster that c_{RID} belongs to is one.
2. The cluster includes the replaceable color, together with the four precedent neighbors of $X(i,j)$. These act together as a complete input to the cluster-mapping function $F_{\text{cluster-map}}$. This gives a binary output value equal to the secret bit.

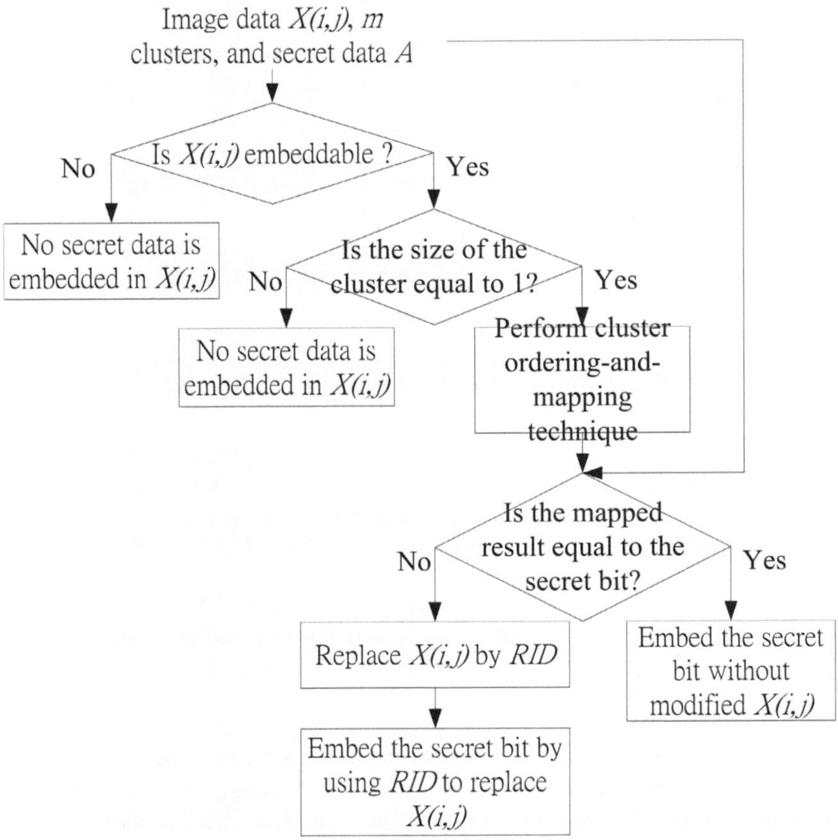

Fig. 5.6. Flowchart of the cluster ordering-and-mapping technique.

3. The color c_{RID} is an embeddable pixel.

The image data $X(i, j)$ of the nearest color is used for the modification.

Let D_{om} denote the hiding capacity of the cluster ordering-and-mapping technique. The formula for calculating D_{om} is,

$$D_{om} = \sum_{i=1}^{h} \sum_{j=1}^{w} \left| f(c_{X(i,j)}) \right|, \quad \text{if} \quad \left| f(c_{X(i,j)}) \right| = 1. \tag{5.7}$$

Here $\left| f(c_{X(i,j)}) \right|$ is the size of the cluster to which the color $c_{X(i,j)}$ belongs.

An example of the cluster ordering-and-mapping technique is shown in Fig. 5.7. Assume the cover image I with the image data $\{X_{1,1}, X_{1,2}, \cdots, X_{4,4}\}$ is as shown in Fig. 5.7(a). We have six clusters that are shown in Fig. 5.7(b). Let $A = (101101 \cdots 1)_2$ be the secret data.

In this example, the image data $X(2,2)$, $X(2,4)$, $X(2,4)$, and $X(4,4)$ shown in Fig. 5.7(c) are embeddable and they satisfy $|f(c_{X(i,j)})| = 1$. We then try embedding four bits into those image data. Since the cluster ordering-and-mapping functions of $X(2,2)$, $X(3,1)$, and $X(4,4)$ are equal to the secret bits, this image data is that of the secret bits which already exist. While the cluster ordering-and-mapping function of $X(2,4)$ is not equal to the secret bit, we modify this color using the closest color that satisfies the replacement conditions. Therefore, color c_{13} is used to replace color c_8, and this result is shown in Fig. 5.7(d).

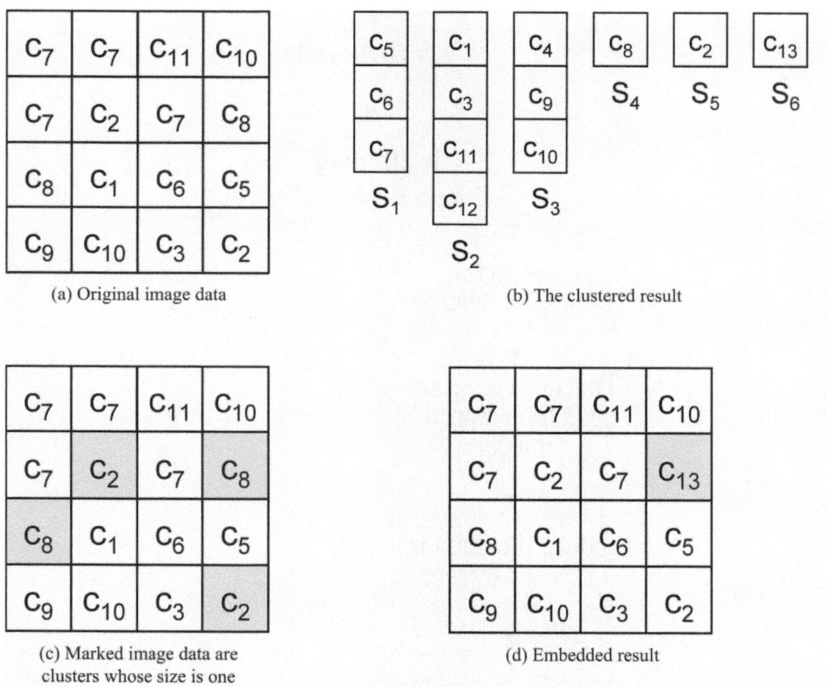

Fig. 5.7. An example of the cluster ordering-and-mapping technique.

On the second round, the combination technique is employed to embed the secret data into the image data. The flowchart of the combination technique is shown in Fig. 5.8. The combination technique was first proposed by Du et al. [15] to embed the secret data into the compressed codes of VQ. The combination technique uses the ordered list formed by element combination of the clusters which each color of the cover image I. The secret data represented by a bit stream can be transformed to a corresponding unsigned integer. The unsigned integer is represented by the order of element combination.

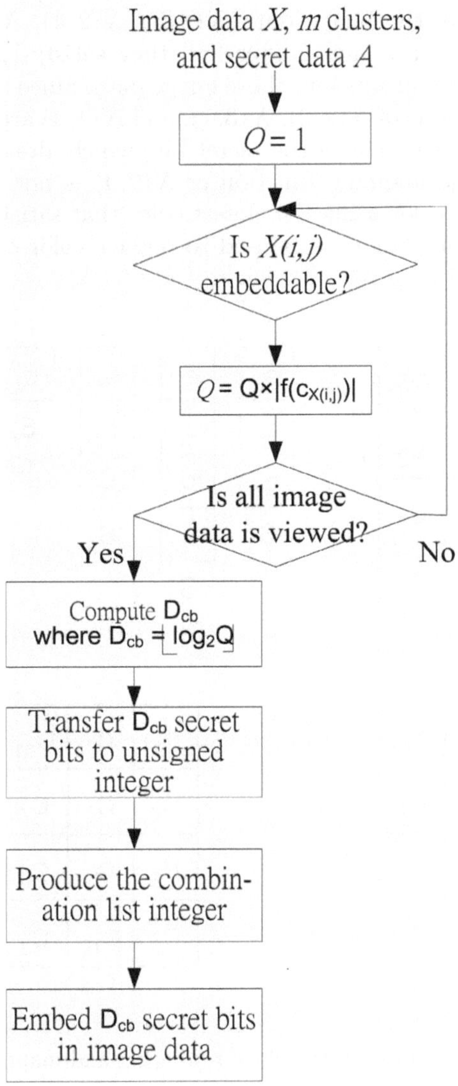

Fig. 5.8. An example of the cluster ordering-and-mapping technique.

To determine the size of the secret bits that can be embedded in cover image, we need to calculate the product value Q,

$$Q = \prod_{i=1}^{h} \prod_{j=1}^{w} \left| f(c_{X(i,j)}) \right| . \tag{5.8}$$

We can then calculate the hiding capacity D_{cb} of the combination technique,

$$D_{cb} = \lfloor \log_2 Q \rfloor . \tag{5.9}$$

According to the embedding capacity D_{cb}, we are able to embed D_{cb} secret bits into the image data. An example of how D_{cb} is derived and how the embedding method works is shown in Fig. 5.9. This uses the result of the example in Fig. 5.7(d). That is, D_{cb} is calculated using Eq. (5.8) and Eq. (5.9). D_{cb} is 20[1]. Then, a bit stream with 20 secret bits is used in the secret data A is embedded in this cover image. Assume a bit stream with 20 secret bits that is transformed to a corresponding unsigned integer to become 916667. The clusters, S_1, S_1, S_2, S_3, S_1, S_1, S_2, S_1, S_1, S_3, S_3, and S_2, to which the colors belong, are selected in order to produce the combinations of the elements. In Fig. 5.9(a) the final combination result is the 916667-th combination. The Stego-Image is shown in Fig. 5.9(b).

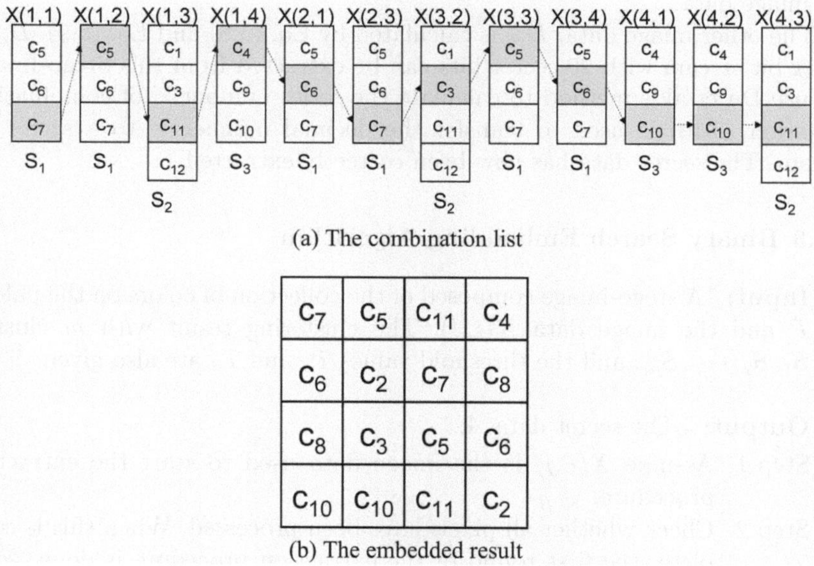

Fig. 5.9. An example of the combination technique.

5.3.2 The Extraction Procedure

The extraction procedure is used to extract the secret data from the Stego-Image. The extraction procedure in the traversing order is similar to that in the embedding procedure. For all of the embeddable image data X, we extract the secret bit when $\left|f(c_{X(i,j)})\right| = 1$. The product data Q is calculated when

[1] $D_{cb} = \lfloor \log_2(3 \times 3 \times 4 \times 2 \times 3 \times 1 \times 3 \times 1 \times 1 \times 4 \times 3 \times 3 \times 3 \times 3 \times 4 \times 1) \rfloor = \lfloor \log_2 1259712 \rfloor = 20$

$|f(c_{X(i,j)})| > 1$ on the first round. As a result, we obtain a bit stream with D_{om} bits and the product Q. The embedding capacity D_{cb} is then calculated using Eq. (5.9).

On the second round, we use Du et al.'s method to calculate the series number of combination Y from the image data $X(i,j)$ that are embeddable pixels $|f(c_{X(i,j)})| > 1$. Then, we transfer the series number to a secret bit stream by Eq. (5.10). Finally, the total secret data is obtained by connecting the secret bit stream on the first round with the secret bit stream on the second round:

$$a_i = (Y \ / \ 2^{D_{cb}-i}) \mod 2. \tag{5.10}$$

An example of the extraction procedure using Fig. 5.9(b) is now described. The image data $X(2,2)$, $X(2,4)$, $X(3,1)$, and $X(4,4)$ are embeddable and the size of the cluster they belong to is one, four secret bits are extracted from the image data.

The other image data, D_{cb} is calculated by Eq. (5.8) and Eq. (5.9). D_{cb} is 20. A bit stream with 20 secret bits can be extracted from this Stego-Image. We use Du et al.'s method to calculate the series number Y of combination. Equation (5.10) is used to transfer the decimal number Y to a secret bit stream. The secret data has now been correctly extracted.

5.3.3 Binary Search Embedding Algorithm

1. **Input:** A stego-image composed of the collection of colors on the palette P and the image data $X(i,j)$. The clustering result with m clusters $S_1, S_2, \cdots, S_m$, and the threshold values T_α and T_β are also given.

2. **Output:** The secret data A.

   Step 1. Assume $X(i,j)$ is the image data used to start the extraction procedure.

   Step 2. Check whether all pixels have been processed. When this is complete, the first round of the extraction procedure is done, go to Step 6. Otherwise, go to the next step.

   Step 3. Check whether the color $c_{X(i,j)}$ corresponding to $X(i,j)$ is embeddable. If $c_{X(i,j)}$ is not embeddable, $X(i,j)$ is skipped. Go to Step 2. Otherwise, go to the next step.

   Step 4. If $|f(c_{X(i,j)})| = 1$, go to the next step. Otherwise, calculate the product Q. Here $Q = Q \times |f(c_{X(i,j)})|$.

   Step 5. Take the color $c_{X(i,j)}$ of $X(i,j)$ and the sorted centers of the clusters z'_1, z'_2, z'_3, and z'_4 of $X(i,j)$'s four preceding neighbors as the input to the cluster mapping function $F_{\text{cluster-map}}$ to obtain an extracted secret bit a. Then, go to Step 2.

   Step 6. Calculate the embedding capacity D_{cb} with Q. Then, go to next step.

Step 7. Perform Du et al.'s method to extract the serial number Y using all image data $X(i,j)$ satisfying that $|f(c_{X(i,j)})| > 1$.

Step 8. Transform the serial number Y into a bit stream. Then, combine these two bit streams as the secret data A to be the output.

5.4 Experimental Results

In this chapter, we present some experiments and their results to help evaluate the performance of the proposed method. In our experiments, six palette images were used as test images. These are shown in Fig. 5.10. These images are at most 256 different colors. Fig. 5.10(a) to (d) show the downloaded images from several homepages on the Internet. Fig. 5.10(e) and Fig. 5.10(f) are of comic pictures.

To evaluate the image quality of a processed image of $h \times w$, the peak-signal-noise ratio (PSNR) was used. The formula of PSNR is defined as follows:

$$\mathrm{PSNR} = 10 \log_{10} \frac{255^2}{\mathrm{MSE}} \quad (\mathrm{dB}), \tag{5.11}$$

$$\mathrm{MSE} = \frac{1}{h \times w} \prod_{i=0}^{h-1} \prod_{j=0}^{w-1} \prod_{k=1}^{3} (\alpha_{i,j,k} - \beta_{i,j,k})^2, \tag{5.12}$$

where $\alpha_{i,j}$ and $\beta_{i,j}$ denote the original and compressed color pixels, respectively. Typically, a larger PSNR value stands for a better image quality.

Table 5.1 shows how Tzeng et al.'s method and our proposed method compare when the same thresholds T_α and T_β ($T_\alpha = 1$ and $T_\beta = 30$) are used to embed the secret data. As shown in the results, our proposed method can offer a bigger embedding capacity than Tzeng et al.'s, and the image quality our proposed method provides is either better or about the same as Tzeng et al.'s.

The Stego-Images are shown in Fig. 5.11. According to our experimental results, using our proposed method, the secret data can be embedded into the cover image without introducing visual artifacts. The secret data embedded in the stego-image can be extracted correctly.

Furthermore, Table 5.2 confirms the high embedding capacity and good image quality that our proposed method is able to provide. Those experimental results were based on the fixed threshold values T_α and T_β ($T_\alpha = 1$ and $T_\beta = 30$) and a variable threshold value of T_γ. According to the threshold value T_γ, the maximum merged clusters could be obtained by our clustering scheme, and those results could be used to embed secret data. Therefore, the threshold value T_γ was set as $10, 15, \cdots, 50$, and the resultant cluster sizes, embedding capacities, and PSNR values obtained are shown in Table 5.2.

Fig. 5.12(a) shows the relationship between the number of clusters and the corresponding embedding capacity. Fig. 5.12(b) shows the relationship

Images \ Schemes	Tzeng et al.'s method		Our proposed method	
	Capacity	PSNR	Capacity	PSNR
(a) Midnight	20012	40.75	38102	41.67
(b) CCU-Logo	4333	42.90	5631	42.84
(c) CCU-Upbar	10349	42.22	17472	42.24
(d) Palette	6160	40.04	7342	40.07
(e) Garfield-a	8168	40.65	12104	40.24
(f) Garfield-b	21405	41.12	40265	41.26

Table 5.1. Embedding performance comparisons (at $T_\alpha = 1$ and $T_\beta = 30$).

Images \ Thresholds	T_γ	10	15	20	25	30	35	40	45	50
(a) Midnight	Clusters	215	155	115	92	72	60	45	40	36
	Capacity	38102	73681	112173	110847	136081	133010	179387	170356	179014
	PSNR	41.67	39.77	38.33	38.26	37.19	37.15	36.43	36.51	36.35
(b) CCU-Logo	Clusters	60	49	40	30	28	24	21	17	16
	Capacity	7126	22003	33133	35426	43391	44445	58077	58737	59687
	PSNR	41.90	40.23	38.20	37.94	36.98	36.90	35.74	35.73	35.48
(c) CCU-Upbar	Clusters	40	31	22	18	14	11	9	9	9
	Capacity	36568	42630	46991	68556	69792	70350	77798	74971	61980
	PSNR	41.48	40.82	39.84	37.68	37.49	37.40	36.70	36.81	37.08
(d) Palette	Clusters	31	30	29	27	26	24	23	23	23
	Capacity	5893	7342	10112	12814	11431	17299	17442	17442	17442
	PSNR	40.40	40.07	39.33	39.41	38.76	36.50	36.44	36.44	36.44
(e) Garfield-a	Clusters	255	254	200	160	125	107	88	71	62
	Capacity	19158	19196	20022	22766	46450	57091	56021	54939	60805
	PSNR	39.84	39.83	39.82	39.36	36.53	35.67	35.69	35.73	35.06
(f) Garfield-b	Clusters	255	253	188	152	127	110	91	79	70
	Capacity	40265	59336	63576	73269	112435	124237	128344	139762	145543
	PSNR	41.26	40.04	39.94	39.25	36.76	36.24	36.10	35.83	35.13

Table 5.2. Embedding capacity and image quality of our proposed method using different threshold values.

between the number of clusters and the corresponding PSNR value when the Midnight image was used as the cover image.

According to the experimental results, as the number of clusters drops, the embedding capacity tends to increase, and the PSNR value will decrease progressively. Since the embedability factor has been taken into account, our proposed method has a good tradeoff between the embedding capacity and image quality.

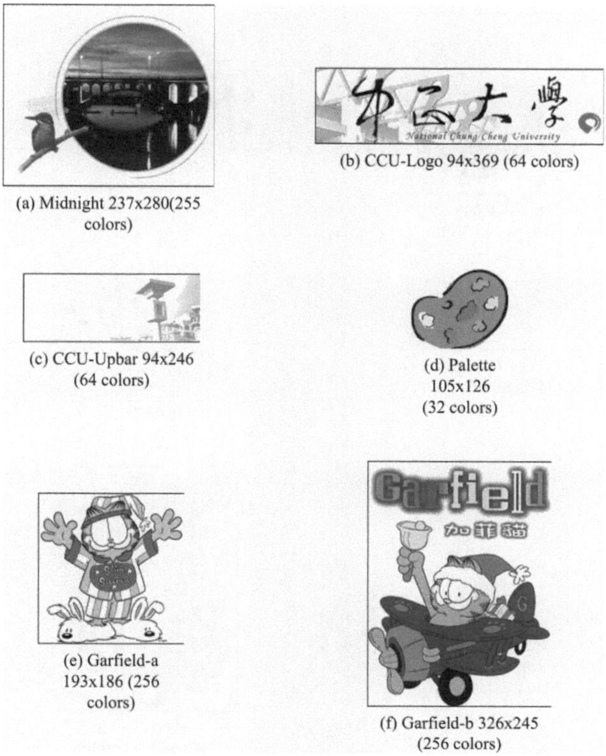

(a) Midnight 237x280(255 colors)

(b) CCU-Logo 94x369 (64 colors)

(c) CCU-Upbar 94x246 (64 colors)

(d) Palette 105x126 (32 colors)

(e) Garfield-a 193x186 (256 colors)

(f) Garfield-b 326x245 (256 colors)

Fig. 5.10. Six test palette images.

5.5 Conclusions

In this section, we discuss our proposed method and our experimental results. Generally speaking, Tzeng et al.'s method can be regarded as one special case of clustering where the number of clusters is equal to the number of colors on the palette. In this case, the total capacity includes only the capacity D_{om}, while the capacity D_{cb} is zero. In other words, D_{om} is the maximum embedding capacity of Tzeng et al.' method. With the help of the clustering technique, our proposed method gains a larger embedding capacity, and it also maintains quite good image quality by taking in the concept of embeddability. As a result, when the number of clusters decreases, the embedding capacity increases, and the PSNR value drops progressively.

Since the result of the clustering depends on the threshold value T_γ, the number of merged clusters is small, and the maximum cluster size is two when the threshold value T_γ is small. Here, the embedding capacity D_{cb} is equal to the number of embeddable pixels with $\left|f(c_{X(i,j)})\right| = 2$. For this reason, only one secret bit is embedded into a pixel. When the maximum cluster size of all examples is larger than two, the embedding capacity will increase. More than

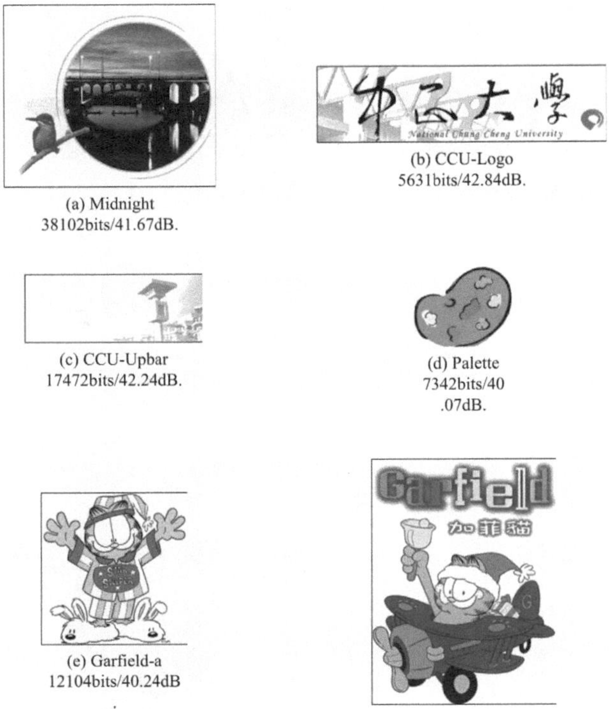

(a) Midnight
38102bits/41.67dB.

(b) CCU-Logo
5631bits/42.84dB.

(c) CCU-Upbar
17472bits/42.24dB.

(d) Palette
7342bits/40
.07dB.

(e) Garfield-a
12104bits/40.24dB

(f) Garfield-b
40265bits/41.26dB.

Fig. 5.11. The embedding results (stego-images) of the proposed method.

one secret bit can then be embedded in one pixel. These results can be seen from our experimental results.

Some fluctuations are shown in Fig. 5.12. This phenomena is produced by the clustering result and the conditions of embeddability. The threshold values T_α, T_β, and T_γ affect the embedding capacity and the image quality. Changes of the threshold value T_γ lead to changes of the clustering result. When the threshold value T_γ is larger, most color occurrence frequencies are more likely to gather around the same cluster. The embedding capacity will therefore increase. When the threshold value T_γ is larger, the difference between clusters becomes larger. Some of the image data will become non-embeddable, which may lead to a drop of the embedding capacity.

To sum up, we have proposed an embedding scheme for palette images that can offer a higher embedding capacity with better image quality than the currently existing methods. We adopt the concept of clustering to obtain high capacity, and include the concept of embeddability in order to maintain the image quality. The two-round embedding procedure is used to embed adequate

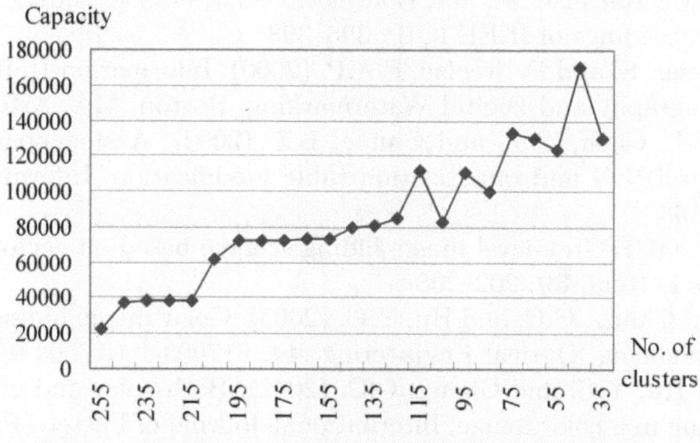

(a) Numbers of clusters vs. embedding capacity

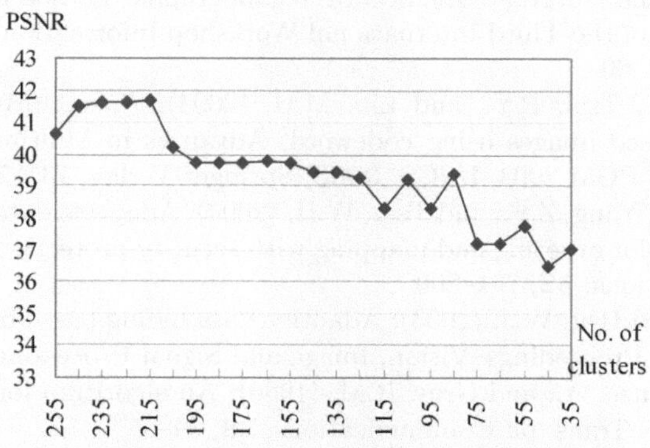

(b) Numbers of clusters vs. PSNR values

Fig. 5.12. Result of the embedding capacity and the PSNR value (cover image: Midnight).

secret data in the cover image. The experimental results have confirmed that our new scheme is capable of confirming our claims.

References

1. Anderson, R.J., and Petitcolas F.A.P. (1998): On the limits of steganography. IEEE Journal on Selected Areas in Communications, **16**, 474–481
2. Bender, W., Gruhl D., and Lu, A.: Techniques for data hiding. IBM Systems Journal, **35**, 313–336
3. Petitcolas F.A.P., Anderson R.J., and Kuhn, M.G. (1999): Information hiding — A survey. Proceedings of the IEEE, **87**, 1062–1078

4. Marvel, L.M., Retter C.T., and Boncelet, C.G.J. (1998): Hiding information in images. Proceedings of IEEE ICIP, 396–398
5. Katzenbeisser, S. and Petitcolas, F.A.P. (2000): Information Hiding Techniques for Steganography and Digital Watermarking. Boston, MA: Artech House.
6. Chang, C.C., Chen, T.S., and Chung, L.Z. (2002): A steganographic method based upon JPEG and quantization table modification. Information Sciences, **141**, 123–138
7. Hu, Y.C. (2003): Grey-level image hiding scheme based on vector quantisation. Electronics Letters, **39**, 202–203
8. Chan, C.S., Chang, C.C. and Hu, Y.C. (2005): Color image hiding scheme using image differencing. Optical Engineering, **44**, 017003-1–017003-9
9. Lin, M.H., Hu, Y.C. and Chang, C.C. (2002): Both color and gray scale secret image hiding in a color image. International Journal of Pattern Recognition and Artificial Intelligence, **16**, 697–713
10. Kwan, M. (1998): GIF colormap steganography. [Online] Available: `http://www.darkside.com.au/gifshuffle/`
11. Fridrich, J. and Du, R. (1999): Secure steganographic method for palette images, Proceedings of the Third International Workshop Information Hiding, Dresden, Germany, 47–60
12. Chang, C.C., Tsai, P.Y., and Lin, M.H. (2004): An adaptive steganography for index-based images using codeword, Advances in Multimedia Information Processing – PCM 2004, LNCS, **3333**, Springer Verlag, 731–738
13. Tzeng, C.H., Yang, Z.F., and Tsai, W.H. (2004): Adaptive data hiding in palette images by color ordering and mapping with security protection. IEEE Trans. on Communications, **52**, 791–800
14. Du, W.C. and Hsu, W.J. (2003): Adaptive data hiding based on VQ compressed images. IEE Proceedings–Vision, Image and Signal Processing, **150**, 233–238
15. Linde, Y., Buzo, A., and Gray, R.M. (1980): An algorithm for vector quantizer design. IEEE Trans. on Communications, **28**, 84–95
16. Gray, R.M. (1984): Vector quantization. IEEE ASSP Magazine, **1**, 4–29

6

GIS Watermarking: Hiding Data in 2D Vector Maps

XiaMu Niu[1], ChengYong Shao[2], and XiaoTong Wang[2]

[1] Information Security Technique Research Center, ShenZhen Graduate School, Harbin Institute of Technology, P. R. China
xiamu.niu@hit.edu.cn

[2] Department of Navigation, Dalian Naval Academy, P. R. China
chengyong.shao@dsp.hit.edu.cn
rfrm@dlut.edu.cn

Summary. The application of digital vector maps faces some yet to be resolved issues such as digital copyright protection, data authentication, data source tracing, for example. This chapter focuses on the topic of 2D vector map data hiding which provides potential solutions to above issues. The particularities of vector map watermarking are first summarized. The state-of-the-art of the research on the vector map watermarking is then reviewed by categorizing the current research into three sub areas. In addition, three schemes are presented towards resolving some open issues of three sub areas. We outline some future works at the end of the chapter.

6.1 Introduction

The rapid development of computer communication and Internet techniques makes it very easy to exchange data via networks. Correspondingly, it also becomes harder to protect the digital copyrights of various digital medias. The technique of watermarking provides a potential solution to the issue. Watermarking can also play many other roles such as hidden communication, data authentication, data tracing (fingerprint), for example. Data sets can be used as the cover data of watermark, for example digital image, audio, video, text, bar-code, 3D model, CAD data, 2D polygonal data, softwares, and VLSI. Among these data types, the watermarking for some general multimedia data, such as digital images, audio, videos and 3D models, has been given much more attention than other data types. This chapter focuses on the techniques of watermarking Geographical Information System (GIS) data, namely 2D vector map watermarking. This has attracted relatively less attention than other areas in the research field.

X. Niu et al.: *GIS Watermarking: Hiding Data in 2D Vector Maps*, Studies in Computational Intelligence (SCI) **58**, 123–155 (2007)
www.springerlink.com

6.1.1 The Necessities of GIS Data Watermarking

Generally, GIS data is of great value. The acquisition of vector maps is a high cost process, in which the high precision instruments and a large amount of physical and labour resources are required. The digitization and the vectorization of original data also represent hard work to produce the required vector maps. Consequently, digital maps in GIS normally cannot be used without cost. The application of GIS has to share its geographical data within the user group in many ways. For example by the via web, or by CD. It means that the map owner must provide some map copies to the users and consumers. This makes the protection of the distributed data sets a crucial issue. There are some special environments, where extra security requirements are needed, especially for sensitive usage. For instance, the application of secret military digital maps requires the capability of authenticating the source of map data as well as confirming the integrity. Digital vector maps are still unable to take the place of traditional paper maps until these requirements can be met. Watermarking can provide solutions to the above issues. A map owner can embed the product ID into the vector maps before distribution in order to protect the copyright. The sources of military maps can be traced by hiding unique identifications in them. Data hiding can also be a feasible method of integrity verification or secret communication by using the hash value or the secret message for the hidden data. Compared with general multimedia data types, there are relatively few research works done in the area of vector map watermarking. To our knowledge, a corporation in Uruguay named *The Digital Map Ltd* is going to patent a copyright protection scheme for vector maps where a watermarking scheme for polygonal data is utilized. A commercial software called *MapSN* has also been developed for digital map producers [1].

6.1.2 Characteristics of 2D Vector Map Data Hiding

The data structure and the application of 2D vector maps are also distinguished from the pixel images as well as other multimedia data types. This results in the differences between the vector map watermarking and the general multimedia watermarking in many aspects. For example these concern the basic principle for data embedding, and the criteria for fidelity evaluating. All above features should be considered when hiding data in vector maps.

Vector Maps: Data Structure and Basic Embedding Principle

Generally, a vector map is formed by Spatial Data, Attribution Data, and some additional data used as indices or extra descriptions. Spatial data normally takes the form of a sequence of 2D coordinates which describe the geographical locations of the map objects which represent the geographical objects in the real world. All map objects can be categorized into three basic geometrical elements. That is points, polylines and polygons. These geometrical elements are composed by organized vertices, and the spatial data is the coordinates of these vertices based on a particular geographical coordinate system. Attribution data describes the properties of map objects such as their names, categorizations and some other information. It is obvious that the information recorded by attribution data is very important and normally cannot be modified arbitrarily, as does the other additional data mentioned above. Until now, all proposed watermarking schemes embedded the watermark into the spatial data of the cover map, namely the coordinates of vertices. Every vector map has a precision tolerance which are denoted as τ. This gives the maximum amplitude of the permissible distortions for the coordinates. Any coordinate distortions definitely below τ will not degrade the validity of the map. The precision tolerance of a cover map plays a similar role as the *visual cover model* in digital image watermarking. It provides a little redundancy for hiding extra information. The basic principle of vector map watermarking is that the coordinate distortions induced by data hiding should not exceed the tolerance τ.

Fidelity of Vector Map Data

A common principle followed by all watermarking schemes is that the embedding of a hidden message should not degrade the validity of the cover data. The term fidelity is often used as a measure of the data's validity in the watermarking world. According to the different data types and their respective usages, the term fidelity could have different meanings. For digital images, videos, audio and other general multimedia data sets, direct use of the data is by the use of human sense organ. In that sense, human eyes can be used to measure the fidelity of images. If the human eyes cannot distinguish between two images, those two images then can be considered as having the same use value. That is, having the same fidelity. Some quantified parameters are defined in order to measure the difference between two data sets such as PSNR, MSE, for example. With respect to evaluating the fidelity of vector map data, neither human perception nor PSNR can provide an appropriate measure. Firstly, the direct user of vector maps are no longer human sense organs but are computers. In a typical scale, even two digital maps are quite similar when judged by the eye. It is still possible that coordinate differences between two maps could exceed the precision tolerance τ. Secondly, the term PSNR mainly reflects the energy of the errors. It is much more appropriate to evaluate images but not vector maps. That is because even a high PSNR of a vector map can not ensure that all vertex errors are within the map's precision tolerance. When we evaluate the fidelity of a vector map, some other factors must be taken into account. That is the shape and the topology of the map objects which cannot be directly reflected by PSNR. In other words, a low fidelity map with obviously distorted shapes or topologies could also have a high PSNR. Due to these factors, it is difficult to perfectly watermark a vector map. At present, there is no appropriate quantified measure of vector map fidelity proposed.

6.1.3 Ways of Possible Attacks

A successful attack means that the watermark could be removed whereas the validity of the cover data could be preserved. Unlike pixel images, the spatial data of vector maps is a series of floating-point values with a certain precision. Consequently, the manners and the features of the possible attacks on vector map watermarking are also different from that of general multimedia watermarking.

Geometrical Attacks

Some geometrical transforms such as translation, rotation, and scaling are the main forms of geometrical attacks. For digital image watermarking, geometrical attacks are very difficult to defend against because these transforms need to permit interpolation of pixel values. It is a irreversible process and always causes the loss of information. However, for vector maps, such attacks are virtually reversible transformations of coordinates where almost little or no information would be lost. Geometrical attacks are relatively easier to defend against in vector map watermarking schemes.

Vertex Attacking

Vertex attacking means the attacks in vertex level. That is by adding new vertices into map (interpolation), or removing vertices from map (simplification or cropping). Such attacks could possibly disturb the synchronization of the detector by changing the number of the vertices. They are therefore very serious to vector map watermarking. Map simplification is a common operation in daily work to enhance the speed of handling the map data. It does cause information lost whereas and to keep the validity of the handled map. As a result, the ability of surviving the map simplification is very important for a robust watermarking scheme.

Object Reordering

Object reordering is an attack in the object level. The spatial data of a vector map contains many objects which are composed by arranged vertices. All objects are stored in the map file in a certain sequence. Either changing the saving sequence of map objects, or reordering the vertices within an object can produce a new map file without degrading data's precision. For the watermarking schemes which are dependent to the objects' order, this operation is a fatal attack.

Noise Distortion

There are mainly two sources which can introduce noise into vector maps. The first one is by some kind of daily work. For example, there are several popular file formats in the GIS world. The transformation among those formats could slightly distort the data. The other is a malicious attack. Attackers attempt to destroy the watermark by adding noise into data sets. Noise distortion is a serious attack but it is generally not a good choice by an attacker because the imposition of noise could possibly degrade the map's validity.

6.2 Robust Watermarking

According to the location where the watermark is embedded, the existing robust methods for vector map watermarking can be categorized into two classes. These are the algorithms in spatial domain and the algorithms in transform domain. In this section, a representative schemes of each class is introduced. After this a shape-preserving algorithm is presented to improve the previous methods.

6.2.1 Spatial Domain Schemes

Watermarking a vector map in spatial domain is to embed a watermark by directly modifying the coordinate values of the vertices. The hidden bits could be represented by some spatial features of vertices. That is the locational relationship between vertices, or the statistical property of coordinates, for example.

Based on Locational Relationship between Vertices

The algorithm proposed by Sakamoto et al. [2] is a typical scheme based on the concept of modifying the locational relationship between vertices. Kang [3] enhanced its robustness to noise attacks. The basic idea of those two schemes is to shift the vertices within a predefined mask and make their locational relationship follow specific patterns representing '0' or '1'. Taking the enhanced scheme proposed by Kang [3] as an example, two vertex patterns and the embedding procedure are shown in Fig. 6.1. Firstly, the original map is segmented into blocks and a mask is defined for each of them. Next, the mask is divided into an upper triangle and a lower triangle by its diagonal line connected by the south-east and the north-west vertices. To embed a bit '1', all vertices in lower triangle are shifted to their mirror positions in the upper triangle with respect to the diagonal line, as shown in Fig. 6.1(a). To embed a bit '0' is just an inverse process shown in Fig. 6.1(b). The hidden data can be extracted by finding which triangle both with the most of the vertices in a mask. The scheme is blind and robust to noise and simplification attacks.

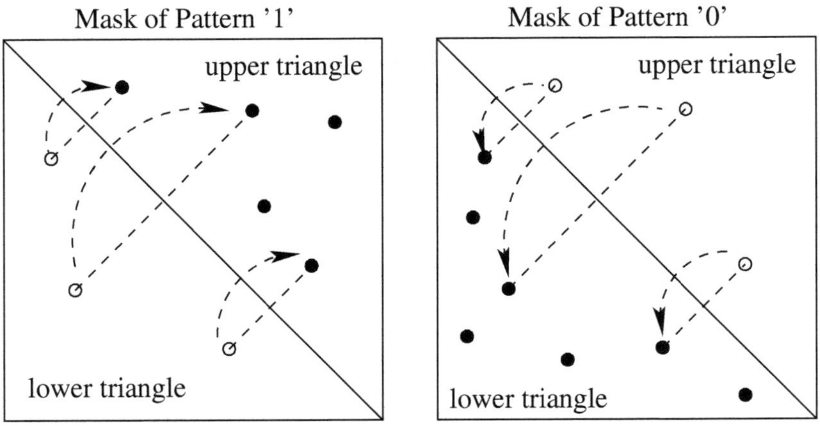

(a) Vertex pattern of bit '1'

(b) Vertex pattern of bit '0'

Fig. 6.1. Two patterns representing '1' and '0' (algorithm in [3]).

Schulz and Voigt [4] proposed a high capacity scheme which is robust to noise and simplification attacks. In the scheme, the original map is divided into many vertical and horizontal strips. The width of the strips could be $\frac{4}{3} \cdot \frac{\tau}{\sqrt{2}}$ to ensure the max distortion below the tolerance τ. The vertices within a strip are shifted to the reference line which is used to represent bit '1' or '0'. Figure 6.2 demonstrates the shifting process. The extraction of the hidden bit will depend on the half of the strip where most vertices located. The algorithm could survive additive noises with the amplitude less than 1/4 of the stripe width.

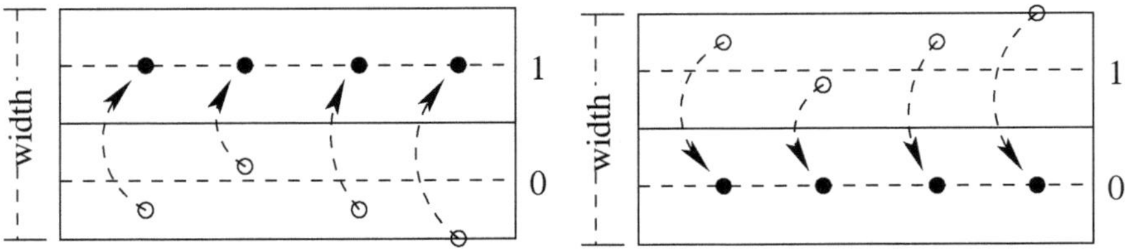

(a) Embed '1' in a strip

(b) Embed '0' in a strip

Fig. 6.2. Embedding data in a strip.

The algorithm proposed by Huber [5] also uses the locational relationship between vertices to hide bits. The scheme is different from those mentioned previously, in which new vertices are interpolated for data embedding. Figure 6.3 is an example of this scheme.

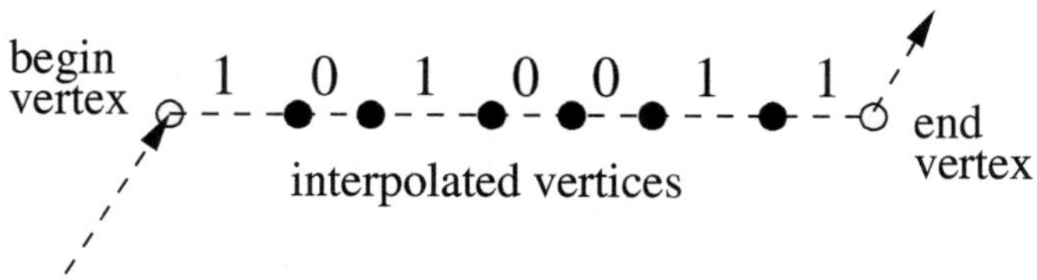

Fig. 6.3. A simple illustration of Huber's scheme.

In Figure 6.3, the Begin Vertex and the End Vertex represented by two white circles are two adjacent vertices in the original map. All black filled points are interpolated new vertices obtained during the embedding procedure. Suppose the distance between the begin vertex and the first interpolated vertex represents a bit '1' and half of the distance represents a bit '0', the data embedded in the line segment is then '1010011'. The scheme has no distortion and it is robust to geometric attacks. Embedding the watermark enlarges the size of the cover data. The scheme is also fragile to map simplification.

Based on Statistical Property

In a scheme proposed by Voigt and Busch [6], the statistical property of the coordinates is utilized for hiding data. A rectangular region in the original map is selected as the cover data to embed a watermark bit. Firstly, the region is divided into patches. Then a pseudo-noise sequence is used to divide all patches into two disjunctive sets A and B. Next, every patch in two sets is further divided into subpatches. For each subpatch, the coordinates of the vertices within it are transformed into new relative values by taking the south-west corner as the origin. If there is no embedded data, the relative coordinates in set A and B are both uniformly distributed with similar properties such as the expectation and the variance. If a bit '1' is to be embedded, the modification of the vertices is done within every subpatch as shown in Fig. 6.4. After the modification, the sample variance of coordinate values in set A (denoted as S_A) is increased and that of set B (denoted as S_B) is decreased. A random variable $F = S_A/S_B$ which follows F-distribution is then used for detection based on a threshold.

By utilizing the statistical property of coordinates, the algorithm has proved to be robust to many attacks such as map shifting, data interpolation, simplification, additive noise, for example.

Correlation Related

Ohbuchi et al. [7] presented a scheme based on correlation detection. A Pseudo Noise Sequence (PNS) is used to improve the security and the detecting reliability in the scheme. The cover map is first segmented into rectangular blocks

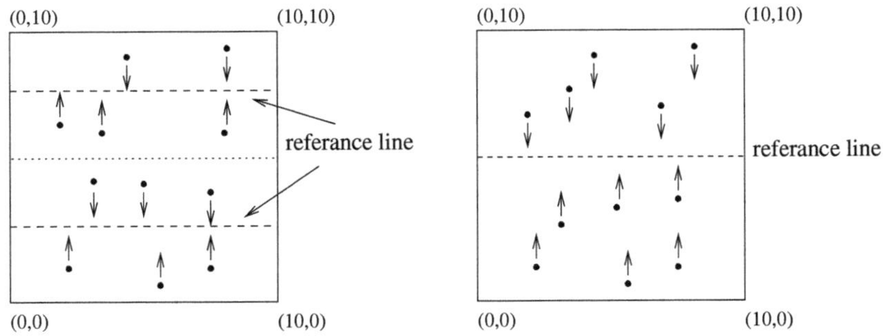

(a) Subpatch in Set A (b) Subpatch in Set B

Fig. 6.4. The modification of vertices in set A and B (algorithm in [6]).

containing like numbers of vertices. One block hides one watermark bit. For an arbitrary block, a hidden bit can be embedded by Eqn. (6.1),

$$V_i^{'} = V_i + b_i \cdot p_i \cdot \alpha, \tag{6.1}$$

where V_i and $V_i^{'}$ are the original coordinates and the watermarked coordinates of the vertices respectively within the ith block. The watermark bit b_i is the ith and p_i is the ith bit of a PNS. The amplitude factor is α. In the watermark extraction procedure, the original map is needed and the same PNS is used for decoding, which can be seen as a correlation based detecting procedure. The scheme is robust to kinds of attacks however it is not a blind scheme. A watermarking scheme with informed detection generally could not be practically used.

Voigt and Busch [8] proposed an algorithm based on a direct sequence spread spectrum. Watermark embedding and extraction are restricted to the specific decimal digital positions of the raw coordinates. Suppose a single bit is to be embedded. The bit is first replaced by a pseudo noise sequence (PNS) in order to form the watermark data, which is in essence a procedure of direct sequence spread spectrum. The PNS is then embedded in the coordinates by modifying the lower 2 decimal digital values of the coordinates. The amplitudes of the modifications are equal to the tolerance of the map data. In the data extraction stage, a modified correlation between the PNS and the lower 2 decimal digital values of watermarked coordinates is calculated and used for judgement. The algorithm is robust to additive noise. Adding or removing vertices could destroy the synchronization of the detector.

6.2.2 Transform Domain Schemes

A watermark is embedded by modifying the transform coefficients of the coordinates. The typical schemes are implemented in following domains: DFT domain, DWT domain, and Mesh-Spectral Domain.

DFT Domain Schemes

Nikolaidis et al. [9, 10] proposed a blind watermarking scheme consisting of embedding a single bit into a polyline by modifying the discrete Fourier coefficients of the polyline's coordinate sequence. Taking a polyline with N vertices as the cover data, a hidden bit can be embedded as follows. Firstly, given the coordinates $\{(x_k, y_k) \mid k = 1, 2, \cdots, N\}$ of the vertices, a complex sequence $z(k)$ is obtained by combining x and y coordinates as $z(k) = \{x_k + j \cdot y_k \mid k = 1, 2, \cdots, N\}$. After DFT is performed on $z(k)$, we get the coefficient sequence of $\{Z(k) \mid k = 1, 2, \cdots, N\}$. Secondly, by denoting a N-length Pseudo Noise Sequence as $\{W_0(k) \in \{-1, +1\} | k = 1, 2, \cdots, N\}$, the generation of the watermark $W(k)$ is a spread spectrum procedure as shown in Eqn. (6.2). Here

$$W(k) = \begin{cases} W_0(k) & ; \quad aN < k < bN, \text{ or }, (1-b)N < k < (1-a)N, \\ 0 & ; \quad \text{otherwise}, \end{cases} \tag{6.2}$$

where two parameters a, b $(0 < a < b < 1)$ are used to select the spectrum range for data embedding. Next, the generated watermark $W(k)$ is embed by modifying the amplitude of $Z(k)$ using either an additive operation (Eqn. (6.3)) or a multiplicative operation (Eqn. (6.4)),

$$|Z'(k)| = |Z(k)| + pW(k), \tag{6.3}$$

$$|Z'(k)| = |Z(k)| + p|Z(k)|W(k). \tag{6.4}$$

To extract the hidden data, the linear correlation (denoted as c) of $|Z'(k)|$ and $W(k)$ is calculated. Then the normalized correlation $c' = c/\mu_c$ is used for a judgement based on a threshold, where μ_c is the theoretical mean value of c. The scheme is inherently robust to many types of attacks such as map translating, rotating, scaling and the start vertex shifting in the watermarked polyline. Change of the vertex number such as simplification or interpolation could disturb the synchronization of the detector.

To improve the reliability of the detector, Nikolaidis et al. [11] also proposed an enhanced algorithm where multiple polylines are used for watermarking. The hidden bit is embedded in each polyline using the same method as in their former works [9, 10]. When detecting the hidden bit, each polyline will get a normalized correlation value $c'_i (i = 1, 2, \cdots, M)$, where M is the number of polylines. A data fusion function $f(\cdot)$ is then chosen to calculate a combined parameter $c = f(c'_1, c'_2, \cdots, c'_M)$, which will be used for the final judgement based on a threshold.

Based on the former works [9, 10], Kitamura et al. proposed a modified scheme [12] embedding multi-watermark bits in the DFT domain. The watermark is a meaningful bit sequence instead of a single bit represented by PNS. The embedding procedure is similar to the former works whereas the extracting procedure is different because the original map would be needed. Consequently, it is not a blind scheme, and this limits its application.

DWT Domain Schemes

Li and Xu proposed a blind scheme [13], which consists of embedding multiple bits into a vector map in DWT domain. The main idea of the scheme is described as follows.

(I) Similar to works [9, 10], the coordinates of the vertices are first combined to a complex sequence. Then a three level wavelet decomposition is performed on the sequence, which results in four sub-bands, i.e. HH1, HH2, HH3, LL3. Considering map's precision tolerance, HH2 and HH3 are selected for embedding data.

(II) Taking the coefficients in HH2 as an example, the embedding method is shown in Fig. 6.5.

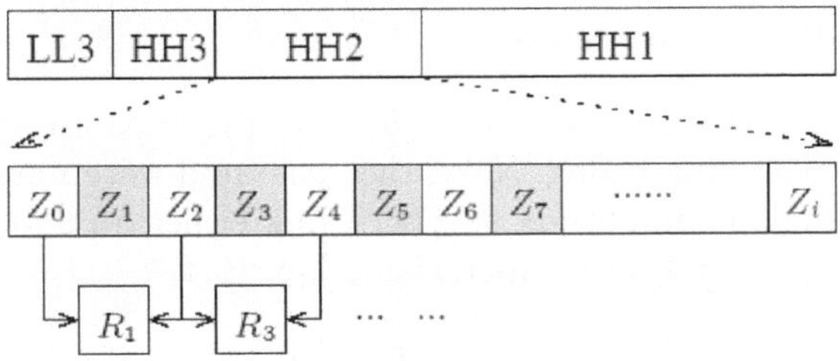

Fig. 6.5. An illustration of the DWT scheme in [13].

The values $Z0, Z1, \cdots, Zi$ are the coefficients in HH2. Starting with $Z1$, the watermark bits will be embedded into every other coefficient. That is, the coefficients with odd index (shadowed) $Z1, Z3, Z5, \cdots$. For example, suppose embedding the first watermark bit $w_1 \in \{0, 1\}$ into $Z1$. A reference value R is calculated by $R_1 = \left(\frac{|Z_0|+|Z_2|}{2}\right) \cdot \alpha$. Two neighboring coefficients Z_0 and Z_2 are used and α is the power factor controlling the embedding amplitude. Calculate $K_1 = \text{round}(|Z_1|/R_1)$ and use the parity of K_1 as the representation of a watermark bit. If $w_1 = 0$, modify $|Z_1|$ to make K_1 be an even number. If $w_1 = 1$, modify $|Z_1|$ to make K_1 be an odd number. The other watermark bits $w_2, w_3, \cdots$ are embedded into $Z_3, Z_5, \cdots$ in the same way.

(III) The data extraction can be performed without using the original map. Wavelet decomposition and $K_i'(i = 1, 3, \cdots)$ are calculated and watermark bits can be extracted according to the parity of each K_i'.

In this scheme, the amplitude of the coordinates' DWT coefficients are modified to specific modes for representing the watermark bits. The scheme is robust to noise and some geometrical attacks. Like other algorithms in transform domains, it is fragile to vertex attacks such as map simplification or interpolation.

Mesh-Spectral Domain Schemes

Although the application of 2D vector maps and 3D models are very different, there are still many similarities between the two data types. They are both vector data and composed of many vertices. It is possible to apply some 3D model watermarking methods to 2D vector maps. Ohbuchi et al. proposed a 2D vector map watermarking scheme [14] in mesh-spectral domain. This was originally used on 3D models [15]. In the algorithm, some techniques in 3D world can be adapted to process 2D vector data. Firstly, all vertices in the original map are connected to establish a 2D mesh using *Delaunay Triangulation*. The whole map is adaptively divided into many blocks using the rule *k-d* tree. For each block, a mesh-spectral analysis is performed on the 2D mesh within the block. The mesh-spectral coefficients are obtained and have the same size as the original coordinate sequence in the block. The spectral coefficient sequence is then considered as the cover data for watermarking. The method of data embedding is similar to the work [7] described in Section 6.2.1. And the scheme is also a non-blind scheme. Owing to the use of the original data, the scheme is robust to many attacks such as map rotating, translating, rotating, map interpolation, simplification, additive noise, and cropping.

6.2.3 Shape-Preserving Method

The algorithms mentioned above are the typical methods for robustly watermarking 2D vector maps in the spatial or transform domain. By analyzing the shortcoming of the former works, a statistic based scheme will be further presented in the remaining part of this section.

Motivation

Considering the main defects of the former works, the proposed scheme will focus on the following two aspects.

1. Shape Distortion and Cover Data Selection.

A principle used in most former works is to enhance the robustness. This is done by strictly controlling the distortion of every vertex under the precision tolerance τ for the sake of keeping the fidelity of the watermarked map. All former works take the 2D coordinates or their frequency coefficients as the cover data to control the distortions of vertices. This criteria is not enough to meet the requirements of the vector map watermarking. This is because the detail shape of the map objects is apt to be modified even if the fidelity of map data is well preserved. An experiment can be done to illustrate the problem. Figure 6.6(a) is an enlarged part of the original map. Fig. 6.6(b) is its corresponding watermarked part. Here the raw coordinates were selected as the cover data and the embedding procedure didn't take account of the map shape. Although the induced distortion of every vertex in Fig. 6.6(b) is under the precision tolerance τ, the local shape of the objects in the map has been modified. The distorted shape degrades the quality of the watermarked map, and the invisibility of the hidden watermark. This could possibly attract the attention of attackers. The main causes of the problem is that the algorithms choose the coordinates or their transform coefficients such as the cover data. This is an inconvenient form to present the shape information of the map objects. Consequently, new cover data, which can be directly related with the map's shape information, have to be selected instead of the raw coordinates in order to conveniently control the shape distortions induced by data embedding.

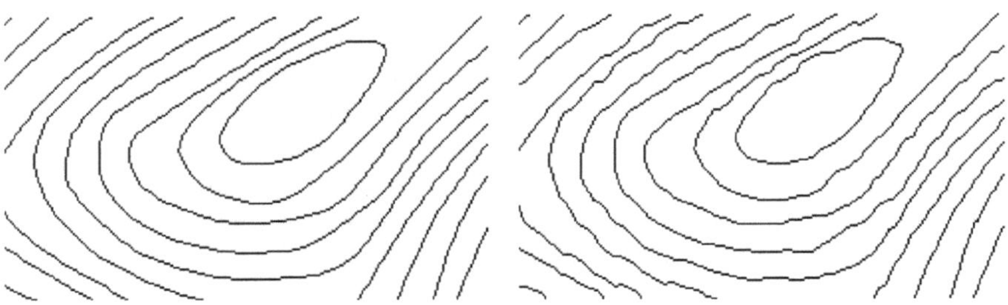

(a) Original map (b) Watermarked map

Fig. 6.6. An example of the distorted shape.

2. Robustness to Attacks

A successful attack generally has to remove the hidden message from the watermarked data while retaining its fidelity. Due to the critical application environment of 2D vector maps, even slight adjustment to the coordinates could possibly destroy the map's fidelity. It is not a good choice for an attacker to manipulate the watermarked map by rotating, translating, scaling, adding random noise, etc. However, most existing algorithms used these attacks. Some operations that can manipulate the map data without losing its fidelity, including map interpolation, simplification and data reordering, should be regarded as the more dangerous attacks. This will be emphasized in the following scheme.

Cover Data Extracting

To reduce the shape-distortions, the cover data adopted in the scheme is expected to explicitly represent the shape information of the map objects, which can not be directly satisfied by the raw coordinates. A distance sequence is extracted from the original map and used as the new cover data. Given the original map M_o, its feature points $F = \{f_1, f_2, \cdots\}$ are detected. These separate M_o into n subsets denoted as $C_1, \cdots, C_i, \cdots, C_n$. The Douglas-Peucker algorithm [16] is used in this scheme for feature point detection based on a threshold T_{DP}. The selection of T_{DP} will be discussed later. For each $i \in \{1, 2, \cdots, n\}$, suppose the subset C_i contains k_i vertices denoted as $v_1^i, v_2^i, \cdots, v_{k_i}^i$. It is clear that the first vertex v_1^i and the last vertex $v_{k_i}^i$ are two adjacent feature points in set F and the other vertices are non-feature points between them. Firstly, two vertices v_1^i and $v_{k_i}^i$ are connected to become a line segment L_i. Then a distance sequence $D_i = \{d_2^i, \cdots, d_{k_i-1}^i\}$ is calculated, where $d_2^i, \cdots, d_{k_i-1}^i$ are distances from every non-feature point $v_2^i, \cdots, v_{k_i-1}^i$ to the line segment L_i. The local shape of C_i can be directly related to set D_i. The middle point of the segment L_i(denoted o_i) is also calculated for further use. Repeat this process for all subsets $C_1, \cdots, C_i, \cdots, C_n$, and obtain a final data set composed of the distance set $D_o = \{D_1, \cdots, D_n\}$. A corresponding middle point set $O = \{o_1, \cdots, o_n\}$ will be extracted from M_o. Set D_o will be used as the cover data for watermarking. The main advantage is that D_o is directly related with the local shapes of the original map M_o and it is invariant to map translation or rotation.

Figure 6.7 demonstrates the above procedure using a simple polyline as the example.

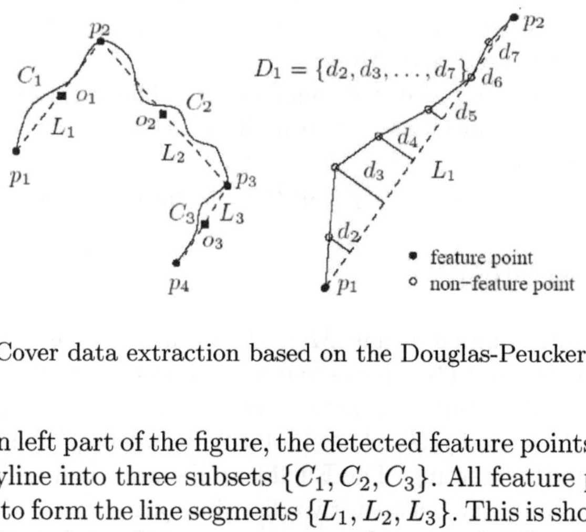

Fig. 6.7. Cover data extraction based on the Douglas-Peucker algorithm.

As shown in left part of the figure, the detected feature points $\{p_1, p_2, p_3, p_4\}$ divide the polyline into three subsets $\{C_1, C_2, C_3\}$. All feature points are connected in turn to form the line segments $\{L_1, L_2, L_3\}$. This is shown as a dotted line. The middle points of the segments are $\{o_1, o_2, o_3\}$. The right part of the Fig. 6.7 then indicates the procedure of calculating the distance by taking the segment L_1 as the example. Suppose there are six non-feature points between the feature points p_1 and p_2, the distance from each non-feature point to the line segment L_1 is calculated as $D_1 = \{d_2, \ldots, d_7\}$. The complete calculation of the whole polyline will obtain a distance sequence $D_o = \{D_1, D_2, D_3\}$.

Watermark Embedding

The watermark is embedded by changing the distributions of the cover data.

The cover data D_o is divided into two subsets D_A and D_B by following steps:

1) Divide the original map M_o into patches of uniform size, using a superimposed rectangular grid cover.
2) Based on a key k, generate a pseudo-random bit sequence whose length is equal to the number of the map patches. Every one bit is assigned to one patch as its flag. The key k can be used as the secret key for watermark detecting.
3) For each $i \in \{1, 2, \cdots, n\}$, check the bit flag of the patch where o_i is situated, and then assign D_i to the subset D_A or D_B according to the flag value '0' or '1'. For a certain map, two subsets D_A and D_B always have similar distributions.

Secondly, to embed a bit '0', just leave D_A and D_B unchanged. To embed a bit '1', leave D_A unchanged and multiply D_B with a factor α $(0 < \alpha < 1)$ as $D'_B = D_B \cdot \alpha$. The goal of the procedure is to introduce enough difference between the distributions of D_A and D'_B, which can then be regarded as a feature to represent a watermark bit.

Finally, combine the subsets D_A and D'_B into a watermarked distance sequence D_W. It is used to calculate the new positions of the map vertices and get the watermarked map M_W.

Let τ denote the precision tolerance of M_o. The location-distortions induced by embedding must below τ to maintain the fidelity of the map M_W. To meet the condition, $T_{DP} \cdot (1 - \alpha) \leq \tau$, where T_{DP} is the threshold used for feature point detection. Thus T_{DP} can be determined as $T_{DP} = \tau/(1 - \alpha)$.

Watermark Detecting

Given the possibly tampered map $\widetilde{M_W}$, the data set $\widetilde{D}_o$ is extracted from it and divided into $\widetilde{D}_A$ and $\widetilde{D}_B$. Here same parameters are used such as T_{DP} and secret key k. The distribution functions of $\widetilde{D}_A$ and $\widetilde{D}_B$ are then calculated, and denoted as $f_a(k)$ and $f_b(k)$. The similarity between $f_a(k)$ and $f_b(k)$ can be used for watermark detecting. The Euclidean distance is used as the measure to evaluate the similarity between two distributions:

$$\mathrm{dis}(f_a, f_b) = \sqrt{\sum_k (f_a(k) - f_b(k))^2}.$$

Note that lower $\mathrm{dis}(f_a, f_b)$ means higher degree of similarity between $f_a(k)$ and $f_b(k)$. Taking $\mathrm{dis}(f_a, f_b)$ as the similarity measure, the detecting procedure is a judgement based on a threshold T. The map is not marked if $\mathrm{dis}(f_a, f_b) < T$. If $\mathrm{dis}(f_a, f_b) \geq T$, the map should have been watermarked because the embedding procedure could degrade the similarity between $f_a(k)$ and $f_b(k)$.

Threshold Determination

The distribution of dis(f_a, f_b) is used to determine the threshold T. A 1000 different blocks of a big contour map are used as the original maps and dis(f_a, f_b) is then calculated for each of them before and after watermarking. Figure 6.8 indicates the resulting distributions of dis(f_a, f_b). The left curve in the figure is the distribution of dis(f_a, f_b) in original maps, and the right is the distribution in watermarked maps. As shown in the figure, if is T selected as 0.078, minimum detection error could be achieved with the false-positive-error of 6.15×10^{-6} and the false-negative-error of 4.33×10^{-5}. To enhance the robustness to additive noise attack, a smaller T should be selected. In this scheme, T is selected as 0.068 for the purpose of resisting the low amplitude noises. The experimental results in the remaining part will indicate that the selection is reasonable.

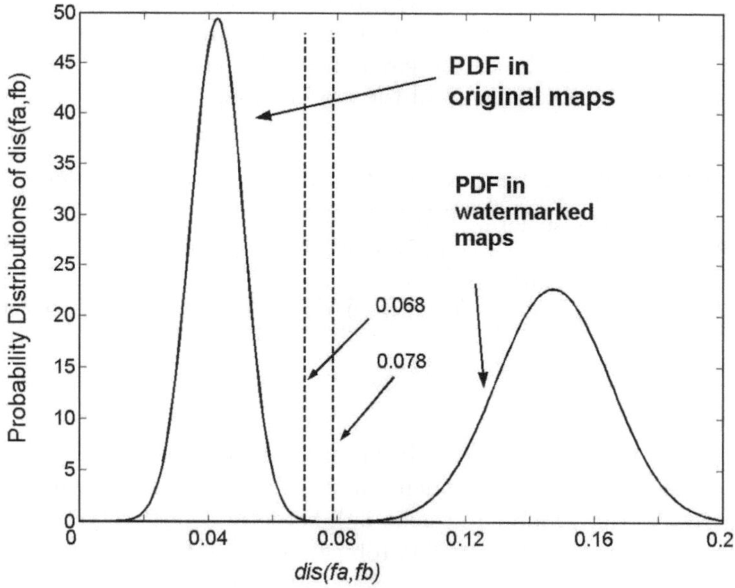

Fig. 6.8. The distribution of dis(f_a, f_b).

Performance

The original map shown in Fig. 6.6 is used for experiments. It is part of a contour map with the scale 1:10000. The tolerance (τ) of the coordinates is 1 meter(m). The size of the divided map patch is 20m$\times$20m. The factor α is chosen as 0.6. The threshold for feature point detection can be calculated as $T_{DP} = \tau/(1-\alpha) = 2.5$m. The threshold T is set to 0.068. The performance of the scheme is discussed in following aspects.

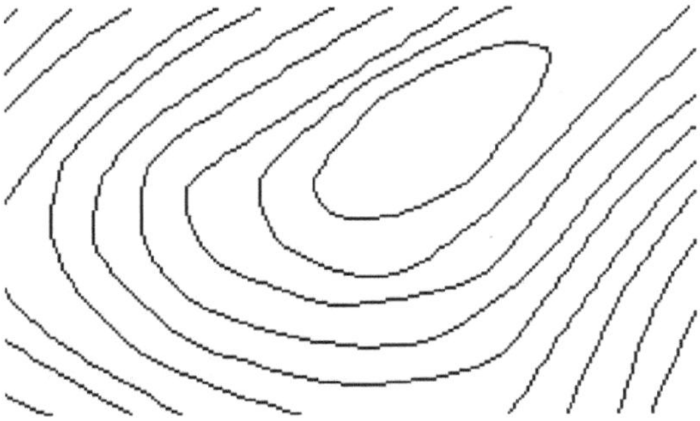

Fig. 6.9. Watermarked map.

1. *Invisibility*
   The resulting map watermarked by the scheme is shown in Fig. 6.9. This indicates the scheme's better invisibility. Comparing with Fig. 6(b), the shape-distortions induced by the algorithm are obviously lower than former works. By choosing D_o as the cover data, the data embedding procedure can preserve the local shapes of the original map.

Table 6.1. Results of robustness tests for map simplification and interpolation.

simplification	Threshold(m)	0.2	0.4	0.6	0.8	1.0
	$dis(f_a, f_b)$	0.14593	0.20967	0.18385	0.21114	0.32018
Interpolation	Stepwidth(m)	1.0	0.8	0.6	0.4	0.2
	$dis(f_a, f_b)$	0.087374	0.094742	0.093985	0.092177	0.092762

2. *Robustness*
   The selected cover data D_o is invariant to map translation and rotation. The division of D_o is independent on the storage order of the map objects. As a result, the proposed scheme is inherently robust to translation, rotation and data reordering. The robustness tests then focus on the most serious forms of attacks to vector map watermarking schemes such as map simplification, interpolation and low-amplitude noise. For map simplification, Douglas-Peucker algorithm is used with the threshold range $[0, \tau]$. The Cubic Spline Algorithm is adopted for map interpolation with a series of stepwidths. All detecting results are shown in Table 6.1. Taking the threshold $T = 0.068$, the watermark can be successfully defended under each attack. This demonstrates the scheme's robustness to above attacks.

Additive noise attack mainly comes from some daily works (e.g. map format transformation) and generally has small amplitude. Given a map for detecting, a series of imposed additive noises with the amplitudes from 0.01m to 0.1m to it to simulate the noise attack procedures. For each noise amplitude, the attacking and the corresponding detecting procedures are repeated for 1000 times. Suppose that the probability of a watermarked map is 0.5, we can calculate the average detection rate of the scheme with certain threshold T.

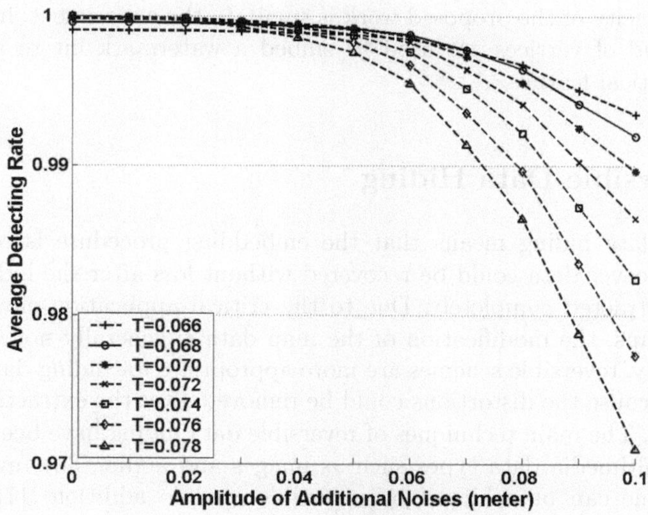

Fig. 6.10. The average detection rate under noise attacks.

The curves in Figure 6.10 are the average detection rates under noise attacks with a series of threshold T from 0.066 to 0.078. It is indicated that the proposed algorithm is robust to the additive noises within the given range of the amplitude. If the threshold T is decreased from 0.078 to 0.068, the noise resisting performance could be enhanced simultaneously. T should not be more small because the detecting rate under lower noise amplitudes could be significantly decreased, as shown by the curve $T = 0.066$ in Figure 6.10. The threshold T used in the scheme is 0.068, and the detecting rate is shown by the solid curve in the figure.

6.2.4 Summary

In this section, the technique of robust vector map watermarking is introduced. A brief review of the typical methods implemented in either the spatial domain or the transform domain is presented. According to the common weakness of the former works, a shape-preserving scheme is proposed. By taking into account the local shapes of the map objects, the scheme can robustly watermark a 2D vector map while introducing low shape-distortions. Experimental results indicate the performance of the scheme in invisibility and robustness. The original map used in the experiments is a contour map with smooth shape feature. We also tested the algorithm on some other map types such as river maps, and boundary maps for example. In most cases the algorithm works well. However, the algorithm can not work on maps composed of straight lines, rectangles representing streets and blocks because there are usually few non-feature points in this type of maps. It should also be noticed that the capacity of the proposed work is small. In the experiment, more than two thousand of vertices are used to embed a watermark bit to achieve a stable statistical feature.

6.3 Reversible Data Hiding

Reversible data hiding means that the embedding procedure is reversible. That is the cover data could be recovered without loss after the hidden data has been extracted completely. Due to the critical application environment of vector maps, the modification of the map data is generally not expected. Consequently, reversible schemes are more appropriate for hiding data in vector maps because the distortions could be removed after the extraction of the hidden data. The main techniques of reversible data hiding have been studied on some multimedia data types such as images and audio. The reversibility of the scheme can be achieved by invertible modulo addition [17], lossless compression [18], histogram shifting [19, 20], difference expansion [21], and companding [22]. However, few works have concerned the topic of reversibly hiding data in 2D vector maps. In this section two reversible data hiding schemes for 2D vector maps based on the techniques of amplitude addition and difference expansion respectively are discussed.

6.3.1 Amplitude Addition Scheme

Voigt et al. designed a reversible watermarking scheme [23] embedding watermark bits in the integer Discrete Cosine Transform (DCT) domain. The main idea of the scheme is to utilize an important feature of map data. That is the high correlation of vertex coordinates. Generally, owing to the continuous and smooth shape of the map objects, the coordinates of the consecutive vertices within an object are always highly correlated. It is well known that the Discrete Cosine Transform has the property of energy compaction for highly correlated data. After the DCT, the energy of the transformed data will be concentrated on DC and low frequency AC coefficients. Taking advantage of the above characteristics, the proposed algorithm combines every eight vertices into an unit and for each unit a single watermark bit will be embedded into it by changing its eight points integer DCT coefficients. The basic embedding method is shown in Fig. 6.11.

The vertical axis in the figure represents the absolute values of the eight DCT coefficients of a unit. D is the DC coefficient and A_1 to A_7 are AC coefficients. Due to the high correlation of the coordinates, the absolute value

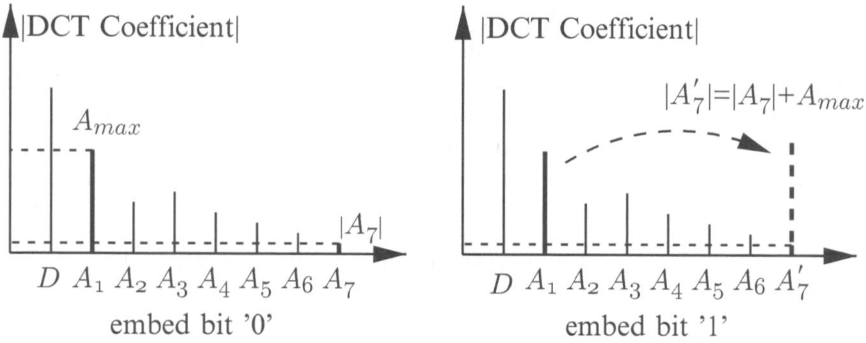

Fig. 6.11. The embedding method of [23].

of the highest frequency coefficient, $|A_7|$, is the smallest in most cases. It is generally smaller than the maximum absolute value from A_1 to A_6 (denoted as $A_{\max} = \max\{|A_1|, \cdots, |A_6|\}$). If the embedded bit '0', the unit remains unchanged. If the embedded bit '1', the coefficient A_7 is modified to $|A_7'| = |A_7| + A_{\max}$. The above embedding method is reversible because the original A_7 could be obtained by subtracting $A_{\max}$ from A_7' after the extraction of the hidden bit. This scheme is the first algorithm where the idea of reversible data hiding is introduced into watermarking digital vector maps. A drawback of the scheme is that the distortions induced by watermarking is relatively too large. The authors have made some compensation.

6.3.2 Difference Expansion Scheme

Basic Idea of Difference Expansion

Difference expansion is a method of reversibly hiding data in pixel images, and was first proposed by Tian [21]. The basic idea of difference expansion is to utilize the high correlation of the cover data. For a pair of adjacent elements denoted as integers x_1 and x_2, which are highly correlated cover data, an integer transform is defined to calculate their difference (d) and integer-mean (m). It is shown in Eqn. (6.5):

$$\begin{cases} d = x_1 - x_2, \\ m = \text{floor}\left(\frac{x_1+x_2}{2}\right). \end{cases} \tag{6.5}$$

The transform is strictly invertible and the Eqn. (6.6) is the inverse transform:

$$\begin{cases} x_1 = m + \text{floor}\left(\frac{d+1}{2}\right), \\ x_2 = m - \text{floor}\left(\frac{d}{2}\right). \end{cases} \tag{6.6}$$

To hide data bits, x_1 and x_2 are transformed to d and m by Eqn. (6.5). The high correlation of the cover data means that two elements x_1 and x_2

are generally very close. That is, their difference d could be very small in most cases. It is possible to provide i bits for placing the hidden data by left shifting d by i bits. This done by expanding d to its 2^i times while keeping the induced distortions an acceptable level. Suppose the expanded difference carrying i hidden bits is denoted as d', the watermarked elements x_1' and x_2' could be calculated by d' and m via Eqn. (6.6). Difference expansion has the following properties when used for reversible data hiding:

1) The cover data should be integers for using difference expansion.
2) The total error $(d' - d)$ induced by expansion will be shared by two elements x_1 and x_2.
3) Highly correlated cover data is recommended for data hiding because higher correlation generally means lower distortions and higher capacity.

Correlation of Coordinates and an Outline of the Scheme

Difference expansion is appropriate for hiding data in the cover data with a high correlation. A natural image is always highly correlated because most adjacent pixels have similar values. This is grayscales or colors, for example. A vector map is composed of a sequence of the coordinates of the vertices. Due to the density of the vertices, the positions of two adjacent vertices are usually very close and the differences between their coordinates are very small. Consequently, coordinate sequence can also be considered as having high correlation. In the following scheme, the raw coordinates of the cover map are taken as the cover data for hiding data by difference expansion. The algorithm begins with the division of the original map in which every two adjacent vertices are grouped into a vertex pair. An embedding condition is then used to judge whether a certain pair is suitable for hiding data by difference expansion. For all suitable pairs, the hidden bits are embedded by expanding the differences of coordinates. Otherwise, the hidden bits are embedded by replacing the Least Significant Bit (LSB) of the differences.

Map Division and Embedding Condition

1. Map Division

Generally, the coordinates of a vector map are floating-point numbers with a fixed precision. In order to perform difference expansion, all coordinates are firstly transformed to integers by multiplying 10^p where p is the number of digits after the decimal point. Then the original map is divided into groups. Each group contains two adjacent vertices. For example, supposing a map object (polyline or polygon) is composed by vertices $\{v_1, v_2, v_3, v_4, \cdots\}$, then the divided object should be $\{(v_1, v_2), (v_3, v_4), \cdots\}$. Repeat the procedure for all map objects (except points), the original map can be divided into N vertex pairs which can be denoted as

$$(v_1^i, v_2^i) = \{(x_1^i, y_1^i)\,,\ (x_2^i, y_2^i)\}\,; \quad i \in [1, N]$$

where (x_1^i, y_1^i) and (x_2^i, y_2^i) are 2D coordinates of the vertices v_1^i and v_2^i. Each vertex pair will be used as an embedding unit. Within a pair, the difference d and the integer-mean m of two vertices are calculated for x and y, respectively,

$$\begin{cases} d_x^i = x_1^i - x_2^i, \\ m_x^i = \text{floor}\left(\frac{x_1^i + x_2^i}{2}\right), \end{cases} \quad i \in [1, N].$$

$$\begin{cases} d_y^i = y_1^i - y_2^i, \\ m_y^i = \text{floor}\left(\frac{y_1^i + y_2^i}{2}\right), \end{cases} \quad i \in [1, N].$$

For N vertex pairs, following N-length sequences could be obtained by the procedure, that is D_x, M_x, and D_y, M_y, which are the difference sequence and the integer-mean sequence respectively for coordinates x and y.

$$\begin{cases} D_x = \{d_x^1, d_x^2, \cdots, d_x^N\}, \\ M_x = \{m_x^1, m_x^2, \cdots, m_x^N\}. \end{cases}$$

$$\begin{cases} D_y = \left\{d_y^1, d_y^2, \cdots, d_y^N\right\}, \\ M_y = \left\{m_y^1, m_y^2, \cdots, m_y^N\right\}. \end{cases}$$

The hidden data can then be embedded into x (or y) coordinates by applying difference expansion to the sequence D_x (or D_y). Namely, by left shifting (expanding) the suitable elements in D_x (or D_y), some extra space could be provided for placing the hidden bits. The selection of the suitable elements in D_x (or D_y) is based on an embedding condition which is related to the precision tolerance of the original map.

2. Embedding Condition

The maximum distortion that is tolerated in a vector map is called the map's precision tolerance, and is denoted as τ. To ensure the validity of the map data, the maximum distortion induced by data hiding should not exceed the tolerance τ. Taking the situation of embedding data in x coordinates as the example, a vertex pair could be suitable for hiding data by bitwise shifting the difference value d_x^i but only when an embedding condition has been satisfied. This section considers the case of left shifting 1 bit that is to expand d_x^i to double. Suppose a hidden bit $w_i \in \{0, 1\}$ is embedded into the x coordinates of the vertex pair (v_1^i, v_2^i) by difference expansion, the modified difference $d_x^{i\,\prime}$ containing w_i is then

$$d_x^{i\,\prime} = 2 \times d_x^i + w_i. \tag{6.7}$$

The watermarked coordinates $x_1^{i\,\prime}$ and $x_2^{i\,\prime}$ are calculated by using $d_x^{i\,\prime}$ and m_x^i in Eqn. (6.6),

$$\begin{cases} x_1^{i\,\prime} = m_x^i + \text{floor}\left(\frac{d_x^{i\,\prime} + 1}{2}\right), \\ x_2^{i\,\prime} = m_x^i - \text{floor}\left(\frac{d_x^{i\,\prime}}{2}\right). \end{cases} \tag{6.8}$$

To ensure the validity of the map data, it must simultaneously satisfy $\left|x_1^{i\prime} - x_1^i\right| \leq \tau$ and $\left|x_2^{i\prime} - x_2^i\right| \leq \tau$. Substitute Eqn. (6.7) and (6.8) into the condition, and an equivalent condition is obtained

$$\begin{cases} \left| \text{floor}\left(\left(\frac{2\times d_x^i + w_i + 1}{2}\right) - \text{floor}\left(\frac{d_x^i + 1}{2}\right)\right| \leq \tau, \\ \left| \text{floor}\left(\left(\frac{2\times d_x^i + w_i}{2}\right) - \text{floor}\left(\frac{d_x^i}{2}\right)\right| \leq \tau. \end{cases} \tag{6.9}$$

According to the parity of d_x^i and the value of w_i (0 or 1), the two sub-conditions in Eqn. (6.9) can be simplified. Their intersection is taken to be the final condition (Eqn. (6.10)) which determines whether the vertex pair (v_1^i, v_2^i) is suitable for difference expansion:

$$-2\tau + 1 \leq d_x^i \leq 2\tau - 2. \tag{6.10}$$

Eqn. (6.10) is then used to check the suitability of all N vertex pairs. A N-length flag F is generated to record the results. Here $F = \{f_i \mid f_i \in \{0, 1\}, i = 1, \cdots, N\}$. When $f_i = 1$ the ith vertex pair (v_1^i, v_2^i) meets the embedding condition. A hidden bit will then be embedded by expanding the difference d_x^i. Accordingly, $f_i = 0$ means that $\left(v_1^i, v_2^i\right)$ does not meet the embedding condition. In this scheme, a hidden bit will also be embedded in such $\left(v_1^i, v_2^i\right)$ by replacing the LSB of d_x^i. The original LSB of d_x^i should not be discarded for the sake of ensuring the reversibility of the scheme. A bit sequence L is generated to record all replaced LSBs to avoid information loss. Both F and L are necessary information which will be needed later for data recovery. They are embedded in the cover map as a part of the hidden data.

Data Embedding and Extraction

1. Structure of Hidden Data

To ensure reversibility and to improve the capacity, the hidden data (denoted as W) should be composed as follows:

$$W = H + \text{comp}(F) + \text{comp}(L) + P,$$

where comp(·) is the lossless compression algorithm. The meaning of each component is listed below.

H: The header information recording the lengths of the other three components. It is useful for reliably separating each data component from W during the procedure of data extraction.

comp(F): Lossless compressed flag F. The flag is necessary for recovering the original data because we must know the embedding method of each vertex pair. That is, by the difference expansion or by LSB replacement. F is compressed to save space for the payload.

comp(L): Lossless Compressed L. To recover the original data when the hidden bit is embedded by LSB replacing, the original LSB of d_x^i must be known. This is recorded in L.

P: The payload of the scheme. It could be the hash for example either MD5in the cover map for data authentication, the meta data of the cover map, or where the secret message is transmitted by users (Hidden Communication).

Comp(F) and comp(L) are both used for lossless data recovering. P is the real payload which is referred to as the capacity of the scheme. The final W is a N-length binary sequence which can be denoted as $W = \{w_1, \cdots, w_N\}$.

2. Data Embedding
We will use the method of hiding data in the x coordinates as an example. The method is exactly the same for the y coordinates. Until now, three N-length sequences could be obtained by former methods. That is the difference sequence D_x, the flag F, and the hidden data W. The embedding task is to hide W in the x coordinates by modifying the difference sequence D_x. Each element d_x^i of D_x is modified as shown in Eqn. (6.11) according to the flag f_i:

$$d_x^{i\,\prime} = \begin{cases} 2 \times d_x^i + w_i & , f_i = 1; \\ 2 \times \text{floor}\left(\frac{d_x^i}{2}\right) + w_i & , f_i = 0; \end{cases} \quad i = 1, \cdots, N. \tag{6.11}$$

For d_x^i when $f_i = 1$, the value w_i is embedded by difference expansion. That is left shift d_x^i by 1 bit and place w_i at the lowest bit of the shifted d_x^i. Otherwise for d_x^i where $f_i = 0$, the value w_i is embedded by directly replacing the LSB of d_x^i. Denoting the modified difference sequence as $D_x' = \{d_x^{1\,\prime}, \cdots, d_x^{N\,\prime}\}$, the watermarked x coordinates could be calculated with D_x' and M_x by the inverse transform as shown in Eqn. (6.6).

3. Data Extraction and Original Map Recovering
Given the watermarked map containing hidden data in its x coordinates, the same methods used in the embedding procedure are used to group the map data and to calculate both the difference sequence D_x' and the integer-mean sequence M_x. The hidden data W can be obtained by extracting the lowest bits of all elements of D_x'. The payload P and two compressed sequence comp(F) and comp(L) may be separated from W with the help of the header information H.

In order to recover the original x coordinates, it is necessary to obtain the original difference sequence D_x. Two sequences comp(F) and comp(L) are uncompressed, obtaining the flag F and the original LSB L. Then D_x is obtained by using D_x', F and L. For $i = 1, \cdots, N$, each element d_x^i of D_x is calculated using Eqn. (6.12),

$$d_x^i = \begin{cases} \text{floor}\left(\frac{d_x^{i\,\prime}}{2}\right), & f_i = 1; \\ 2 \times \text{floor}\left(\frac{d_x^{i\,\prime}}{2}\right) + L(j), & f_i = 0. \end{cases} \tag{6.12}$$

Here $d_x^{i\,\prime}$ and f_i are respectively the elements of D_x' and F. For $f_i = 1$, d_x^i is obtained by discarding the lowest bit of $d_x^{i\,\prime}$ and right shifting it by 1 bit. For $f_i = 0$, d_x^i is recovered by directly replacing the LSB of $d_x^{i\,\prime}$ by the original LSB $L(j)$, where j is the index of L.

Finally, the original x coordinates can be completely recovered by the use of Eqn. (6.6) and the restored difference sequence D_x and the integer-mean sequence M_x.

Experiments

The performance of the scheme was tested by experiments using a river map (Fig. 13(a)) with the scale 1:4000000 as the cover data. The total number of the vertices in the map is 252000. There are 6 digits after the decimal point of every coordinate value. All coordinates are first converted into integers by multiplying 10^6. The precision tolerance of the map is $\tau = 0.5$ kilometer.

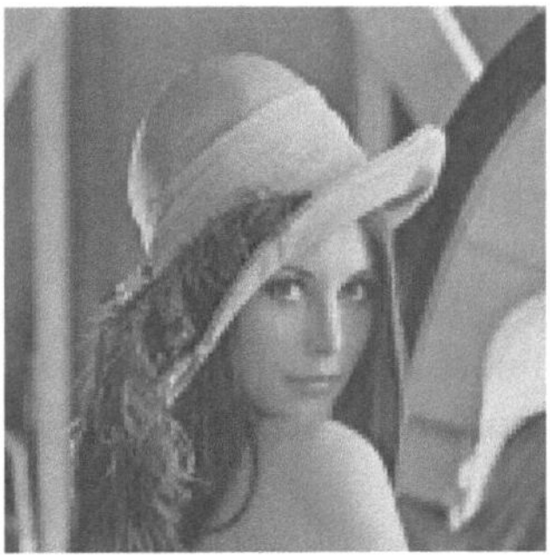

Fig. 6.12. Grayscale image (Lena, 130 × 130).

Both the x and y coordinates are used to hide data in order to improve the capacity. Although the induced distortions of some vertices could exceed the tolerance τ, the validity of the map data can be ensured as the original map can be exactly recovered after the hidden data has been extracted. Hidden data with a max length of 146550 bits can be embedded. Here the max capacity of the scheme is about 0.58bit/vertex. The MD5 hash of the cover map (128 bits) and a grayscale image with a size of 130 × 130 (135200 bits, Fig. 6.12) is taken as the hidden data and is embedded into the cover map. The remaining space of the payload could also be utilized to hide other user data. For example the meta data of the cover map. Figure 6.13(b) is the watermarked map which indicates that the distortions induced by data hiding can be well controlled

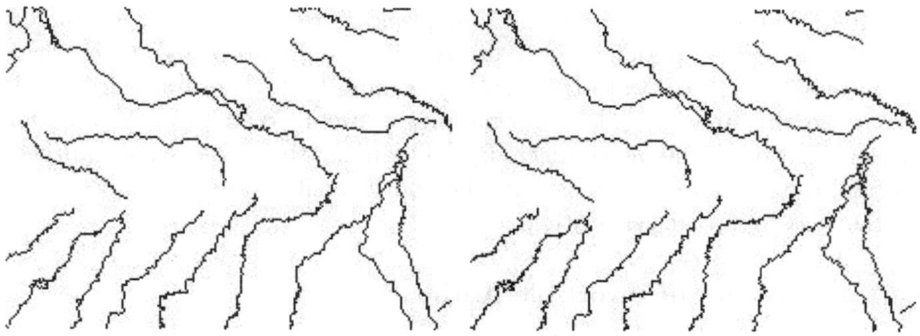

(a) Original map of river (b) Watermarked map

Fig. 6.13. Original map and watermarked map.

by use of this scheme. After the hidden data has been successfully extracted, the cover map is recovered. Experimental results indicate that the recovered map is exactly the same as the original map as their MD5 hashes matched exactly.

6.3.3 Summary

This section discusses the issue of Reversible Data Hiding in vector maps. Two algorithms are introduced. The first is implemented in the integer DCT domain. The high correlation of the map coordinates and the energy compaction property of DCT are utilized by the scheme. The hidden data is embedded by modifying the amplitude of the integer DCT coefficients. The distortions in this scheme are not easy to control. The second scheme is implemented in the spatial domain and are based on Difference Expansion. A relatively high capacity can be achieved and the induced distortions can be well controlled.

Some defects are apparent in the analyzing powers of the algorithm. Firstly, the invisibility of the scheme could not be good. Since the hidden data is embedded into the x (or y) coordinates, the movement directions of the vertices are restricted to the x or y directions. Consequently, the shape of the watermarked map has disturbed appearance. This degrades the invisibility of the scheme. Secondly, the payload of the scheme depends to some extent on the type of map. The type of the cover map determines the correlation of its raw coordinates. Some maps do not have highly correlated coordinates. For example the contour maps with large scales. The low correlation of the coordinates could result in a reduced capacity.

6.4 Fragile Watermarking

As described in Section 6.1.1, there are some special applications where a higher security level is required. As an instance, secret military maps must be strictly authenticated before use. If a map known to be modified, it is necessary to know which part has been altered. The ability to verify the integrity of the map data and locate the changes is important. There has been little activity in this area. Fragile watermarking is useful for data authentication and localization of the interference. By introducing the idea of image authentication, this section introduces a fragile and reversible watermarking scheme for 2D vector map authenticating.

6.4.1 Framework of Invertible Authentication

Figure 6.14 is a block diagram of the general methods of invertible authentication. The basic idea is simple. For the original data to be protected, its authentication information is first calculated and used as the hidden data (watermark). The authentication information may be a hash, message authentication code, or digital signature computed over the original data. The obtained information is then inserted back into the original data by an invertible watermarking method (Fig. 6.14(a)). The original data can now be transmitted because it has been protected by watermarking. Accordingly, to verify the integrity of the received data which is suspected to have been modified (Fig. 6.14(b)), the embedded authentication information is extracted. The original data is then reconstructed because the adopted watermarking method is invertible. Then the authentication information of the recovered data is calculated. Finally, the integrity of the received data can be verified by comparing the extracted signature with the calculated signature of the recovered data. If two signatures are exactly matched, the received data is deemed to be authentic.

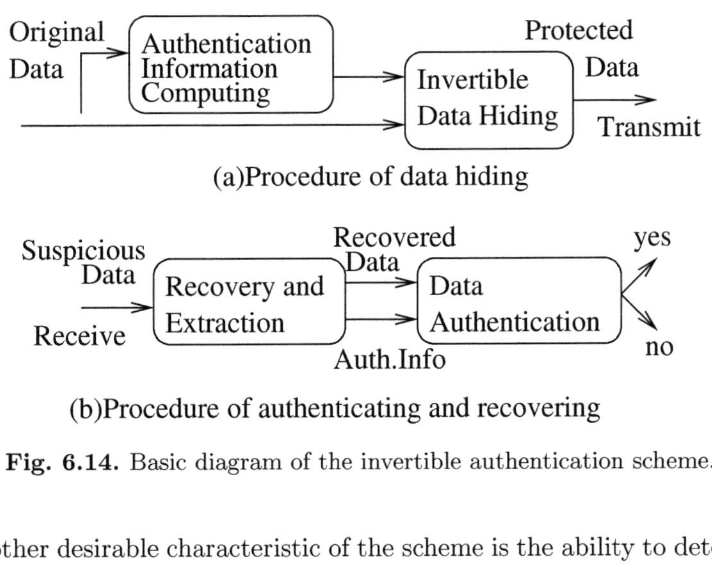

Fig. 6.14. Basic diagram of the invertible authentication scheme.

Another desirable characteristic of the scheme is the ability to detect tampering. In image authentication, this characteristic could be obtained by dividing the original image into blocks and authenticating each block independently. The precision of the localization is determined by the size of the blocks. Based on the basic idea, the tamper locating ability of 2D vector maps could be achieved by dividing the cover map into segments and performing authentication on each segment.

The authentication scheme for vector maps should be fragile to any attempt to tamper. The change of a single bit is a critical application environment in a map data. The remaining part of the section presents a fragile and invertible watermarking scheme for 2D vector map authentication.

6.4.2 To Authenticate Vector Map by the Use of Invertible Fragile Watermarking

The Vector Map Authenticating Scheme described here is based on the method proposed by Fridrich et al. [18], used for image authentication. In this scheme, the Least Significant Bit (LSB) plane of the original image is replaced by a bit-string containing the authentication information and the compressed form of the original LSB. The additional capacity is provided by lossless compression of the original LSB, which enables the reconstruction of the original image.

For 2D vector maps, we create space for storing the hash digest by losslessly compressing the bit-plane of the coordinates. These are chosen according to the distortion tolerance (τ) of the map data. The selected bit-plane is then replaced by the watermark. This is composed by the hash digest of the original data and the compressed form of the selected bit-plane. In the watermark extraction procedure, the same bit-plane is extracted from the map data. The compressed original bit-plane is decompressed and used to reconstruct the original map data. By comparing the extracted hash digest and the calculated hash digest of the restored map, the integrity of the data can be authenticated. To obtain the information and the location of the tamper, the original map should be divided into segments. The above procedure is performed for each segment. The scheme is quite fragile. Any distortions of the protected data will definitely indicate the failed authentication area.

Detail of the Scheme

Authenticating a contour map with the scale 1:10000 is used as an example. Supposing the tolerance of the map data is $\tau = 1$ (meter), the detail of the authentication scheme is as follows.

1. Embedding Procedure

1) Divide the original vector data into segments. Each segment contains 128 vertices, $I_n = \{(x_i, y_i) \mid i = 1, 2, ..., 128\}$. Then translate the coordinates from decimal to binary.

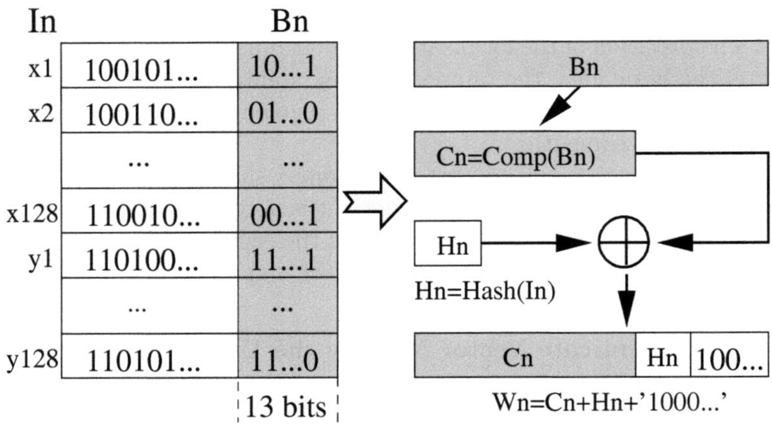

Fig. 6.15. The procedure of watermark generation.

2) To ensure the induced distortions not exceed the tolerance τ, choose the last 13 bit-plane of x and y coordinates as the positions used for embedding watermark. This can be denoted as $B_n = \{b_i \in \{0,1\} \mid i = 1, 2, \cdots, 128 \times 13 \times 2\}$. Compress the selected bit-plane without loss. Then denote the compressed bit-plane as $C_n = \text{Comp}(B_n)$. Here $\text{Comp}(\cdot)$ is the lossless compression function.
3) Calculate the hash digest of the original map as $H_n = \text{Hash}\,(I_n)$. Then the watermark data can be constructed as $W_n = H_n + C_n$. The length of W_n is extended to equal the length of B_n by appending an ending mark followed by enough zero's to complete the row to the end of W_n. The procedure of watermark generation is shown in Fig. 6.15.
4) Replace the selected bit-plane of I_n with the watermark W_n to get a watermarked segment I_{wn}. Repeat the procedure for all segments. Then the original map is protected by watermarking.

2. Extracting and Authenticating Procedure

1) Divide the suspect map into the same number of segments I'_{wn}.
2) For each I'_{wn}, extract the watermark W'_n. Then separate W'_n into the Hash Digest H'_n and the Compressed Bit-Planes C'_n. Decompress C'_n to B'_n.
3) Replace the selected bit-plane with B'_n and calculate the hash digest H''_n of the recovered map.
4) If the two hashes H'_n and H''_n exactly match, the map data in current segment is deemed authentic and the original data has been recovered as part of the process. If the two hashes differ, then the segment under consideration has been tampered with.

Experiment Results

Some experiments are done to test the performance of the proposed algorithm. The adopted hash function is MD5. It is a one-way function which can take an arbitrary length input and return a signature with the fixed length of 128 bits. Fig. 6.16 shows the results of the experiment. The differences between the original map [Fig. 6.16(a)] and the watermarked map [Fig. 6.16(b)] are well controlled. If there has been no tampering, the original vector map can be exactly restored during the extraction procedure. To check the scheme's localization ability, we tampered several coordinates of an arbitrary segment in the watermarked map. Fig. 6.16(c) is the restored map of the tampered watermarked map. The tampered segment can be reliably detected and has been marked in the figure. The other segments are restored without loss.

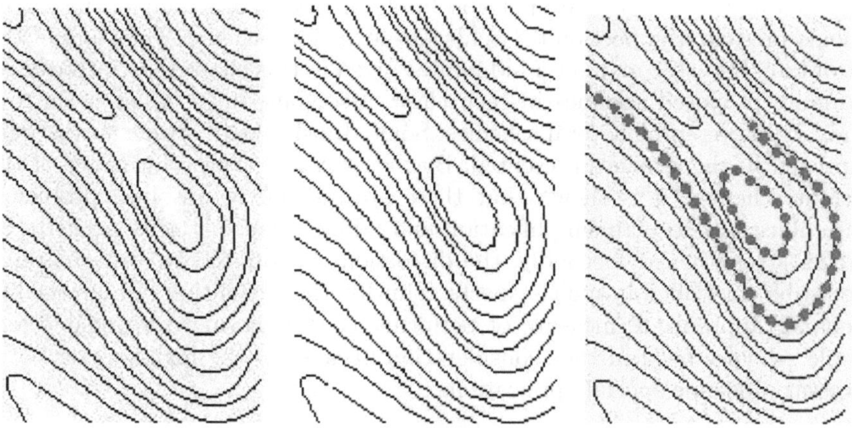

(a) Original map (b) Watermarked map (c) Authenticated map

Fig. 6.16. Experiment results.

The scheme is fully fragile, where authentication will definitely fail even if there is only a single bit of the protected data has been altered. Note that the tamper locating precision of the scheme is limited to the length of the map segments. The selection of the segment length should ensure that every segment can provide enough space for inserting the authenticating information. This is highly related to the type of the cover map and the method of lossless compression. For maps with highly correlated coordinates, the segment length could be selected shorter than that in the maps with lower correlation. The type of the cover map could have an important influence on the precision of the scheme's tamper locating ability. The lossless compression algorithm adopted in the experiment is the Huffman coding algorithm which is popularly used for data compression. Since the coordinates of the original contour map are highly correlated, enough space could be provided by compressing the LSB of the segment containing 128 vertices. However, as the scheme can not be practically applied as the Huffman code book was not considered.

6.5 Summary and Future Works

The Digital Vector Map is an important part of geographical information system(GIS) and has been widely used in many regions. In this chapter the topic of GIS watermarking has been considered. That is, the techniques of hiding data in 2D vector maps. This has many potential usages in the applications of vector map data. According to the properties and the purpose of the schemes, related works in this field were categorized into three classes. That is, robust watermarking, reversible data hiding and fragile watermarking. The boundaries among these classes are not absolutely distinct. For example, the fragile scheme presented in Section 6.4 is also an invertible scheme. The state of the art of the 2D vector map data hiding was given in this chapter by introducing the main proposed schemes in each class. Also some open issues in current study were presented several schemes. Some drawbacks of former works were improved in the schemes presented. By investigating the performance of the current schemes, it is shown that there are still many unsolved problems. The robustness to map simplification and additive noise attacks needs to be further strengthened. Secondly, the distortions introduced by watermarking should be controlled in multi-aspects. Thirdly, the evaluation of map quality needs an appropriate measure of performance. Furthermore, reversible and fragile schemes need further consideration because of the high security level necessary in some special applications.

6.5.1 Robustness to Certain Attacks

Most proposed algorithms have good performance to resist geometrical attacks, but are less robust against additive noise attack. Most schemes are fragile to map simplification or cropping. This is especially for attacks implemented in the transform domain. It is understandable that the more information lost during the attack, the more dangerous it is. Maliciously imposing noise on map data is not a good choice for an attacker, small noise distortions do occur in some daily works such as map format transformation. Consequently, a robust scheme should at least be robust to noises with low amplitudes. Map simplification is a common operation in GIS and can cause information lost without degrading the validity of the map data. It is very important for a watermarking scheme to resist this attack. This can be considered an open issue and needs to be enhanced.

6.5.2 Fidelity: Error, Shape, Topology, etc.

The most important principle, which must be strictly followed by vector map watermarking schemes, is that distortions induced by data hiding must be strictly controlled in order to ensure the quality of the marked map. With respect to vector maps, the term distortion has many meanings. One is that distortions may mean the coordinate errors of vertices. Almost all existing algorithms have taken this factor into account. It is a well known rule that the errors of vertices induced by watermarking should not exceed the cover map's precision tolerance τ. For the schemes in the spatial domain, data embedding directly modifies coordinates, and it is convenient to control the errors. In the case of transform domains, the situation is different. Those Transform Domain Based Schemes directly modify the transform coefficients instead of the coordinates. It is not convenient to control the introduced errors. In addition to vertex errors, distortions also mean the errors of many other features such as the shape or topology of map objects. This kind of distortion is of great importance to map quality. They have been ignored by almost all former works. Even slight distortions of vertices can also induce unacceptable changes in shape or topology information. For example by destroying the smoothness of map objects, or making the originally separated objects overlapped. It is one of the future work needed to control distortions in vector map watermarking schemes.

6.5.3 Fidelity Evaluation

Although kinds of algorithms for watermarking vector maps have been proposed, there is still no appropriate measure for evaluating the fidelity of watermarked maps. Such a measure could be important for a watermarking scheme in order to evaluate the extent of the distortion introduced by the embedding procedure. An ideal measure of the map fidelity should take into account not only the errors of coordinates, but also the distortions of the map shapes. We have described that both human perception and PSNR are not appropriate candidates. A method to rationally evaluate vector map's fidelity remains a topic for a future work.

6.5.4 Reversible and Fragile Schemes

Until now, few works in current world literatures have considered the topic of designing reversible watermarking schemes for vector maps. Since the most important restriction of vector map watermarking is the precision of the cover data, reversible schemes provide the best solution to this requirement. In addition, most former works focused on designing robust schemes, but few have considered the fragile schemes. Map data authentication is still a crucial issue for many special applications, especially for the military applications. Designing fragile schemes for the purpose of map data authentication is another important future work.

Acknowledgment

This work is supported by the Foundation for the Author of National Excellent Doctoral Dissertation of P. R. China (Project Number FANEDD-200238), the National Natural Science Foundation of China (Project Number 60372052), the Multidiscipline Scientific Research Foundation of Harbin Institute of Technology. P. R. China (Project Number HIT.MD-2002.11), National Program for New Century Excellent Talents in University (NCET-04-0330), the Foundation for the Excellent Youth of Heilongjiang Province, and the Natural Science Foundation of GuangDong province.

References

1. `http://www.thedigitalmap.com`
2. Sakamoto, M., Matsuura, Y., and Takashima, Y. (2000): A scheme of digital watermarking for geographical map data. Symposium on cryptography and Information security
3. Kang, H. (2001): A vector watermarking using the generalized square mask. Proc. International Symposium on Information Technology: Coding and Computing, 234–236
4. Schulz, G. and Voigt, M. (2004): A high capacity watermarking system for digital maps. Proceedings of the 2004 multimedia and security workshop on Multimedia and security, 180–186
5. Huber, B.: Gis & steganography – part 3: Vector steganography. Available: `http://www.directionsmag.com/`
6. Voigt, M. and Busch, C. (2003): Feature-based watermarking of 2d-vector data. Proceedings of SPIE, Security and watermarking of Multimedia Content, **5020**, 359–366
7. Ohbuchi, R., Ueda, H., and Endoh, S. (2002): Robust watermarking of vector digital maps. Proc. IEEE International Conference on Multimedia and Expo, (ICME '02), **1**, 577–580
8. Voigt, M. and Busch, C. (2002): Watermarking 2d-vector data for geographical information systems. Proceedings of SPIE, Security and watermarking of Multimedia Content, **4675**, 621–628
9. Nikolaidis, N., Pitas, I., and Solachidis, V. (2000): Fourier descriptors watermarking of vector graphics images. Proc. IEEE International Conference on Image Processing, **3**, 9–12
10. Solachidis, V., Nikolaidis, N. and Pitas I. (2000): Watermarking polygonal lines using Fourier descriptors. Proc. IEEE International Conference on Acoustics, Speech and Signal Processing (ICASSP'2000), 1955–1958
11. Nikolaidis, N., Pitas, I., and Giannoula, A. (2002): Watermarking of sets of polygonal lines using fusion techniques. Proc. IEEE International Conference on Multimedia and Expo (ICME '02), **2**, 549–552
12. Kitamura, I., Kanai, S. and Kishinami, T. (2001): Copyright protection of vector map using digital watermarking method based on discrete Fourier transform. Proc. IEEE International Geoscience and Remote Sensing Symposium (IGARSS '01), **3**, 1191–1193

13. Li, Y. and Xu, L. (2003): A blind watermarking of vector graphics images. Proc. Fifth International Conference on Computational Intelligence and Multimedia Applications (ICCIMA 2003), 424–429
14. Ohbuchi, R., Ueda, H., and Endoh, S. (2003): Watermarking 2d vector maps in the mesh-spectral domain. Proc. International Conference on Shape Modeling and Applications, 216–225
15. Ohbuchi, R., Takahashi, S., Miyazawa, T., and Mukaiyama, A. (2001): Watermarking 3d polygonal meshes in the mesh spectral domain. Proc. Graphics Interface, 9–17
16. Douglas, D.H. and Peucker, T.K. (1973): Algorithms for the reduction of the number of points required to represent a digitized line or its caricature. Canadian Cartographer, **10**, 112–122
17. Honsinger, C., Jones, P., Rabbani, M., and Stoffel, J. (1999): Lossless recovery of an original image containing embedded data. U.S. Patent 6 278 791
18. Fridrich, J., Goljan, M., and Du, R. (2001): Invertible authentication. Proc. SPIE, Security and Watermarking of Multimedia Contents, **3971**, pp. 197–208
19. Ni, Z., Shi, Y., Ansari, N., and Su, W. (2003): Reversible data hiding. Proceedings IEEE of ISCAS'03, **2**, II-912–II-915
20. Leest, A., Veen, M. and Bruekers, F. (2003): Reversible image watermarking. Proc. IEEE International Conference on Image Processing, **2**, 731–734
21. Tian, J. (2002): Reversible watermarking by difference expansion. Proc. of Workshop on Multimedia and Security, 19–22
22. Veen, M., Bruekers, F., Leest, A., and Cavin, S. (2003): High capacity reversible watermarking for audio. Proceedings of the SPIE, **5020**, 1–11
23. Voigt, M., Yang, B., and Busch, C. (2004): Reversible watermarking of 2d-vector data. Proceedings of the 2004 Multimedia and Security Workshop on Multimedia and Security, 160–165

7

Adaptive Embedding and Detection for Improved Video Watermarking

Isao Echizen[1], Yasuhiro Fujii[1], Takaaki Yamada[1], and Satoru Tezuka[1], and Hiroshi Yoshiura[2]

[1] Systems Development Laboratory, Hitachi, Ltd., Kawasaki, Japan
{iechizen, fujii, t-yamada, tezuka}@sdl.hitachi.co.jp

[2] Faculty of Electro-Communication, The University of Electro-Communications, Tokyo, Japan
yoshiura@hc.uec.ac.jp

Summary. Video watermarks must maintain picture quality and withstand video processing. Resolving the tradeoff between these conflicting requirements has been one of the central problems of video watermarking. Previous video watermarking methods, however, have trouble satisfying these conflicting quality and survivability requirements because they utilize the watermarking methods for still picture and neglect the properties of motion pictures. To resolve this tradeoff, we describe adaptive video embedding and detection techniques that utilize the properties of motion pictures. Motion-adaptive embedding can allocate watermarks to picture areas which are adaptively based on motion properties of video and, statistically adaptive detection can control the accumulation of watermarks based on the statistical properties of video to prevent degradation in the watermark signal by video processing. Experimental evaluations using actual motion pictures have shown that these techniques can be effective for resolving the tradeoff and can be widely used in the pixel-based watermarking.

7.1 Introduction

Because of its advantages over analog video, digital video is now being provided through the Internet and digital broadcasting and on various types of media, such as DVDs. It requires less space, is easier to process, and does not degrade with time or repeated use. The copyrights of digital video are easily violated because digital video can be easily copied and delivered through the Internet or on various types of media. Video watermarking is thus becoming an important means of copyright protection for digital video.

Video watermarking can be used to embed copyright and copy-control information in video pictures and is expected to be used in DVD players and recorders as well as in digital broadcasting equipment such as set-top boxes [1, 2]. Video watermarks must survive video processing and not degrade

I. Echizen et al.: *Adaptive Embedding and Detection for Improved Video Watermarking*, Studies in Computational Intelligence (SCI) **58**, 157–187 (2007)
www.springerlink.com

picture quality. Resolving the tradeoff between these conflicting requirements has been one of the main objectives in research on video watermarking. The video watermarking methods reported so far have trouble doing this because they simply utilize the techniques developed for still pictures and neglect the properties of motion pictures.

In this chapter we present two adaptive video watermarking techniques that utilize the properties of motion pictures. One is Motion-Adaptive Embedding in which watermarks are allocated to picture areas adaptively based on motion vectors and deformation quantities among adjacent frames. The other technique is Statistically Adaptive Detection in which the accumulation of watermarks is controlled to prevent degradation in the watermark signal by video processing.

Methods of video watermarking can be classified into two types: those operating in the pixel domain and those operating in the frequency domain. In this chapter, we focus on the former and describe representative methods that operate the luminance values.

In Sect. 7.2 we briefly review the concept of video watermarking and give an overview of the two techniques that utilize the properties of motion pictures. We describe the first, Motion-Adaptive Embedding using motion estimation, and discuss its effectiveness in Sect. 7.3. In Sect. 7.4 we describe Statistically Adaptive Detection using inferential statistics and discuss its effectiveness.

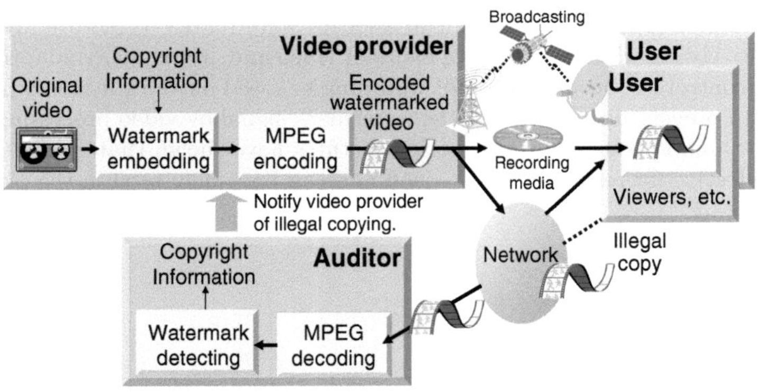

Fig. 7.1. An example of the use of video watermarking.

7.2 Video Watermarking

7.2.1 Typical Use

As shown in Fig. 7.1, watermarks (WMs) representing copyright information are typically embedded into video pictures that are then compressed using an MPEG encoder. The video provider broadcasts the encoded pictures or distributes them over a network or on recording media, such as DVD-ROMs. When the encoded watermarked pictures are received, they are decoded, and a user can watch them on a TV set or a personal computer. If a user illegally copies and redistributes the pictures (for example, by placing them on a web page), the auditor detects the copyright information embedded in the pictures and notifies the video provider of the illegal copying. The video provider could even identify the illegal copier if the pictures contained embedded information identifying the user to whom they had originally been provided.

7.2.2 Overview of Two Techniques

As mentioned above, watermarks must survive video processing and not degrade picture quality. That is, they must be detectable even after the pictures have gone through image-processing procedures such as MPEG compression and resizing, and they must not interfere with picture enjoyment. These requirements conflict because survivability is ensured by embedding more WMs, which in turn degrades picture quality. As mentioned above, resolving this tradeoff has been a major objective of the research on watermarking, and numerous studies have focused on both watermark embedding and detection. However, the methods reported so far are not always effective because they simply utilize watermarking methods developed for still pictures and neglect the properties of motion pictures. We have been studying video watermarking in the pixel domain and previously proposed improved embedding and detection techniques using motion picture properties [3, 4, 5, 6]. These motion-adaptive embedding and statistically adaptive detection techniques resolve the tradeoff in requirements.

Motion-adaptive embedding [3, 4]: Taking into consideration the properties of the pictures enables adaptive allocation of the watermarks. Picture quality is degraded less by embedding the watermarks in areas where they are easily perceived; survivability is improved by embedding them more heavily in areas where they are hard to perceive. Conventional methods consider only the properties of each frame and neglect the inter-frame properties. We have found that watermarks are less perceptible when embedded in areas where the picture contents are moving, and we have developed watermark imperceptibility criteria based on motion information. We also developed an embedding technique that uses this criteria to allocate watermarks to picture areas adaptively.

Statistically adaptive detection [6]: It is common in conventional watermarking to embed identical watermark patterns in different regions. That is known as redundant coding and is used to improve resistance to video processing without degrading picture quality. The watermarks can then be detected by accumulating those from each region of interest. Some video processing methods remove watermark signals from specific regions of the frames. This degrades the combined signal of the accumulated watermarks and thus reduces the detection ratio. Our statistically adaptive detection technique sets up a scale for estimating the bit-error rates of the WMs for each frame region by using statistical properties of motion pictures and uses those rates to identify the best regions to detect the watermarks and thus improve the detection ratio.

In the following section, we describe the above video watermarking methods in detail and show their effectiveness.

7.3 Motion-Adaptive Embedding Using Motion Estimation

Because video watermarks must not degrade picture quality and must survive video processing, the properties of the pictures are generally taken into consideration so that the watermarks can be allocated adaptively. Picture quality degradation is avoided by embedding watermarks sparsely in plain areas, where they are easily perceived; survivability is ensured by embedding them heavily in messy areas, where they are hard to perceive [1, 7, 8]. Conventional watermarking methods have trouble satisfying these conflicting quality and survivability requirements simultaneously. That is because they consider only the properties of each frame. That is of each still picture and neglect the inter-frame properties of motion. In this section, we explain how watermark perceptibility is affected by inter-frame motion and distortion and describe our adaptive watermarking technique which employs motion estimation.

7.3.1 Conventional Methods

Conventional methods for maintaining picture quality can be classified into two types:

(a) those that reduce the quantity of embedded WMs by making a small number of WMs robust enough to be reliably detected [9, 10, 11], and
(b) those that embed WMs where they will be less perceptible [1, 7, 8, 12].

Type (a) methods maintain picture quality by reducing the luminance change while maintaining WM robustness. One such method is an improvement of the patchwork algorithm [11] reported by Bender and coworkers [13]. It embeds WMs by creating a statistically meaningful difference between the average luminance of pixels (ζ_i, η_i), $\frac{1}{P}\sum_{i=1}^{N} y_{\zeta_i,\eta_i}^{(f)}$, and the average luminance of pixels (ξ_i, ψ_i), $\frac{1}{P}\sum_{i=1}^{N} y_{\xi_i,d_i}^{(f)}$. Here each frame consists of $2P$ pixels and $y_{\zeta_i,\eta_i}^{(f)}$ and $y_{\xi_i,\psi_i}^{(f)}$ represent the luminance values of pixels (ζ_i, η_i) and (ξ_i, ψ_i) of the f-th frame. The locations of pixels (ζ_i, η_i) and (ξ_i, ψ_i) are randomly determined in each frame without overlapping. Small luminance changes in these pixels result in a statistically meaningful difference if (ζ_i, η_i) and (ξ_i, ψ_i) are in neighboring areas for each i [11]. Type (b) methods, on the other hand, maintain picture quality directly and are usually more effective. Most of them use the "masking effects" found in the human visual system [1, 7, 8]. Because picture content masks the WMs, these methods strongly embed WMs in messy areas and weakly in plain areas. The methods select as "messy areas" regions with large luminance differences and many high-frequency elements. The quality of motion pictures is still degraded, however, because when these methods select messy areas they consider only the properties of each frame or still picture. They neglect inter-frame properties of motion.

7.3.2 Criteria for Watermark Imperceptibility Using Motion Picture Properties

Our motion-adaptive embedding technique adjusts the strength of the embedded WMs based on their estimated imperceptibility. It embeds them more strongly in areas where they are estimated to be relatively imperceptible. This section describes the criteria used for measuring WM imperceptibility that is used to take motion into account.

Analysis of WM Imperceptibility

Analyzing the relationship between WM Imperceptibility (WMIP) and motion picture properties (Fig. 7.2), we observed the following:

- WMIP depends on the velocity of object movement between frames — the higher the velocity, the less perceptible the WMs.
- WMIP also depends on the degree of object deformation between frames — the greater the deformation, the more imperceptible the WMs.

These observations indicate that WMIP depends not only on the properties of the still pictures making up the sequence of images constituting a motion picture, but also on the motions of the objects in those images. That is their velocities and their degrees of deformation. These can be estimated as a motion vector and a deformation quantity by using a motion-estimation technique, such as block-matching. The following subsections describe the block-matching techniques widely used for motion estimation in MPEG encoders and present our criteria for measuring WMIP that uses these techniques.

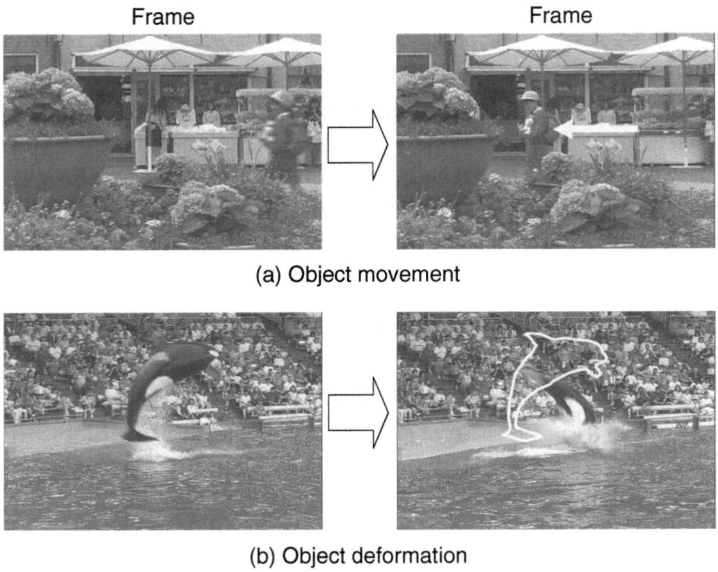

Fig. 7.2. The relationship between WM Imperceptibility and Motion Picture Properties.

Block-Matching Techniques

Block-matching techniques [14] are based on between-frame matching of MPEG macro-blocks (16×16-pixel blocks) and determine one motion vector for each macro-block. The following procedure is done for all macro-blocks in a frame:

Step 1: The luminance set of the f-th frame consisting of $W \times H$ pixels is $\mathbf{y}^{(f)} = \{y_{i,j}^{(f)} \mid 1 \le i \le W\,,\, 1 \le j \le H\}$. The sum of absolute difference $d(k,l)$ between the macro-block of current frame $\mathbf{y}^{(f)}$ and that of reference frame $\mathbf{y}^{(f-1)}$. This is displaced by (k,l) from the block of $\mathbf{y}^{(f)}$, and is calculated using the following equation (see Fig. 7.3):

$$d(k,l) = \sum_{i,j=0}^{15} \left| y_{b_x+i,b_y+j}^{(f)} - y_{b_x+k+i,b_y+l+j}^{(f-1)} \right| , \tag{7.1}$$

where (b_x, b_y) is the pixel location representing the starting point of the macro-block.

Step 2: The $d(k,l)$'s are calculated within search range k,l. A range of $-15 \le k,l \le 15$ is typically searched [14], and 31×31 $d(k,l)$'s are generated.

Step 3: The motion vector $\mathbf{v}$ is identified as vector (k_0, l_0) for the minimum of 31×31 $d(k,l)$'s. That is, based on the equation

$$d = d(k_0, l_0) = \min_{k,l} d(k, l), \tag{7.2}$$

where d is the inter-frame deformation of the object, and $\mathbf{v} = (k_0, l_0)$ is the motion vector representing the velocity of the movement of the object. If more than one (k_0, l_0) gives the same minimum value, $d(k_0, l_0)$, the shortest (k_0, l_0) vector is then chosen as motion vector $\mathbf{v}$.

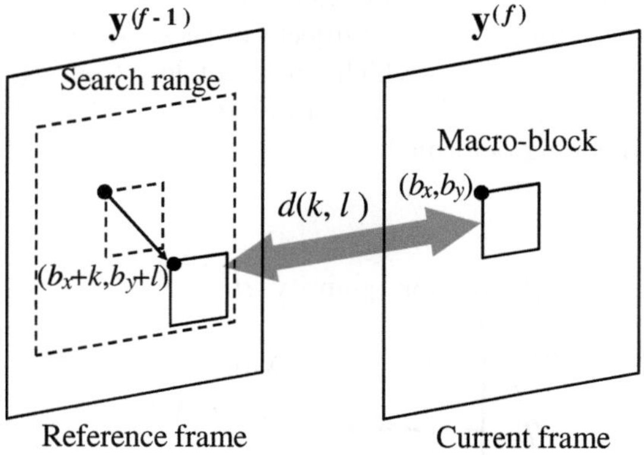

Fig. 7.3. Block-matching method.

Criteria Using Motion Information

We first define the following terminology.

WMIP $r_{i,j}$ of a pixel in a motion picture: It is a measure representing the degree of imperceptibility of a luminance change at a pixel (i, j). If, for example, the WMIP of pixel (1,0) is larger than that of pixel (2,0), a change in luminance at pixel (1,0) is less perceptible than one at pixel (2,0).

As described in the analysis of WM imperceptibility, the element $r_{i,j}$ of a pixel in a motion picture depends on two kinds of motion information and on the still picture properties. Thus, $r_{i,j}$ is a function of d, $\mathbf{v}$, and $s_{i,j}$:

$$r_{i,j} = f(d, \mathbf{v}, s_{i,j}), \tag{7.3}$$

where $s_{i,j}$ is the pixel WMIP based only on the still picture properties[3].

[3] Various methods of determining $s_{i,j}$ have been presented; we use the one reported by Echizen and coworkers [12]. It uses the one-dimensional luminance standard deviation to prevent contour distortion by WMs. See Ref. [12] for details.

There has been little research on the determination of f, but so far there is no known way to determine f optimally. We therefore used a two-step function of motion vector $\mathbf{v}$ and a deformation quantity d. The suitability of this function was demonstrated by our experimental evaluation (see Sect. 7.3.4).

To establish the two-step function specifically, we used the motion estimation results to classify the macro-blocks in each frame into two types. This is shown in Fig. 7.4.

Static areas: Macro blocks in which the length of motion vector $|\mathbf{v}|$ is less than threshold value $T_{\mathbf{v}}$ and deformation quantity d is less than threshold value T_d: $d < T_d$ and $|\mathbf{v}| < T_{\mathbf{v}}$. Objects in these areas are static.

Motion areas: Macro-blocks in which $|\mathbf{v}|$ is not less than $T_{\mathbf{v}}$ or d is not less than T_d. That is, areas where $d \geq T_d$ or $|\mathbf{v}| \geq T_{\mathbf{v}}$. Objects in these areas are moving or being deformed.

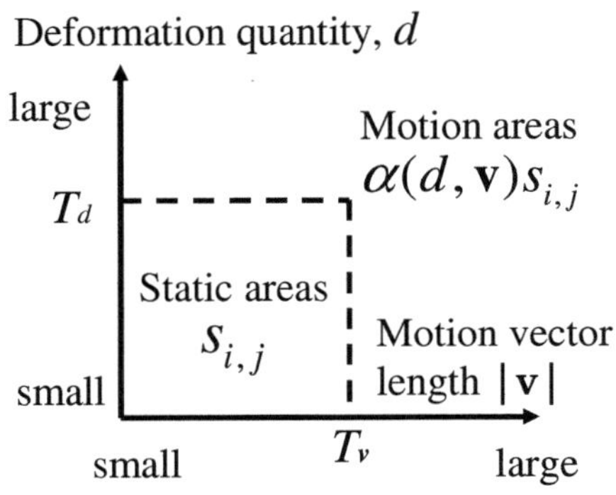

Fig. 7.4. Classification using motion information.

The WMIP $r_{i,j}$ is given by a two-step function:

$$r_{i,j} = f(d, \mathbf{v}, s_{i,j}) = \begin{cases} s_{i,j}, & d < T_d, |\mathbf{v}| < T_{\mathbf{v}}, \\ \alpha(d, \mathbf{v}) s_{i,j}, & \text{otherwise}, \end{cases} \tag{7.4}$$

where coefficient $\alpha(d, \mathbf{v})$ is greater than 1 and increases with d or $|\mathbf{v}|$. $T_{\mathbf{v}}$ and T_d were respectively set to 6 and 5000. This is based on the results of subjective evaluation using standard video samples [15] with five different strengths of embedded WMs. The value of $\alpha(d, \mathbf{v})$ was then set subjectively using the $T_{\mathbf{v}}$ and T_d values. To set the value of $\alpha(d, \mathbf{v})$, we assume that the value of $\alpha(d, \mathbf{v})$ is proportional to the deformation quantity, d. The length of the motion vector, $|\mathbf{v}|$, is as follows:

$$\alpha(d, \mathbf{v}) = \alpha_0 + \gamma_d d + \gamma_{\mathbf{v}} |\mathbf{v}|, \tag{7.5}$$

where coefficients α_0, γ_d, and $\gamma_\mathbf{v}$ are positive. These coefficients were estimated based on subjective evaluation, using standard video samples with five different strengths of embedded WMs. The watermarked pictures had been encoded using MPEG-2. The results are shown in Table 7.1; the values of γ_d and $\gamma_\mathbf{v}$ depend on the bit rate. They increased with a decreasing bit rate. We used these values in our detailed evaluation (see Sect. 7.3.4).

Table 7.1. Values of α_0, γ_d, and $\gamma_\mathbf{v}$ at various bit rates.

	2 Mbps	4 Mbps	6 Mbps	8 Mbps
α_0	1.07	1.12	1.02	1.41
γ_d	7.42×10^{-4}	6.42×10^{-4}	5.37×10^{-4}	3.25×10^{-4}
$\gamma_\mathbf{v}$	0.102	0.085	0.080	0.054

7.3.3 Motion-Adaptive Embedding

Overall Structure

Our motion-adaptive embedding technique is most effective when implemented in MPEG encoders because they already have the necessary motion estimation functions. As shown in Fig. 7.5(a), the watermarking process embeds copyright information into each frame by using the motion information estimated by the MPEG encoder. The watermarked frames are then encoded. As shown in Fig. 7.5(b), the watermarking process is comprised of an embedding process and an embedding control process.

The motion-adaptive embedding method would be most effective when used in MPEG encoders as they already have the necessary motion estimation functions. Figure 7.5 shows the overall system structure of the motion-adaptive method done using a MPEG encoder. As shown in Fig. 7.5(a), the watermarking process embeds copyright information into each frame by using the motion information obtained from the motion estimation of the MPEG encoder. The watermarked frames are then encoded.

Figure 7.5(b) shows the structure of the watermarking process, which has a embedding process and an embedding control process:

Embedding process: Embeds into each frame WMs representing the copyright information. The WM strength is determined using the $r_{i,j}$ calculated in the embedding control process.

Embedding control process: Calculates $r_{i,j}$, WMIP of each pixel, from the original frames. This process consists of two subprocesses:
- (a) Intra-frame analysis: Calculates $s_{i,j}$ for each frame.
- (b) $r_{i,j}$-operation: Calculates $r_{i,j}$ using $s_{i,j}$, $\mathbf{v}$, and d.

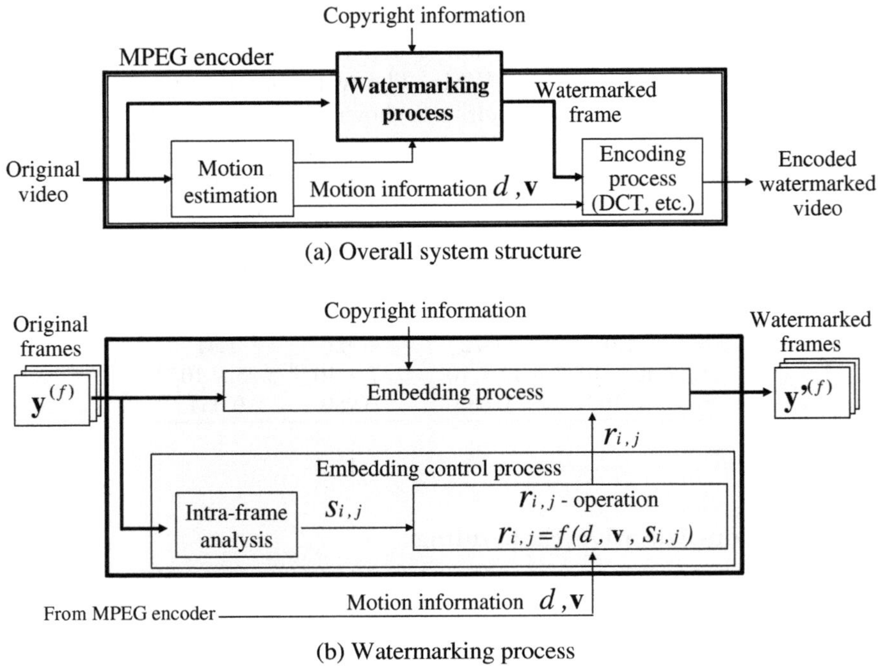

Fig. 7.5. System structure of motion-adaptive embedding technique.

The embedding control process can be used in various WM embedding systems because it is combined with the embedding process only though $r_{i,j}$. This can be calculated independently of the embedding process.

Process Flow

The process flow of the 1-bit-WM embedding is now described. Steps E2 and E3 are embedding control steps, and Steps E4 and E5 are embedding steps. For multiple-bit embedding, each frame is divided into regions, and the 1-bit embedding process is then applied to each region.

Step E1: Do the following steps over the range $f = 1, 2, \cdots$.
Step E2: Calculate $s_{i,j}$ from luminance set $\mathbf{y}^{(f)}$ of the input frame.
Step E3: Calculate $r_{i,j}$ from $\mathbf{v}$, d (calculated by the motion estimation function of the encoder), and $s_{i,j}$.
Step E4: Determine WM strength $\mu_{i,j}^{(f)}$ at pixel (i, j) of frame $\mathbf{y}^{(f)}$:

$$\mu_{i,j}^{(f)} = \frac{r_{i,j}}{\sum_{i,j} r_{i,j}} Q, \tag{7.6}$$

where Q is the embedding quantity for frame $\mathbf{y}^{(f)}$[4]. This means that the Q for a frame is distributed among its pixels in proportion to $r_{i,j}$.

Step E5: Generate watermarked frame $\mathbf{y}'^{(f)}$ by adding WM pattern $\mathbf{m}$ (= $\{m_{i,j} \mid m_{i,j} \in \{-1,+1\}, 1 \leq i \leq W, 1 \leq j \leq H\}$ which comprises a pseudorandom array of ± 1s) to the original frame $\mathbf{y}^{(f)}$. This is dependent on embedding bit b:

$$y'^{(f)}_{i,j} = \begin{cases} y^{(f)}_{i,j} + \mu^{(f)}_{i,j} m_{i,j}, & \text{if } b = 1; \\ y^{(f)}_{i,j} - \mu^{(f)}_{i,j} m_{i,j}, & \text{if } b = 0. \end{cases} \tag{7.7}$$

An example process flow of the corresponding WM detection comprises the following steps:

Step D1: Do the following steps over the range $f = 1, 2, \cdots$.

Step D2: Calculate the correlation value c by correlating the WM pattern $\mathbf{m}$ using the watermarked image $\mathbf{y}'^{(f)}$. That is,

$$\begin{aligned} c &= \frac{1}{HW} \sum_{i,j} m_{i,j} y'^{(f)}_{i,j} = \frac{1}{HW} \sum_{i,j} m_{i,j} (y^{(f)}_{i,j} \pm \mu^{(f)}_{i,j} m_{i,j}) \\ &= \frac{1}{HW} \sum_{i,j} m_{i,j} y^{(f)}_{i,j} \pm \frac{1}{HW} \sum_{i,j} \mu^{(f)}_{i,j}. \end{aligned} \tag{7.8}$$

Step D3: Determine the bit-value b by comparing c with the threshold value $T (> 0)$:

$$b = \begin{cases} 1, & \text{if } c \geq T; \\ 0, & \text{if } c \leq -T; \\ \text{“not detected,”} & \text{if } -T < c < T. \end{cases} \tag{7.9}$$

7.3.4 Experimental Evaluation

Subjective Evaluation of the Watermarked Picture Quality

Procedure

We evaluated the MPEG quality by using five standard motion pictures [15], each of which had 450 frames of 720×480 pixels. We used the motion-adaptive technique and a conventional method to embed WMs into luminance set $\mathbf{y}^{(f)}$ of the motion pictures. After MPEG-2 encoding using a software codec, we compared the visual qualities of the resulting pictures using standard subjective evaluation [16].

---

[4] Q is set by the system designer and is controlled by the users taking account of the intended use.

Motion-Adaptive Method: The WMs were embedded using the procedure described in Sect. 7.3.3 with embedding bit $b = 1$.

Conventional Method: The watermarking procedures were identical except that $s_{i,j}$ was used in Step E4 instead of $r_{i,j}$. The embedding quantity for each frame was the same for both methods. The difference between $r_{i,j}$ and $s_{i,j}$ resulted in different distributions of the WMs among the pixels.

We selected five standard motion pictures based on the Degree of Object Movement between frames and the Degree of Object Deformation between frames (see Fig. 7.6):

(a) Walk through the Square ("Walk"): — People walking in a town square — medium movement and medium deformation.
(b) Flamingos: — Pan-scanned scene of flamingos — much movement and little deformation.
(c) Whale Show ("Whale"): — Spraying whale with audience — little movement and much deformation.
(d) Entrance Hall ("Hall"): — Three people talking in an entrance hall — little movement and little deformation.
(e) Rustling Leaves ("Leaves"): — Fluttering leaves — much movement and much deformation.

The pictures were subjectively evaluated using the procedure described in Recommendation ITU-R BT.500-7 [16]. The original and watermarked pictures after MPEG-2 encoding were simultaneously shown to ten evaluators. They rated the picture quality based on the scale shown in Table 7.2. For each picture, the average of the ten scores was used to determine the quality level.

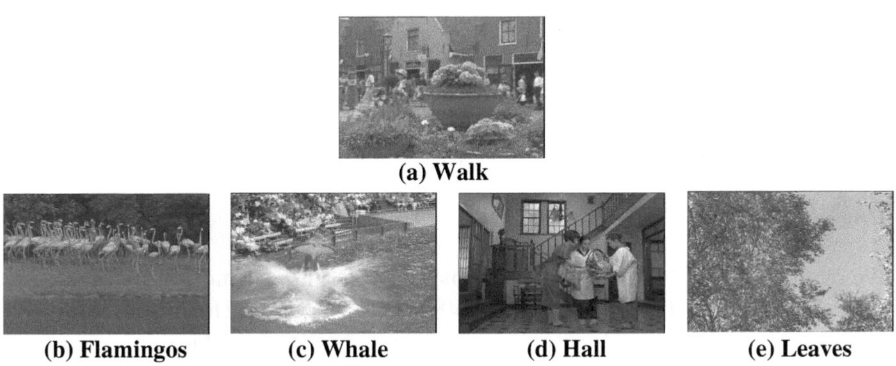

Fig. 7.6. Pictures evaluated.

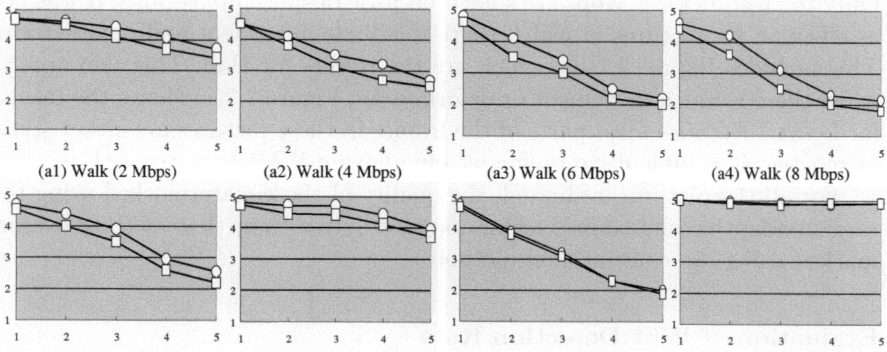

Fig. 7.7. Quality of watermarked pictures. (Here the circles indicate the Motion-Adaptive Technique, and the squares indicate the use of the Conventional Method).

Table 7.2. Level of disturbance and rating scale.

Disturbance	Points
Imperceptible	5
Perceptible but not annoying	4
Slightly annoying	3
Annoying	2
Very annoying	1

Results

Evaluation results are shown in Fig. 7.7, where the horizontal axis is the averaged embedding quantity per pixel, $q = Q/(720 \times 480)$, and the vertical axis is the average picture quality score, here 1 means that the WMs were very annoying, and 5 means that they were imperceptible.

Figures 7.7(a1)–(a4) show the results for the Walk picture at the four different bit rates. The degradation in picture quality was significantly reduced for each of the bit rates because the motion-adaptive technique preferentially allocated the WMs to the moving areas, where they were less perceptible. In the Walk picture, the motion-adaptive method/technique can embed 30 to 40% more WMs while maintaining the same picture quality. Figures 7.7(b) and (c), which are the results for Flamingos and Whale, show that the motion-adaptive technique also significantly reduces degradation in picture quality.

Only the results for 8 Mbps are shown because of space limitations. It was not as effective for pictures in which there was little movement and deformation. This includes Figure 7.7(d), which are the results for Hall. This also applies when there is much movement or deformation. Figure 7.7(e) shows the results for Leaves. Because most parts of the frames in these pictures are either static or moving, it is difficult to preferentially allocate WMs to parts with motion.

For all the pictures evaluated, the quality of those watermarked using the motion-adaptive embedding technique was better than that of those watermarked using the conventional method.

Evaluation of WM Detection Rate

This section describes the results of evaluating the motion-adaptive technique. It considers improvement in WM detection in comparison with rates obtained using the motion-adaptive technique and that of the conventional method. The rates were measured using the same picture quality after the MPEG-2 encoding.

Procedure

We evaluated the detection rate using the five pictures evaluated.

Step 1: Select the level of picture quality, L, at which the evaluation is to be done. For example, $L = 4$ means "Perceptible but not annoying". Then obtain the average embedding quantity $q_{\text{prop}}^{(L)}$ for the motion-adaptive technique corresponding to L. This is done by referring to the relationship between q and picture quality shown in Fig. 7.7. Obtain the corresponding average embedding quantity, $q_{\text{prev}}^{(L)}$, by the conventional method. For Fig. 7.7(a4), Walk at 8 Mbps, $q_{\text{prop}}^{(4)}$ and $q_{\text{prev}}^{(4)}$ were, respectively, 2.2 and 1.5[5].

Step 2: Embed the 64-bit information into each of the 450 frames of the picture using the motion-adaptive and conventional methods. Do this in such a way that the average embedding quantities are, respectively, $q_{\text{prop}}^{(4)}$ and $q_{\text{prev}}^{(4)}$. This results in two watermarked pictures with the same quality.

Step 3: Encode and decode the watermarked pictures using an MPEG-2 hardware codec.

Step 4: Using the process based on WM detection described in Sect. 7.3.3, detect the 64-bit information in each frame of the two watermarked pictures. In order to clarify the improvement in WM detection of the motion-adaptive technique, we did the following.The threshold

---

[5] For Fig. 7.7(e), Hall was at 8 Mbps, because the levels of picture quality for the motion-adaptive and conventional methods were both greater than 4. We set $q_{\text{prop}}^{(L)}$ and $q_{\text{prev}}^{(L)}$ to 5 which is the highest evaluation value.

Table 7.3. Correct detection percentage.

Picture	Scheme	2 Mbps	4 Mbps	6 Mbps	8 Mbps
Walk	Motion-adaptive	98.0	84.2	99.6	100
	Conventional	68.5	51.1	51.6	62.9
Flamingos	Motion-adaptive	40.6	97.5	99.6	99.8
	Conventional	12.1	94.4	98.9	99.6
Whale	Motion-adaptive	15.2	89.5	98.7	99.6
	Conventional	12.7	88.8	96.9	98.7
Hall	Motion-adaptive	100	100	100	100
	Conventional	99.6	100	100	100
Leaves	Motion-adaptive	11.8	90.2	94.0	97.1
	Conventional	10.3	89.7	93.8	96.4

value was set to determine the bit value to zero ($T = 0$). The 64-bit information was always detectable.

Step 5: Count the number of frames in which the information was detected correctly.

This procedure was done for each of the four MPEG-2 bit rates (2, 4, 6, and 8 Mbps).

Results

The results are summarized in Table 7.3, which lists the percentages of the 450 frames from which information was detected correctly. That is the correct detection rates. The percentages for incorrect detection was 100 minus the listed values. These are the false-negative error rates.

For Walk, Flamingos, and Whale, each has both static and motion areas. The motion-adaptive technique improved the detection rates at all four bit rates and especially that at 2 Mbps. For Hall and Leaves, the motion-adaptive technique negligibly improved the detection rates. This is because most parts of the frames in these pictures are either static or moving. As described in Sect. 7.3.4, the motion-adaptive technique was also comparatively ineffective in improving the picture quality of watermarked pictures when WMs could not be preferentially readily allocated to motion areas. These detection reliability results correspond to the results obtained by subjective evaluation of picture quality.

The motion-adaptive embedding technique gave better detection rates for all of the evaluated pictures and yielded an average improvement of 9.5%. The motion-adaptive embedding technique thus improves watermark durability.

7.4 Statistically Adaptive Detection Using Inferential Statistics

Video providers subject watermarked pictures to various kinds of video processing. These include compression using MPEG or other compression technology, resizing, and filtering. These video processing procedures can be exploited by illegal users to remove the embedded information. The watermarks should be robust enough to be reliably detected after any of these processes. Watermark survivability is essential, and methods for improving WM survivability have been actively studied. Methods using redundant coding [17, 18, 19] and spread spectrum coding [20, 21] of the embedded information have been established. Methods for embedding information in elements that will be negligibly affected by the expected image processing have also been developed [22, 23].

Redundant coding is a basic method for improving WM resistance to video processing without degrading picture quality. It embeds watermarks repeatedly in every frame or region. The embedded watermarks are accumulated and detected during watermark detection. The chance of error is reduced. This accumulation, may be problematic after video processing that removes WMs from specific frames or regions. This is because a WM signal could be attenuated due to attempted accumulation from regions from which the WMs had been removed during video processing. The detection method should therefore be used to detect WMs only from those frames and regions where WMs remain.

The statistically adaptive detection technique sets up a scale for estimating the bit-error rates of the WMs for each frame region by using statistical properties of motion pictures. It uses those rate to determine the regions in which to accumulate so as to prevent watermark signal attenuation.

7.4.1 Conventional Methods

Redundant coding methods can be classified into two types.

(a) Redundant Coding within a Frame: Watermark embedding is done by dividing the frame picture into several regions and applying the same watermark to each region. In WM detection, the WMs are extracted by accumulating all the divided pictures in a frame [17, 18].
(b) Redundant Coding over Frames: WM embedding is done by applying the same watermark in each consecutive frame of the video. In WM detection, the WMs are extracted by accumulating all the frames or a specific number of sequential frames [18, 19].

Among these methods, the one proposed by Kalker and coworkers [18] is a basic WM scheme using both types. We briefly describe this method and its problems. For ease of understanding, we first introduce the 1-bit-WM scheme and then describe the multiple-bit-WM scheme.

1-bit-WM Scheme

WM embedding

The luminance set of the f-th frame consisting of N pixels is $\mathbf{y}^{(f)} = \{y_i^{(f)} \mid 1 \leq i \leq N\}$. The process flow of the 1-bit-WM embedding is as follows.

Step E1: Do the following steps over $f = 1, 2, \cdots$.
Step E2: Use the original frame $\mathbf{y}^{(f)}$ and divide $\mathbf{y}^{(f)}$ into R regions $\mathbf{y}^{(f,r)}$s ($r = 1, \cdots, R$) consisting of the corresponding pixels: $\mathbf{y}^{(f,r)} = \left\{y_i^{(f,r)} \mid 1 \leq i \leq \lfloor \frac{N}{R} \rfloor\right\}$, which satisfies $\mathbf{y}^{(f)} = \bigcup_r \mathbf{y}^{(f,r)}$, $\mathbf{y}^{(f,r)} \bigcap_{r \neq r'} \mathbf{y}^{(f,r')} = \emptyset$.
Step E3: Generate each watermarked region $\mathbf{y}'^{(f,r)}$ by adding the WM pattern $\mathbf{m} = \left\{m_i \in \{-1, +1\} \mid 1 \leq i \leq \lfloor \frac{N}{R} \rfloor\right\}$. This comprised of a pseudo random array ± 1s and added to the original region $\mathbf{y}'^{(f,r)}$:

$$\mathbf{y}'^{(f,r)} = \begin{cases} \mathbf{y}^{(f,r)} + \mu^{(f,r)}\mathbf{m}, & \text{if } b = 1, \\ \mathbf{y}^{(f,r)} - \mu^{(f,r)}\mathbf{m}, & \text{if } b = 0, \end{cases} \tag{7.10}$$

where $\mu^{(f,r)}$ is WM strength of the region $\mathbf{y}^{(f,r)}$.
Step E4: Output the watermarked frame $\mathbf{y}'^{(f)}$.

WM detection

The correlation value c is calculated by correlating the WM pattern $\mathbf{m}$ with the accumulated region.

Step D1: Do the following steps over $f_0 = 1, F+1, 2F+1, \cdots$.
Step D2: Input F watermarked frames $\mathbf{y}'^{(f)}$s ($f = f_0, \cdots, f_0 + F - 1$) and divide FR regions $\mathbf{y}'^{(f,r)}$s ($f = f_0, \cdots, f_0 + F - 1, r = 1, \cdots, R$).
Step D3: Accumulate the FR regions $\mathbf{y}'^{(f,r)}$s, in the region: $\tilde{\mathbf{y}} = \{\tilde{y}_i \mid 1 \leq i \leq \lfloor \frac{N}{R} \rfloor\}$. The $\tilde{y}_i$ of the accumulated region $\tilde{\mathbf{y}}$ is given by

$$\tilde{y}_i = \frac{1}{FR} \sum_{f=f_0}^{f_0+F-1} \sum_{r=1}^{R} y'^{(f,r)}_i. \tag{7.11}$$

Step D4: Calculate the correlation value c, which is obtained by correlating the WM pattern $\mathbf{m}$ with the accumulated region $\tilde{\mathbf{y}}$. That is,

$$c = \frac{1}{\lfloor \frac{N}{R} \rfloor} \sum_{i=1}^{\lfloor \frac{N}{R} \rfloor} m_i \tilde{y}_i = \frac{1}{FR \lfloor \frac{N}{R} \rfloor} \sum_{f,r,i} m_i y_i^{(f,r)} \pm \mu, \tag{7.12}$$

where μ is WM signal given by $\mu = \frac{1}{FR} \sum_{f,r} \mu^{(f,r)}$. Since $m_i y_i^{(f,r)}$ is considered to be an independent stochastic variable with mean 0 [13], each c follows the normal distribution with mean $\pm\mu$ and variance σ^2 if the number of $m_i y_i^{(f,r)}$s, $FR\lfloor\frac{N}{R}\rfloor$ is large enough. That is,

$$c \sim \begin{cases} N(\mu,\sigma^2), & \text{if } b=1; \\ N(-\mu,\sigma^2), & \text{if } b=0. \end{cases} \tag{7.13}$$

In the case of detection from original frames, c follows $c \sim N(0,\sigma^2)$. The transition of the normal distribution due to WM embedding is shown in Fig. 7.8: the normal distribution of the original frames $N(0,\sigma^2)$ is shifted to either $N(\mu,\sigma^2)$ or $N(-\mu,\sigma^2)$ according to embedded bit b.

Step D5: Determine the embedded bit b by comparing c with a threshold value $T(>0)$:

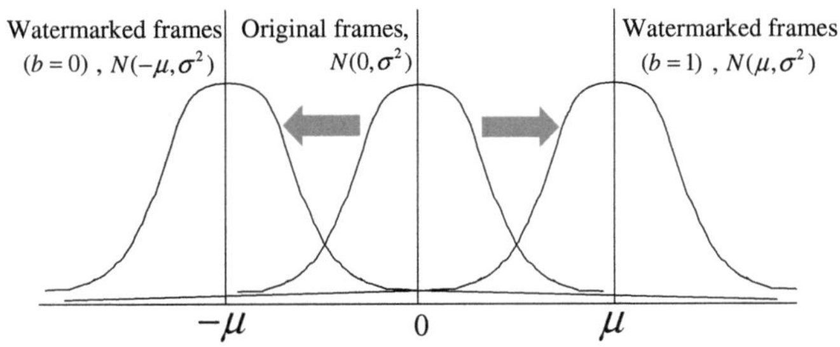

Fig. 7.8. Transition of distribution in WM embedding.

$$b = \begin{cases} 1, & \text{if } c \geq T; \\ 0, & \text{if } c \leq -T; \\ \text{"not detected,"} & \text{if } -T < c < T. \end{cases} \tag{7.14}$$

Multiple-bit-WM Scheme

WM embedding

Each region $\mathbf{y}^{(f,r)}$ is divided into K subregions $\mathbf{y}^{(f,r,k)}$s $(k = 1, \cdots, K)$ and the 1-bit embedding scheme is then applied to each subregion:

Step E1: Do the following steps over $f = 1, 2, \cdots$.

Step E2: Input the original frame $\mathbf{y}^{(f)}$ and divide $\mathbf{y}^{(f)}$ into RK subregions $\mathbf{y}^{(f,r,k)}$s $(r = 1, \cdots, R, k = 1, \cdots, K)$ consisting of the corresponding pixels: $\mathbf{y}_k^{(f,r)} = \left\{ y_{k,i}^{(f,r)} \mid 1 \leq i \leq \left\lfloor \frac{N}{(RK)} \right\rfloor \right\}$, which satisfies $\mathbf{y}^{(f)} = \bigcup_{r,k} \mathbf{y}^{(f,r,k)}$, $\mathbf{y}^{(f,r,k)} \bigcap_{r \neq r'} \mathbf{y}^{(f,r',k)} = \emptyset$, and $\mathbf{y}^{(f,r,k)} \bigcap_{k \neq k'} \mathbf{y}^{(f,r,k')} = \emptyset$ (See example shown in Fig. 7.9).

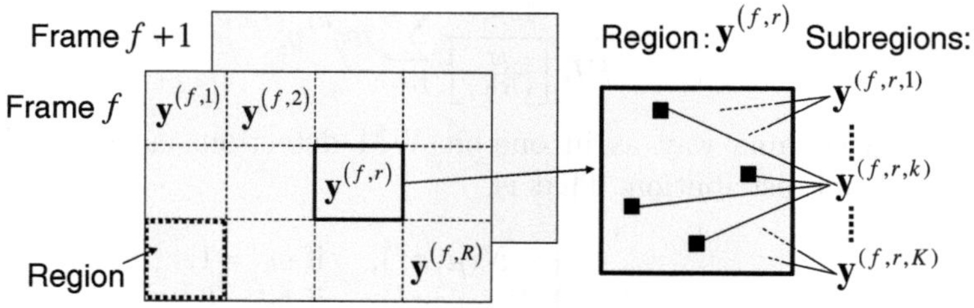

Fig. 7.9. An example of video partitioning.

Step E3: Generate each watermarked region $\mathbf{y}'^{(f,r,k)}$ by adding the WM pattern $\mathbf{m}^{(k)} = \left\{m_i^{(k)} \in \{-1,+1\} \mid 1 \le i \le \left\lfloor \frac{N}{(RK)} \right\rfloor\right\}$. This is a pseudo random array ± 1s and introduced into the original region $\mathbf{y}'^{(f,r,k)}$:

$$\mathbf{y}'^{(f,r,k)} = \begin{cases} \mathbf{y}^{(f,r,k)} + \mu^{(f,r)}\mathbf{m}^{(k)}, & \text{if } b_k = 1, \\ \mathbf{y}^{(f,r,k)} - \mu^{(f,r)}\mathbf{m}^{(k)}, & \text{if } b_k = 0, \end{cases} \tag{7.15}$$

where $\mu^{(f,r)}$ is WM strength of the region $\mathbf{y}^{(f,r)}$.

Step E4: Output the watermarked frame $\mathbf{y}'^{(f)}$.

WM detection

K correlation values c_k's are calculated by correlating the WM pattern, $\mathbf{m}^{(k)}$, with the accumulated subregion.

Step D1: Do the following steps over $f_0 = 1, F+1, 2F+1, \cdots$.

Step D2: Input F watermarked frames $\mathbf{y}'^{(f)}$s ($f = f_0, \cdots, f_0+F-1$) and then divide FRK subregions $\mathbf{y}'^{(f,r,k)}$s ($f = f_0, \cdots, f_0+F-1, r = 1, \cdots, R, k = 1, \cdots, K$).

Step D3: For each k, where $k = 1, \cdots, K$, accumulate the FR subregions $\mathbf{y}'^{(f,r,k)}$s in the subregion $\tilde{\mathbf{y}}^{(k)} = \left\{\tilde{y}_i^{(k)} \mid 1 \le i \le \left\lfloor \frac{N}{(RK)} \right\rfloor\right\}$. The $\tilde{y}_i^{(k)}$ of the accumulated subregion $\tilde{\mathbf{y}}^{(k)}$ is given by

$$\tilde{y}_i^{(k)} = \frac{1}{FR} \sum_{f=f_0}^{f_0+F-1} \sum_{r=1}^{R} y_i'^{(f,r,k)}. \tag{7.16}$$

Step D4: Calculate the set consisting of the K correlation values

$$\mathbf{c} = \{c_k \mid 1 \le k \le K\}. \tag{7.17}$$

Each correlation value c_k is obtained by correlating the WM pattern $\mathbf{m}^{(k)}$ with the accumulated subregion $\tilde{\mathbf{y}}^{(k)}$. That is,

$$c_k = \frac{1}{FR\left\lfloor \frac{N}{(RK)} \right\rfloor} \sum_{f,r,i} m_i^{(k)} y_i^{(f,r,k)} \pm \mu. \tag{7.18}$$

In the same way as in one-bit WM detection, each c_k follows a normal distribution. That is,

$$c_k \sim \begin{cases} N(\mu, \sigma^2), & \text{if } b_k = 1; \\ N(-\mu, \sigma^2), & \text{if } b_k = 0. \end{cases} \tag{7.19}$$

Step D5: Determine K embedded bits b_ks by comparing c_k with a threshold value of $T(> 0)$, where

$$b_k = \begin{cases} 1, & \text{if } c_k \geq T; \\ 0, & \text{if } c_k \leq -T; \\ \text{"not detected,"} & \text{if } -T < c_k < T. \end{cases} \tag{7.20}$$

Problem with Kalker's Method

WMs on pictures must be able to survive several kinds of video processing procedures. Kalker's accumulation operation (7.16) is not always effective because the WM signal μ in formula (7.18) could be attenuated. This is due to an attempted accumulation from regions from which the WMs had been removed during video processing. If accumulation or averaging is done on two regions with the same noise level and WM signal level, the noise level for region σ is reduced to $1/\sqrt{2}\sigma$. WM signal μ is reduced to $1/2\mu$ if the WMs for one of the two regions is removed. The S/N ratio is worsened by the accumulation. Kalker's accumulation operation could cause the signal of the WMs, μ, to decrease so much that the embedded bits could not be reliably detected.

The statistically adaptive detection technique solves this problem by identifying the accumulated regions remaining in WMs and detecting the WMs from the accumulated region.

7.4.2 Statistically-Adaptive Detection

Principle

The statistically adaptive detection technique identifies the accumulated regions with a minimal degree of WM removal. It detects the WMs from the accumulated regions. We use the Bit-Error Rate (BER) as the measure of the degree of WM removal. The BER is estimated for each watermarked region, and the estimated BERs are used to control the accumulation operation so that the BER of the accumulated region is minimized. This prevents a decrease in the S/N ratio.

Fig. 7.10 shows the structure of the process of the statistically adaptive technique, which comprises a correlation-value calculation, a BER estimation, a sorting operation, an accumulation control, and a bit-value determination:

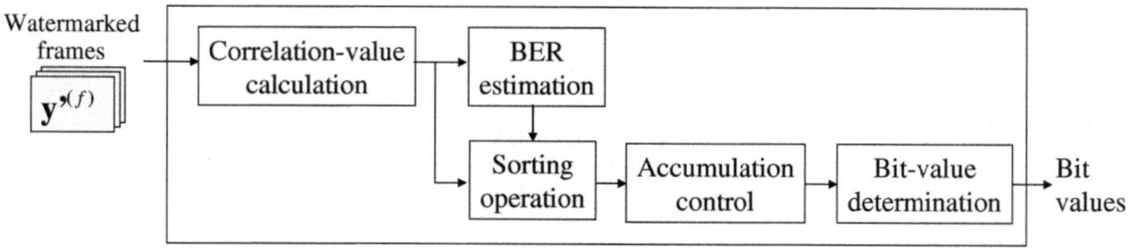

Fig. 7.10. System structure of a statistically adaptive detection technique.

Correlation-value calculation: Calculates the correlation values from the region.
BER estimation: Estimates the BER from the correlation values of the region.
Sorting operation: Sorts the regions, which are the corresponding set of correlation values by the corresponding BERs.
Accumulation control: Accumulates, one by one, regions that is sets of correlation values in ascending order of their BERs, It re-estimates the BER for the accumulated region at each step. The accumulated region having the smallest BER is selected.
Bit-value determination: This determines the bit values. It is done by comparing a threshold value with the set of correlation values of the accumulated region and it selects the smallest BER.

The statistically adaptive technique can be applied to the various kinds of correlation-based WM scheme described in Sect. 7.4.1.

Process Flow

The process flow of the statistically adaptive detection technique is shown in Fig. 7.11. Step D3 represents the flows of the correlation-value calculation and the BER estimation. Step D4 represents the flow of the sorting operation, and Steps D5 through D7 represent the flow of the accumulation control. Step D8 represents the flow of the bit-value determination.

Step D1: Do the following steps over $f_0 = 1, F+1, 2F+1, \cdots$.
Step D2: Input F watermarked frames $\mathbf{y}'^{(f)}$s ($f = f_0, \cdots, f_0+F-1$) and divide FRK regions $\mathbf{y}'^{(f,r,k)}$s ($f = f_0, \cdots, f_0+F-1, r = 1, \cdots, R, k = 1, \cdots, K$).
Step D3: For each region $\mathbf{y}'^{(f,r)}$ ($f_0 \le f \le f_0+F-1, 1 \le r \le R$), calculate the set consisting of the K correlation values,

$$\mathbf{c}^{(f,r)} = \{c_k^{(f,r)} \mid 1 \le k \le K\}, \tag{7.21}$$

and estimate BER $p(\mathbf{c}^{(f,r)})$ from the set $\mathbf{c}^{(f,r)}$. The correlation value $c_k^{(f,r)}$ of the region $\mathbf{y}'^{(f,r,k)}$ is given by correlating the WM pattern $\mathbf{m}^{(k)}$ with the region $\mathbf{y}'^{(f,r,k)}$. That is,

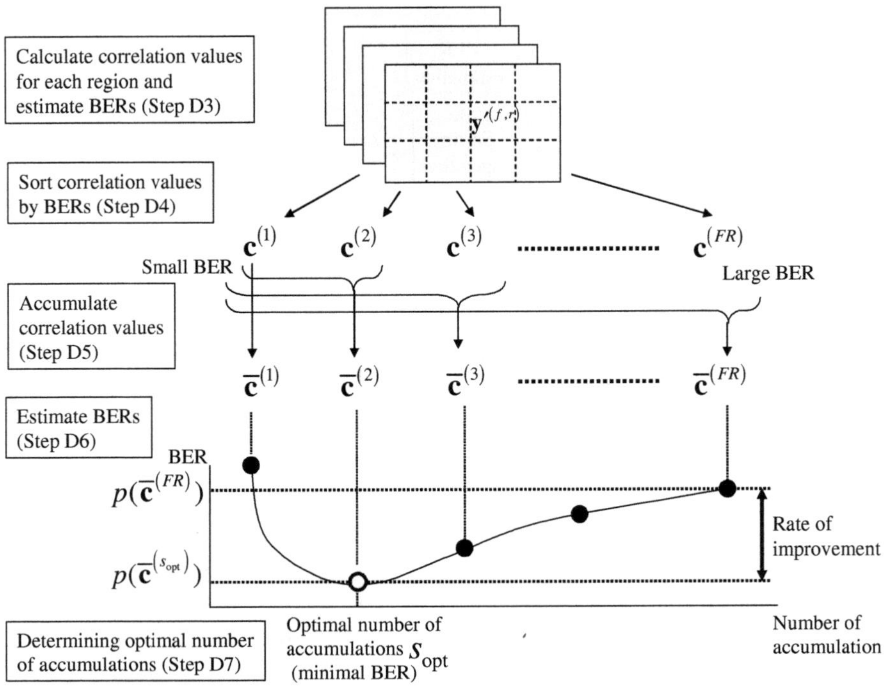

Fig. 7.11. Overview of Statistically Adaptive Detection.

$$c_k^{(f,r)} = \frac{1}{\left\lfloor \frac{N}{(RK)} \right\rfloor} \sum_{i=1}^{\lfloor fracN(RK) \rfloor} m_i^{(k)} {y'}_i^{(f,r,k)}$$
$$= \frac{1}{\left\lfloor \frac{N}{(RK)} \right\rfloor} \sum_i m_i^{(k)} y_i^{(f,r,k)} \pm \mu^{(f,r)}. \tag{7.22}$$

Doing the above process over FR regions ($f = f_0, \cdots, f_0 + F - 1, r = 1, \cdots, R$), we get FR sets $\mathbf{c}^{(f_0,1)}, \cdots, \mathbf{c}^{(f_0+F-1,R)}$ and the corresponding FR BERs $p(\mathbf{c}^{(f_0,1)}), \cdots, p(\mathbf{c}^{(f_0+F-1,R)})$.

Step D4: Sort the FR sets $\mathbf{c}^{(f_0,1)}, \cdots, \mathbf{c}^{(f_0+F-1,R)}$ by the corresponding BERs and rename the suffixes of the sets and the BERs in ascending order of the BERs. Thus we get the FR sets $\mathbf{c}^{(1)}, \cdots, \mathbf{c}^{(FR)}$ that satisfy $p(\mathbf{c}^{(1)}) \leq \cdots \leq p(\mathbf{c}^{(FR)})$.

Step D5: Generate the accumulated sets $\bar{\mathbf{c}}^{(s)}$s ($s = 1, \cdots, FR$) from the FR sets by

$$\bar{\mathbf{c}}^{(s)} = \{\bar{c}_k^{(s)} = \frac{1}{s} \sum_{i=1}^{s} c_k^{(i)} \mid 1 \leq k \leq K\}. \tag{7.23}$$

Step D6: Estimate the BERs $p(\bar{\mathbf{c}}^{(s)})$ $(s = 1, \cdots, FR)$ from the FR accumulated sets $\bar{\mathbf{c}}^{(s)}$s

Step D7: Select the set of the correlation values having the smallest BER $\bar{\mathbf{c}}^{(s_{\text{opt}})}$, where s_{opt} represents the optimal number of accumulations:

$$s_{\text{opt}} = \arg \min_{1 \le s \le FR} p(\bar{\mathbf{c}}^{(s)}). \tag{7.24}$$

Step D8: Determine K embedded bits b_ks by comparing $\bar{c}_k^{(s_{\text{opt}})}$ with a threshold value $T(> 0)$ as is the case with formula (7.20) of Kalker's WM detection:

$$b_k = \begin{cases} 1, & \text{if } \bar{c}_k^{(s_{\text{opt}})} \ge T; \\ 0, & \text{if } \bar{c}_k^{(s_{\text{opt}})} \le -T; \\ \text{"not detected,"} & \text{if } -T < \bar{c}_k^{(s_{\text{opt}})} < T. \end{cases} \tag{7.25}$$

Note that the set $\bar{\mathbf{c}}^{(FR)}$ of Step D5 is equal to the set $\mathbf{c}$ in formula (7.17) of Kalker's WM detection, meaning that the difference between $p(\bar{\mathbf{c}}^{(s_{\text{opt}})})$ and $p(\bar{\mathbf{c}}^{(FR)})$ represents the rate of BER improvement with the statistically adaptive technique.

7.4.3 BER Estimation

To estimate the BERs of the regions, we use inferential statistics because the correlation values of the regions follow a normal distribution dependant on the WM signal and the image noise. The basic method of the BER estimation described in Sect. 7.4.2 was previously presented [5]. This method can be used to estimate the BER from a watermarked still picture after video processing by using inferential statistics. We expanded this method to handle BER estimation for the regions and implemented it in our statistically adaptive detection technique.

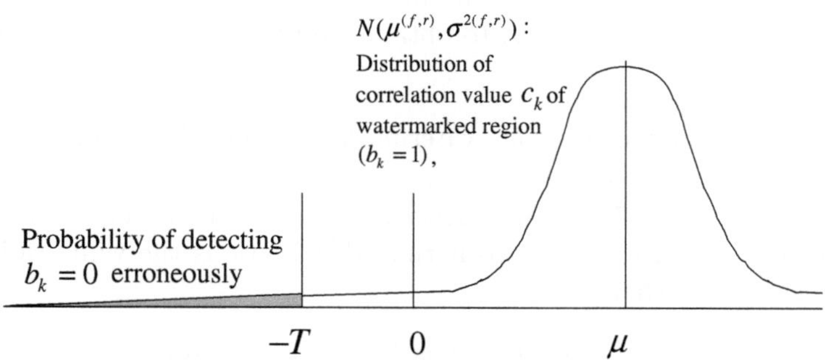

Fig. 7.12. Calculation of BER.

BER of Region

We estimate the BER for each watermarked region from the K correlation values $c_k^{(f,r)}$ in formula (7.22) of the statistically adaptive detection technique. As mentioned in Sect. 7.4.1, in Kalker's WM detection, each correlation value, $c_k^{(f,r)}$, follows a normal distribution with mean $\pm\mu^{(f,r)}$ and variance $\sigma^{2(f,r)}$ if the number of $m_i^{(k)} y_i^{(f,r,k)}$s, $\left\lfloor \frac{N}{(RK)} \right\rfloor$ is large enough:

$$c_k^{(f,r)} \sim \begin{cases} N(\mu^{(f,r)}, \sigma^{2(f,r)}) \text{ if } b_k = 1; \\ N(-\mu^{(f,r)}, \sigma^{2(f,r)}) \text{ if } b_k = 0. \end{cases} \tag{7.26}$$

The calculation of the BER when $b_k = 1$ is embedded is illustrated in Fig. 7.12, where the gray area indicating the probability of erroneously detecting $b_k = 0$ is given by

$$p(\mathbf{c}^{(f,r)})_{\mathrm{BE}|b_k=1} = \int_{-\infty}^{-T} \phi(c; \mu^{(f,r)}, \sigma^{2(f,r)})\, dc, \tag{7.27}$$

where $\phi(c; \mu^{(f,r)}, \sigma^{2(f,r)})$ is the probability density function of $N(\mu^{(f,r)}, \sigma^{2(f,r)})$. The probability of detecting $b_k = 1$ erroneously (when the embedded bit is 0) is correspondingly given by

$$p(\mathbf{c}^{(f,r)})_{\mathrm{BE}|b_k=0} = \int_{\infty}^{T} \phi(c; -\mu^{(f,r)}, \sigma^{2(f,r)})\, dc. \tag{7.28}$$

From formulas (7.27) and (7.28), $p(\mathbf{c}^{(f,r)})_{BE|b_k=1} = p(\mathbf{c}^{(f,r)})_{BE|b_k=0}$. Thus, the BER of the region $\mathbf{y}'^{(f,r)}$ for an arbitrary embedded bit is

$$p(\mathbf{c}^{(f,r)}) = \int_{-\infty}^{-T} \phi(c; \mu^{(f,r)}, \sigma^{2(f,r)})\, dc. \tag{7.29}$$

As shown in formula (7.29), the mean $\mu^{(f,r)}$ and variance $\sigma^{2(f,r)}$ of the normal distribution can be used to obtain the BER. There are, however, two problems.

- The information we get from watermarked region $\mathbf{y}'^{(f,r)}$ is not $\mu^{(f,r)}$ and $\sigma^{2(f,r)}$; it is the K correlation values $c_k^{(f,r)}$.
- As shown in Fig. 7.13, the correlation values are subject to change by video processing, and the two normal distributions the values follow can approach each other.

The $\mu^{(f,r)}$ and $\sigma^{2(f,r)}$ should thus be estimated from correlation values that follow a mixture normal distribution.

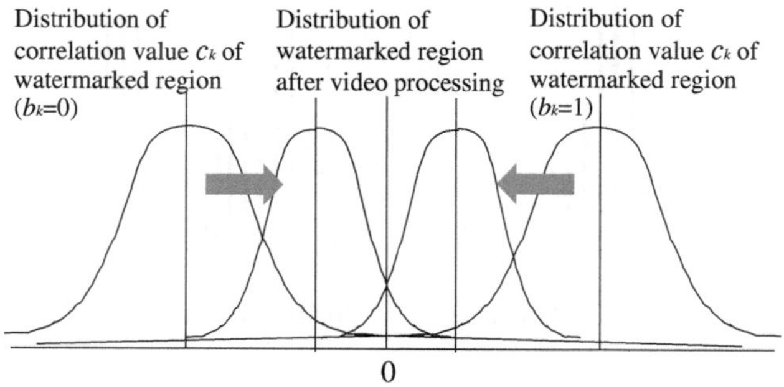

Fig. 7.13. Transition of distribution by video processing.

Estimating Distribution from Correlation Values

To estimate mean $\mu^{(f,r)}$ and variance $\sigma^{2(f,r)}$ from the, K correlation values $c_k^{(f,r)}$s, we consider the case where all embedded bits are known, i.e., $b_k = 1, \forall k$, and the general case where all embedded bits are unknown:

(1) All embedded bits are "1": Fig. 7.14(a) shows the histogram of K correlation values $c_k^{(f,r)}$s. The horizontal axis of the histogram represents the value of $c_k^{(f,r)}$, and the vertical axis represents the frequency of that value. The histogram describes the normal distribution, $N(\mu^{(f,r)}, \sigma^{2(f,r)})$, because K correlation values $c_k^{(f,r)}$s follow on $N(\mu^{(f,r)}, \sigma^{2(f,r)})$ and are independent on each k: the values of $\mu^{(f,r)}$ and $\sigma^{2(f,r)}$ could therefore be estimated using the following formulas if the number of embedded bits, K, is large enough:

$$\mu^{(f,r)} = \frac{1}{K}\sum_k c_k^{(f,r)}, \tag{7.30}$$

$$\sigma^{2(f,r)} = \frac{1}{K}\sum_k c_k^{(f,r)2} - \mu^{(f,r)2}. \tag{7.31}$$

(2) The values of all embedded bits are unknown: As shown in Fig. 7.14(b), the K correlation values independently follow a distribution described by either $N(\mu^{(f,r)}, \sigma^{2(f,r)})$ or $N(-\mu^{(f,r)}, \sigma^{2(f,r)})$ based on the embedded bit. Thus, the histogram describes a mixture normal distribution comprising two normal distributions.

In the following we take up the expectation-maximization (EM) algorithm from inferential statistics supposing the case (2) and use it to estimate the BER for a region.

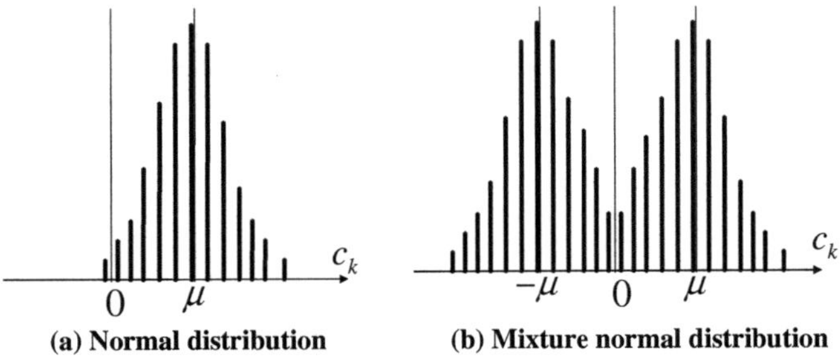

Fig. 7.14. Histogram of correlation values.

EM Algorithm

The expectation-maximization (EM) algorithm is a representative maximum-likelihood method for estimating the statistical parameters of a probability distribution [24, 25]. For a mixture normal distribution comprising two normal distributions that the correlation values, $c_k^{(f,r)}$, follow, the EM algorithm can estimate the probability, $w_k^{(f,r)}$, that each $c_k^{(f,r)}$ follows $N(\mu^{(f,r)}, \sigma^{2(f,r)})$, $\mu^{(f,r)}$, and $\sigma^{2(f,r)}$. The relationship between $w_k^{(f,r)}$, $\mu^{(f,r)}$, and $\sigma^{2(f,r)}$ is given by

$$\mu^{(f,r)} = \frac{1}{K\beta^{(f,r)}} \sum_k w_k^{(f,r)} c_k^{(f,r)}, \tag{7.32}$$

$$\sigma^{2(f,r)} = \frac{1}{K\beta^{(f,r)}} \sum_k w_k^{(f,r)} c_k^{(f,r)2} - \mu^{(f,r)2}, \tag{7.33}$$

where $\beta^{(f,r)} = 1/K \sum_k w_k^{(f,r)}$ is the weighting factor of $N(\mu^{(f,r)}, \sigma^{2(f,r)})$ to the mixture normal distribution. These parameters are sequentially updated from initial values by iterative calculation, and $\mu^{(f,r)}$ and $\sigma^{2(f,r)}$ are used as estimates when they are converged. The $\mu^{(f,r)}$ and $\sigma^{2(f,r)}$ are estimated from K correlation values $c_k^{(f,r)}$s:

Step 1: Set the initial values of the parameters $\beta^{(f,r)}$, $\mu^{(f,r)}$, and $\sigma^{2(f,r)}$ to $\beta^{(f,r)}[0]$, $\mu^{(f,r)}[0]$, and $\sigma^{2(f,r)}[0]$.
Step 2: Do Step 3 through Step 5 over $t = 1, 2, \cdots$.
Step 3: For each k calculate $w_k^{(f,r)}[t]$ from $c_k^{(f,r)}$:

$$w_k^{(f,r)}[t] = \frac{\beta^{(f,r)}[t]\phi(c_k^{(f,r)}; \mu^{(f,r)}[t], \sigma^{2(f,r)}[t])}{g(c_k^{(f,r)}; \beta^{(f,r)}[t], \mu^{(f,r)}[t], \sigma^{2(f,r)}[t])}, \tag{7.34}$$

where $g(c; \beta, \mu, \sigma^2)$ is the probability density function of the mixture normal distribution, that is,

$$g(c;\beta,\mu,\sigma^2) = \beta\phi(c;\mu,\sigma^2) + (1-\beta)\phi(c;-\mu,\sigma^2). \tag{7.35}$$

Step 4: Update $\beta^{(f,r)}[t]$, $\mu^{(f,r)}[t]$, and $\sigma^{2(f,r)}[t]$ by the following formulas:

$$\beta^{(f,r)}[t+1] = \frac{1}{K}\sum_k w_k^{(f,r)}[t], \tag{7.36}$$

$$\mu^{(f,r)}[t+1] = \frac{1}{K\beta^{(f,r)}[t+1]}\sum_k w_k^{(f,r)}[t]c_k^{(f,r)}, \tag{7.37}$$

$$\sigma^{2(f,r)}[t+1] = \frac{\sum_k w_k^{(f,r)}[t]c_k^{(f,r)2}}{K\beta^{(f,r)}[t+1]} - \{\mu^{(f,r)}[t]\}^2. \tag{7.38}$$

Step 5: Stop the process and set

$$\mu^{(f,r)} = \mu^{(f,r)}[t+1], \tag{7.39}$$
$$\sigma^{2(f,r)} = \sigma^{2(f,r)}[t+1], \tag{7.40}$$

if the parameters satisfy the following conditions:

$$|\beta^{(f,r)}[t+1] - \beta^{(f,r)}[t]| < \delta, \tag{7.41}$$
$$|\mu^{(f,r)}[t+1] - \mu^{(f,r)}[t]| < \delta, \tag{7.42}$$
$$|\sigma^{2(f,r)}[t+1] - \sigma^{2(f,r)}[t]| < \delta. \tag{7.43}$$

The BER of the region, $\mathbf{y}'^{(f,r)}$, $p^{(f,r)}$, is calculated from $\mu^{(f,r)}$ and $\sigma^{2(f,r)}$ by using formula (7.29).

7.4.4 Experimental Evaluation

We experimentally compared the ability of the statistically adaptive detection technique to detect watermarks after MPEG-2 encoding for three different bit rates (3, 4, and 5 Mbps) with that of Kalker's method by using the Walk standard motion picture (450 frames of 720×480 pixels) used in the evaluation of the motion-adaptive embedding technique (Sect. 7.3.4).

Procedure

A WM pattern representing 256-bit information ($K = 256$) was generated using a pseudo-random generator [26] and embedded in each of four 360×240-pixel regions ($R = 4$) of every frame by using the multiple-bit-WM scheme described in Sect. 7.4.1.

After MPEG-2 encoding and decoding for three different bit rates (3, 4, 5 Mbps), the 256-bit information was sequentially detected in 30-frame segments of the 450 frames of the watermarked pictures ($F = 30$; the number of detecting points was $450/30 = 15$) and the BERs measured using the statistically adaptive detection technique described in Sect. 7.4.2 were compared with those measured using Kalker's detection method described in Sect. 7.4.1. The above procedure was done using 1000 different random WM patterns. We did not control watermark strength for each pixel, which would minimize the degradation in picture quality, because we focused on evaluating the WM detection method and such control might affect the evaluation. We instead made the watermark strength, $\mu^{(f,r)}$ in formula (7.15), uniform for all pixels. The example strength we used were three, and the corresponding PSNR was 38.6. We also set the threshold value for determining the bit value of the formulas (7.20) and (7.25) to zero ($T = 0$) so that the 256-bit information was always detectable.

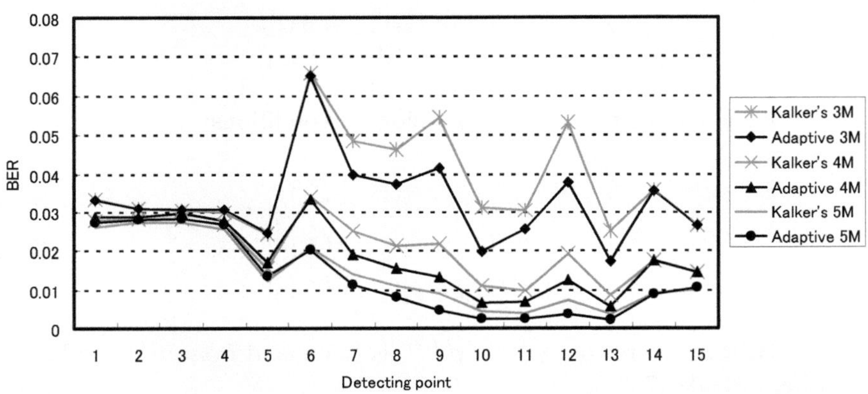

Fig. 7.15. Evaluation results.

Results

The average values (over 1000 WM patterns) of the measured BERs obtained using the statistically adaptive and Kalker's methods are shown for each bit rate in Fig. 7.15, where the horizontal axis represents the detecting points, from 1 to 15, and the vertical axis represents the average BERs. We can see that the BERs with the statistically adaptive technique were better than or equal to those of Kalker's method for each bit rate. For all bit rates, the average ratios of the statistically adaptive BER to the Kalker's BER are 0.903. The statistically adaptive technique thus yielded an average improvement of 9.7%.

From the plots of Fig. 7.15, we sampled two cases for each evaluated sample: effective and non-effective cases of statistically adaptive detection.

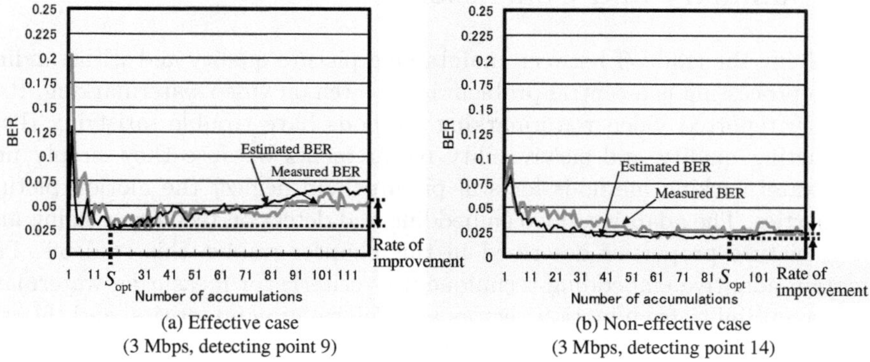

Fig. 7.16. Transitions of BERs.

Example transitions of the BERs estimated using the statistically adaptive technique (corresponding to Fig. 7.11) are shown in Figs. 7.16(a) and 7.16(b), where the horizontal axes represent the number of accumulations (the order of the accumulation follows the ascending order of the estimated BERs), and the vertical axes represent the estimated and measured BERs at the detecting points. From these transitions we can see that the estimated BERs were roughly consistent with the experimentally measured ones. In Fig. 7.16(a) (3 Mbps, detecting point 9), the BER tended to increase with the number of accumulations, and the rate of improvement was about 2.5%. For all bit rates, similar trends were found for detecting points 7 through 13, where most parts of the neighboring frames were messy or moving. We can infer that the strengths of WMs in regions having various picture properties are affected by MPEG-2 encoding so that the BERs of the regions increased with the number of accumulations as a result of the sorting operation of the statistically adaptive detection technique. In Fig. 7.16(b) (3 Mbps, detecting point 14), on the other hand, the plot of BER against the number of accumulations is flat, and the rate of improvement is nearly 0. For all bit rates, similar trends were found for detecting points 1 through 6, 14, and 15, where most parts of the neighboring frames were static. We can infer that the strengths of WMs in the regions were not affected by MPEG-2 encoding so that the BERs of the regions were not changed by the sorting operation.

For all the MPEG-2 bit rates evaluated, the statistically adaptive detection technique produced lower or equal BERs depending on the picture properties and yielded an average improvement of 9.7%. The statistically adaptive detection technique thus improves watermark detection.

7.5 Summary and Conclusion

Resolving the tradeoff between maintaining picture quality and withstanding video processing is a central problem in research on video watermarking. Previously reported video watermarking methods have trouble satisfying these conflicting quality and survivability requirements because they simply utilize watermarking methods for still pictures and neglect the motion picture properties. The adaptive video embedding and detection techniques using motion picture properties described in this chapter resolve this tradeoff. The motion-adaptive embedding technique uses criteria for measuring watermark imperceptibility from motion vectors and deformation quantities, and the statistically adaptive detection technique controls accumulation using inferential statistics so that the error rate of WMs is minimal. Experimental evaluation using actual motion pictures showed that using these two techniques can maintain picture quality and improve watermark survivability after MPEG encoding. They are widely applicable to pixel-based watermarking.

References

1. Swanson, M., Kobayashi, M., and Tewfik, A. (1998): Multimedia data-embedding and watermarking technologies. Proc. IEEE, **86**, 1064–1087
2. Bloom, J., Cox, I., Kalker, T., Linnartz, J., Miller, M., and Traw, C. (1999): Copy protection for DVD video. Proc. IEEE, **87**, 1267–1276
3. Echizen, I., Yoshiura, H., Fujii, Y., and Tezuka, S. (2003): Use of motion estimation to improve video watermarking for MPEG encoders. Proc. Intl. Workshop on Digital Watermarking, LNCS, Springer-Verlag, **2939**, 184–199
4. Echizen, I., Fujii, Y., Yamada, T., Tezuka, S., and Yoshiura, H. (2005): Perceptually adaptive video watermarking using motion estimation. Int'l Journal of Image and Graphics, World Scientific, **5**, 89–109
5. Echizen, I., Yoshiura, H., Fujii, Y., Yamada, T., and Tezuka, S. (2005): Use of inferential statistics to estimate error probability of video watermarks. Security and Watermarking of Multimedia Contents VII, SPIE, **5681**, 391–399
6. Echizen, I., Fujii, Y., Yamada, T., Tezuka, S., and Yoshiura, H. (2005): Improved Video Watermark Detection Using Statistically-Adaptive Accumulation. Proc. Intl. Conf. on Knowledge-Based Intelligent Information and Engineering Systems, Springer-Verlag, LNCS, **3684**, 300–308
7. Delaigle, J., Vleeschouwer, C., and Macq, B. (1998): Watermarking algorithm based on a human visual model. Signal Processing, **66**, 319–335
8. Vleeschouwer, C., Delaigle, J., and Macq, B. (2002): Invisibility and application functionalities in perceptual watermarking – An overview. Proc. IEEE, **90**, 64–77
9. Hartung, F. and Girod, B. (1996): Digital watermarking of raw and compressed video. Proc. SPIE, **2952**, 205–213
10. Kundur, D. and Hatzinakos, D. (1998): Digital watermarking using multiresolution wavelet decomposition. Proc. Intl. Conf. Acoustics, Speech and Signal Processing, 2969–2972

11. Kobayashi, S., Kamijoh, K., and Shimizu, S. (1998): Data hiding based on neighbor pixels statistics. Proc. IPSJ 56th Annual Conf., 1V–03
12. Echizen, I., Yoshiura, H., Arai, T., Kimura, H., and Takeuchi, T. (1999): General quality maintenance module for motion picture watermarking. IEEE Trans. Consumer Electronics, **45**, 1150–1158
13. Bender, W., Gruhl, D., and Morimoto, N. (1995): Techniques for data hiding. Proc. SPIE, **2420**, 164–173
14. Dufaux, F. and Moscheni, F. (1998): Motion estimation techniques for digital TV: a review and new contribution. Proc. IEEE, **83**, 858–876
15. The Institute of Image Information and Television Engineers : Evaluation video sample (standard definition)
16. Rec. ITU-R BT.500-7 (1995): Methodology for the subjective assessment of the quality of television pictures
17. Lin, E. and Delp, E. (2004): Spatial synchronization using watermark key structure. Security and Watermarking of Multimedia Contents VI, Proc. SPIE, **5306**, 536–547
18. Kalker, T., Depovere, G., Haitsma, J., and Maes, M. (1999) Video watermarking system for broadcast monitoring. Security and Watermarking of Multimedia Contents, Proc. SPIE, **3657**, 103–112
19. Kusanagi, A. and Imai, H. (2001): An image correction scheme for video watermarking extraction. IEICE Trans. Fundamentals, **E84-A**, 273–280
20. Cox, I., Kilian, J., Leighton, T., and Shamoon, T. (1997): Secure spread spectrum watermarking for multimedia. IEEE Trans. Image Processing, **6**, 1673–1687
21. Hartung, F., Su, J., and Girod, B. (1999): Spread spectrum watermarking: Malicious attacks and counterattacks. Security and Watermarking of Multimedia Contents, Proc. SPIE, **3657**, 147–158
22. Seo, Y., Choi, S., Park, S., and Kim, D. (2004): A digital watermarking algorithm using correlation of the tree structure of DWT coefficients. IEICE Trans. Fundamentals, **E87-A**, 1347–1354
23. Liang, T. and Rodriguez, J. (2000): Robust watermarking using robust coefficients. Security and Watermarking of Multimedia Contents II, Proc. SPIE, **3971**, 335–356
24. Redner, R. and Walker, H. (1984): Mixture densities, maximum likelihood and the EM algorithm. SIAM Review, **26**, 195–239
25. Xu, L. and Jordan, M. (1996): On convergence properties of the EM algorithm for Gaussian mixtures. Neural Computation, **8**, 129–151
26. Matsumoto, M. and Nishimura, T. (1998): Mersenne Twister: A 623-dimensionally equidistributed uniform pseudorandom number generator. ACM Trans. on Modeling and Computer Simulation, **8**, 3–30

8

Steganographic Methods Focusing on BPCS Steganography

Hideki Noda[1], Michiharu Niimi[1], and Eiji Kawaguchi[2]

[1] Kyushu Institute of Technology, Dept. of Systems Innovation and Informatics, 680-4 Kawazu, Iizuka, 820-8502 Japan
noda@mip.ces.kyutech.ac.jp,
niimi@mip.ces.kyutech.ac.jp
http://www.know.comp.kyutech.ac.jp/

[2] KIT Senior Academy, Kitakyushu, Japan
e-kawagu@alto.ocn.ne.jp

Summary. Steganography is a technique to hide secret information in some other data (we call it a vessel) without leaving any apparent evidence of data alteration. This chapter describes a high capacity steganographic method called bit-plane complexity segmentation (BPCS) steganography. BPCS steganography usually uses an image as the vessel data, and secret information is embedded in the bit-planes of the vessel. This technique makes use of the characteristics of the human vision system whereby a human cannot perceive any shape information in a very complicated binary pattern. We can replace all of the "noise-like" regions in the bit-planes of the vessel image with secret data without deteriorating image quality. The principle and possible applications of BPCS, attacks to BPCS, and BPCS applicable to JPEG2000 images are here addressed. Additionally, histogram preserving JPEG steganography is described, and finally experimental results are given.

8.1 Bit-Plane Complexity Segmentation (BPCS) Steganography

Internet communication has become an integral part of the infrastructure of today's world. In some Internet communication it is desired that the communication be done in secret. Encryption provides an obvious approach to information security, and encryption programs are readily available. However, encryption clearly marks a message as containing "interesting" information, and the encrypted message becomes subject to attack. Furthermore, in many cases it is desirable to send information without anyone even noticing that information has been sent.

Steganography presents another approach to information security. In steganography, data is hidden inside a vessel or container that looks like it

H. Noda et al.: *Steganographic Methods Focusing on BPCS Steganography*, Studies in Computational Intelligence (SCI) **58**, 189–229 (2007)
www.springerlink.com

contains only something else. A variety of vessels are possible, such as digital images, sound clips, and even executable files. In recent years, many steganographic programs have been posted on Internet Web pages. Most of them use image data for the container of the secret information. Some of them use the least significant bits of the image data to hide secret data. Other programs embed the secret information in a specific band of the spatial frequency component of the carrier. Some other programs make use of the sampling error in image digitization. However, all those steganographic techniques are limited in terms of information hiding capacity. They can embed only $5-15\%$ of the vessel image at the best. Therefore, traditional steganography is more oriented to watermarking of computer data than to secret person-person communication applications.

We have invented a new technique to hide secret information in an image. This is not based on a programming technique, but is based on the property of human vision system. Its information hiding capacity can be as large as 50% of the original image data. This could open new applications for steganography leading to a more secure Internet communication age.

Digital images are categorized as either binary (black-and-white) or multi-valued pictures despite their actual color. We can decompose an n-bit image into a set of n binary images by bit-slicing operations [1, 2]. Therefore, binary image analysis is essential to all digital image processing. Bit slicing is not necessarily the best in the standard binary coding system (We call it Pure-Binary Coding system (PBC)), but in some cases the Canonical Gray Coding system (CGC) is much better [3].

8.1.1 The Complexity of Binary Images

The method of steganography outlined in this chapter makes use of the complex regions of an image to embed data. There is no standard definition of image complexity. Kawaguchi discussed this problem in connection with the image thresholding problem, and proposed three types of complexity measures [4, 5, 6]. In this chapter we adopted a black-and-white border image complexity.

The Definition of Image Complexity

The length of the black-and-white border in a binary image is a good measure for image complexity. If the border is long, the image is complex, otherwise it is simple. The total length of the black-and-white border equals to the summation of the number of color-changes along the rows and columns in an image. For example, a single black pixel surrounded by white background pixels has the boarder length of 4.

We will define the image complexity α for an $m \times m$ size binary image by the following.

$$\alpha = \frac{k}{2m(m-1)}, \quad 0 \leq \alpha \leq 1, \tag{8.1}$$

where k is the total length of the black-and-white border in the image and $2m(m-1)$ is the maximum possible border length obtained from an $m \times m$ checkerboard pattern. Eq. (8.1) is defined globally, i.e., α is calculated over the whole image area. It gives us the global complexity of a binary image. However, we can also use α for a local image complexity (e.g., an 8×8 pixel-size area). We will use such α as our local complexity measure in this chapter.

8.1.2 Analysis of Informative and Noise-Like Regions

Informative images are simple, while noise-like images are complex. However, this is only true in cases where such binary images are part of a natural image. In this section we will discuss how many image patterns are informative and how many patterns are noise-like. We will begin by introducing a "conjugation" operation of a binary image.

Conjugation of a Binary Image

Let P be a $2^N \times 2^N$ size black-and-white image with black as the foreground area and white as the background area. W and B denote all-white and all-black patterns, respectively. We introduce two checkerboard patterns W_c and B_c, where W_c has a white pixel at the upper-left position, and B_c is its complement, i.e., the upper-left pixel is black (See Fig. 8.1). We regard black and white pixels as having a logical value of "1" and "0," respectively.

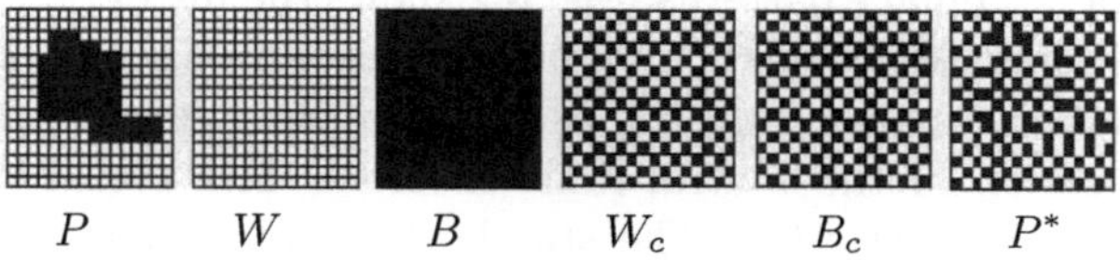

Fig. 8.1. Illustration of each binary pattern ($N = 4$).

P is interpreted as follows. Pixels in the foreground area have the B pattern, while pixels in the background area have the W pattern. Now we define P^* as the conjugate of P which satisfies:

(1) The foreground area shape is the same as P.
(2) The foreground area has the B_c pattern.
(3) The background area has the W_c pattern.

Correspondence between P and P^* is one-to-one, onto. The following properties hold true and are easily proved for such conjugation operation. $\oplus$ designates the exclusive OR operation,

$$P^* = P \oplus W_c; \tag{8.2}$$

$$(P^*)^* = P; \tag{8.3}$$

$$P^* \neq P. \tag{8.4}$$

Let $\alpha(P)$ be the complexity of a given image P, then we have

$$\alpha(P^*) = 1 - \alpha(P). \tag{8.5}$$

It is evident that the combination of each local conjugation (e.g., 8×8 area) makes an overall conjugation (e.g., 512×512 area). Eq. (8.5) says that every binary image pattern P has its counterpart P^*. The complexity value of P^* is always symmetrical against P regarding $\alpha = 0.5$. For example, if P has a complexity of 0.7, then P^* has a complexity of 0.3.

Criterion to Segment a Bit-Plane into Informative and Noise-Like Regions

We are interested in how many binary image patterns are informative and how many patterns are noise-like with regard to the complexity measure α.

Firstly, as we think 8×8 is a good size for local area, we want to know the total number of 8×8 binary patterns in relation to α value. This means we must check all 2^{64} different 8×8 patterns. However, 2^{64} is too huge to make an exhaustive check by any means. Our practical approach is as follows. We first generate as many random 8×8 binary patterns as possible, where each pixel value is set random, but has equal black-and-white probability. Then we make a histogram of all generated patterns in terms of α. This simulates the distribution of 2^{64} binary patterns. Fig. 8.2 shows the histogram for 4,096,000 8×8 patterns generated by our computer. This histogram shape almost exactly fits the normal distribution function as shown in the figure. We would expect this by application of the central limit theorem. The average value of the complexity α was exactly 0.5. The standard deviation was 0.047 in α. We denote this deviation by σ ("Sigma" in Fig. 8.2).

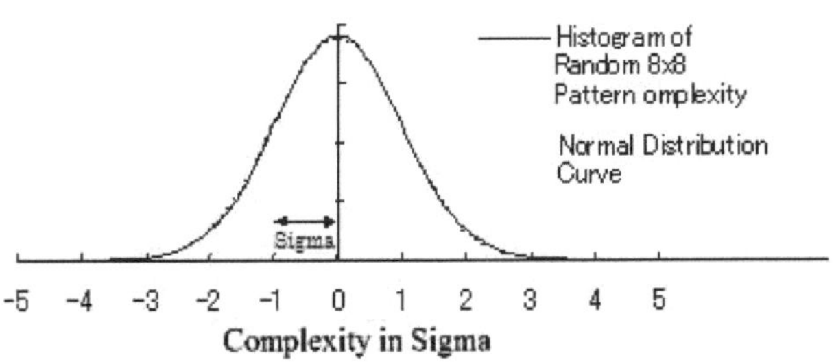

Fig. 8.2. Histogram of randomly generated 8×8 binary patterns.

Secondly, our next task is to determine how much image data we can discard without deteriorating the image quality, or, rather at what complexity does the image data become indispensable. To discard data means to replace local image areas in a bit-plane with random noise patterns. If we replace all the local areas having complexity value $\alpha_L \leq \alpha$, yet the image still maintains good quality, then perhaps we can discard more. If the quality is no longer good, then we can not discard that much. If $\alpha_L = \alpha$ is the minimum complexity value to be good, such α_L is used as the threshold value.

To be indispensable, or rather "informative," for an image means the following. If the image data is still "picture-like" after we have discarded (randomized) a certain amount of image data for such an α that $\alpha \leq \alpha_U$, and if we discard more, then it becomes only noise-like. Then, that α_U is regarded as the limit of the informative image complexity. If α_L and α_U coincide ($\alpha_0 = \alpha_L = \alpha_U$), we can conclude α_0 is the complexity threshold to divide informative and noise-like regions in a bit-plane.

We made a "random pattern replacing" experiment on a bit-plane of a color image. Fig. 8.3 illustrates the result. Fig. 8.3 shows that if we randomize regions in each bit-plane which are less complex than $0.5 - 8\sigma$, the image can not be image-like any more. While, we can randomize the more complex regions than $0.5 - 8\sigma$ without losing much of the image information. This means the most of the informative image information is concentrated in between 0 and $0.5 - 8\sigma$ in complexity scale. Surprising enough, it is only 6.67×10^{-14} % of all 8×8 binary patterns. Amazingly, the rest (i.e., 99.9999999999999333%) are mostly noise-like binary patterns.

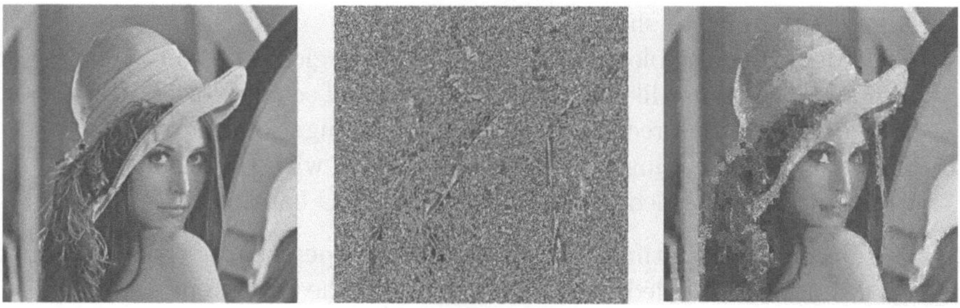

A) Original image B) Randomization (simple side) C) Randomization (complex side)

Fig. 8.3. Randomization of the less and the more complex than $0.5 - 8\sigma$.

The conclusion of this section is as follows. We can categorize the local areas in the bit-planes of a multi-valued image into three portions: (1) Natural informative portions, (2) Artificial informative portions, and (3) Noise-like portions. The reason we categorize the excessively complicated patterns as "informative" is based on our experiments [7]. The most important fact here is that replacing a noise-like portion with any noise-like 8×8 binary blocks does not produce any visual change on the vessel.

8.1.3 Bit-Plane Complexity Segmentation (BPCS) Steganography

BPCS steganography is our new steganographic technique, which has a large information hiding capacity. As have shown in the previous section, the replacement of the complex regions in each bit-plane of a color image with random binary patterns is invisible to the human eyes. We can use this property for our information hiding (or, embedding) strategy. The term information embedding capacity is the same as information hiding capacity.

In our method we call a carrier image a "vessel," "cover" or "dummy" image. It is a color image in BMP file format, which embeds the secret information (files in any format). We segment each secret file (already compressed form) to be embedded into a series of blocks having 8 bytes of data each. These blocks are regarded as 8×8 image patterns. We call such blocks the secret blocks. We embed these secret blocks into the vessel image using the following steps.

(1) Convert the vessel image from PBC to CGC system. This conversion is executed by the exclusive-or operation [3].
(2) Segment each bit-plane of the vessel image into informative and noise-like regions by using a threshold value (α_0). A typical value is $\alpha_0 = 0.25$.
(3) Group the bytes of the secret file into a series of secret blocks.
(4) If a block (S) is less complex than the threshold (α_0), then conjugate it to make it a more complex block (S*). The conjugated block must be more complex than α_0 as shown by Eq. (8.5).
(5) Embed each secret block into the noise-like regions of the bit-planes (or, replace all the noise-like regions with a series of secret blocks). If the block is conjugated, then record this fact in a "conjugation map."
(6) Also embed the conjugation map as was done with the secret blocks.
(7) Convert the embedded vessel image from CGC back to PBC.

The Decoding algorithm (i.e., the extracting operation of the secret information from an embedded vessel image) is just the reverse procedure of the embedding steps.

The novelty in BPCS steganography is itemized in the following.

A) Segmentation of each bit-plane of a color image into "Informative" and "Noise-like" regions.
B) Introduction of the $B - W$ boarder based complexity measure (α) for region segmentation.
C) Introduction of the conjugation operation to convert simple secret blocks to complex blocks.
D) Using CGC image plane instead of PBC plane.

E) There are many variations in implementing a BPCS steganography program. Such variation can be put into an embedding/extraction key. This key is neither included in the program, nor hidden in the vessel image.

8.2 Possible Application Systems of BPCS Steganography

Possible applications of BPCS steganography are categorized into several groups according to its property. The most important properties of BPCS are,

(A) very high embedding capacity,
(B) secure confidentiality of the embedded information,
(C) fragility of the embedded information,
(D) vessel image and embedded data can not be separated in the embedded vessel image. An embedded vessel image is called "stego image."

So, we can categorize the applications in reference to those properties. In the following we will explain three specific applications. The first one is with property (A) and (B), the second one makes use of (C), and the last one owes to property (D). Some application can make use of other steganography than BPCS. We will mention it accordingly.

8.2.1 Web-Based Communication

A web-based confidential corresponding method by BPCS steganography is the most unprecedented realization of secret communication channel. It is the most hard-to-detect communication method. Fig. 8.4 illustrates the scheme, where A and B are two persons having a respective "home-pages" on the Internet. The communication steps are as follows. They have a common key to embed in and extract from the message.

Step-1: A and B decide which key to use
Step-2: A embeds his secret message, that is addressed for B, in A's image to make it a stego image
Step-3: A uploads the stego image on A's home-page
Step-4: B downloads the image and extracts the message by using the common key and read the message
Step-5: B embeds his reply-message in B's image
Step-6: B uploads the image on B's home-page
Step-7: A downloads the image and extracts the reply-message to read the reply-message

In this communication scheme, it is extremely difficult for the third party to check the secret communication. This scheme can be implemented by using

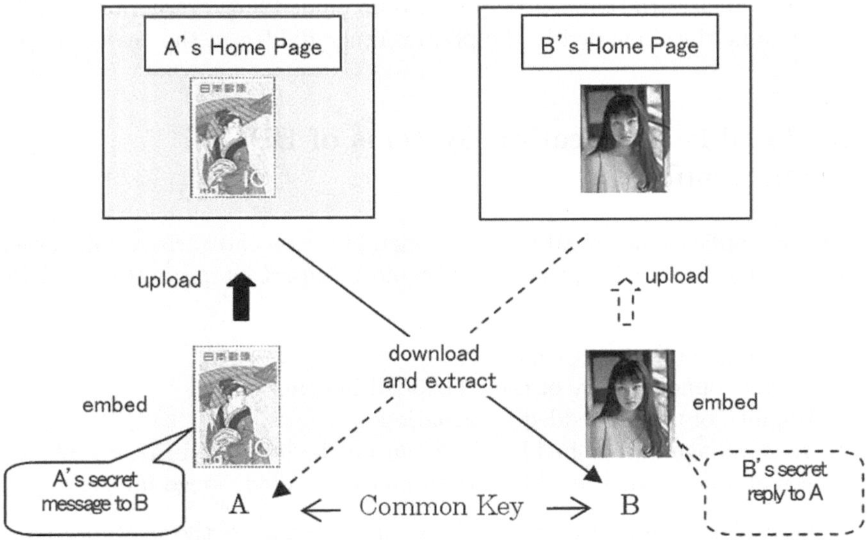

Fig. 8.4. Web-based confidential communication.

BMP or PNG image by BPCS method. But if the message is not so large, using a JPEG image may be better because JPG looks more innocuous than BMP to the third party.

8.2.2 Forgery Detective Digital Certificate System

This application makes use of the fragility of the embedded data in BPCS steganography. Also, a large embedding capacity plays a key role.

Currently, a certification document is "written" or "printed" on a paper surface or on a plastic card surface. No computer data can serve as a certificate document by itself. This is because all computer data today have a "single-layered information structure" in the sense that all information is just as it looks. Computer data are always alterable, and it is impossible to tell whether the given computer data is original or not just by looking. A PDF file is not very easy to alter, but is still editable. Therefore, a digital document is forgeable. It is impossible to decide if it is authentic or counterfeit. This is the reason why we cannot e-mail a digital certification document over the Internet. Currently, a digital signature system is available to make a digital document formally authentic. However, it is based on an extra information-infrastructure, namely, the human authentication bureau. But it is not very handy for our daily use. Therefore, a digital certification system using no extra frameworks, if invented, is very evolutionary. The following is one of such.

We will classify the types of certificate-document forgeries into two categories.

Type-1 Forgery: Altering a part of the authentic certificate
Example: Tampering a driver's permit, credit card, passport, student transcript, etc.
Type 2 Forgery: Creating a new fake certificate
Example: PhD diploma, pedigree, expert evidence, medical certificate, etc.

BPCS steganography can protect both types of forgeries in a digital manner.

Digital documents include several types of data such as plain texts, graphics, images, and motion pictures in some case. When people see them on a computer monitor, they look just image information. People do not care if the original data consist of several different data types or not. So, it does not cause any problem to convert the document data into all image data. However, the converted image still have a single layered information structure.

A multi-layered information structure of media data, such as an image, is as follows. It has an external layer, which is visible, and an internal layer, which is invisible for human eyes. The internal layer can be further structured as sub-external and sub-internal layers. It is very obvious that this kind of multi-layered information structure is implemented by steganographic data embedding method.

In order to make a digital document to serve as a certification document, we will do the following.

Step-1: Convert a given digital document consisting of several data categories into one single image file. We call this file conversion as "vessel image creation." The data size will significantly increases in this step.
Step-2: Embed the original document data in the created vessel image according to a steganographic scheme. This step needs a large data-embedding capacity. So, BPCS method is the best. The external view of the embedded vessel-image, i.e., stego image, is the external information, and the embedded original document is the internal information. The internal information can be extracted only if it is not altered at all.

As it is clear from Step-2, the external and the internal layer have the same visual information. In order for someone to alter this multi-layered digital document successfully, he/she must alter the two layers at the same time. However, this is impossible from the nature of steganography. On top of that, once he/she tries to alter a part of the external layer, they will damage the internal information immediately because the embedded data is so fragile, especially in BPCS steganography. Once the internal layer is damaged, it will never be extracted.

Type-1 forgery detection
Determining whether a given digital certificate having a multi-layered information structure is authentic or not in a Type-1 sense is very easy. If the

extraction fails, it is forged. If the extraction succeeds, but some discrepancy exists between the external and the internal layer, it is apparently tampered. Otherwise, the document is authentic.

Type-2 forgery detection

A Type-2 forgery protective digital certificate needs some additional scheme. It is a "one-way scrambled key" for embedding and extracting the original document data. The detailed scheme is described in other literature [8].

The capability of forgery detection depends on the fragileness of the steganography that we use. We knew, throughout our experiment, that embedding JPG files in a PNG vessel image is the best. However, this is beyond the scope the topic here.

8.2.3 Media Database System Application

Most media database system has varieties of metadata associated with the content of the respective data. They are used for content retrieving. A media database system today handles the media data and the metadata in separate data categories, but tightly associated with each other within the DBMS. One troublesome problem is as follows. When someone creates and edits metadata, he/she must work using an editing system combined with the DBMS. This means the work place for metadata handling is limited around the DBMS. So, editing metadata "off-line" is difficult in some situation.

Another problem is the difficulty of a local database re-organization. This happens when someone wants to download a set of specially localized media data from a large database system and tries to re-organize or merge with another local database. He/she may able to collect and download the media data, but may not able to download the associated metadata easily as he/she wants to do.

These problems are caused by the fact that media data and the metadata are separately handled in the system and associated with media data under the tight control of the DBMS.

One solution to this problem is that each media data carries its own metadata as well as some additional data that may be used in some other system in an embedded form according to a steganography such as BPCS. This application of the steganography makes use of the property (D) above. We are finding a new way to go in this new direction.

8.3 An Attack to BPCS Steganography Using Complexity Histogram and Countermeasure

BPCS allows the replacement of nearly half of cover image in size with secret data without any image degradation that can be perceived by humans. Through several experiments, however, we have confirmed that the shape of the complexity histogram of the image with secret data embedded is, in general, different from that of the original one. Here the complexity histogram represents the relative frequency of occurrence of the various complexities in the binary image. The unnatural distribution of complexity histogram, hence, can be used as a signature or a distinguishing mark between natural images and images with information embedded by BPCS. Since the term "steganography" literally means "covered writing," steganographic techniques should not be distinguishable from cover images.

In this section, we discuss this possible attack to BPCS and present a countermeasure that removes this distinguishing mark. The problem of BPCS is that all bits in noise-like regions are used for secret data. This causes the complexity of secret data to be different from that of the original noisy pattern replaced with secret information. In the proposed method, only half of the bits in noise-like regions are used for secret data. The remaining half of the bits are used to adjust the complexity measure in those regions. The adjustment of complexity is performed by changing the pixel values of the bits in the noise-like regions that are not used for encoding secret data.

8.3.1 Changes in Complexity Histograms

Let P_{ORG} be a block replaced with secret data and P_{EMB} be a squared binary pattern mapped from secret data. From a principle of embedding in BPCS, the complexity of P_{ORG} and P_{EMB} satisfies the following conditions

$$\alpha_{\mathrm{TH}} \leq \alpha(P_{\mathrm{ORG}}) \quad \text{and} \quad \alpha_{\mathrm{TH}} \leq \alpha(P_{\mathrm{EMB}}) \tag{8.6}$$

where "$\alpha(P_{\mathrm{ORG}})$" means the complexity of P_{ORG} and α_{TH} represents the threshold used to determine whether the subimage is noise-like or not. However the following equation is not always satisfied,

$$\alpha(P_{\mathrm{ORG}}) = \alpha(P_{\mathrm{EMB}}). \tag{8.7}$$

This causes a change in the shape of the complexity histogram. In order to explain this fact, we will look at the complexity histogram in greater detail. As mentioned above, the complexity histogram used in this section represents the relative frequency of occurrence of the various complexities in a binary pattern. Because the complexity of an original binary pattern is rarely equal to that of a binary pattern mapped from secret data, a change in shape in the complexity histogram will generally occur. Binary patterns having a complexity value that exceeds the threshold are substituted for noise-like binary patterns (secret data) having the complexity distribution described below.

One might assume that the complexities of random binary patterns of size $n \times n$ would follow a normal distribution, and indeed, this has been experimentally verified [9]. Thus, for BPCS, patterns in bit-plane images that are replaced by secret information generally have a normal distribution of complexities, because the secret information is noise-like.

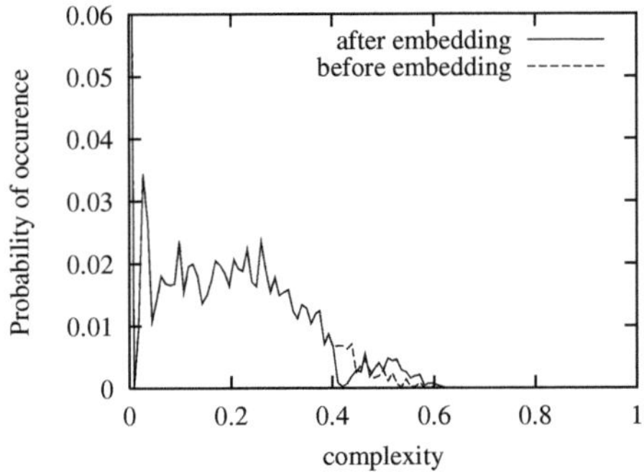

Fig. 8.5. Complexity histogram of 4th bitplane ($\alpha_{TH} = 0.41$).

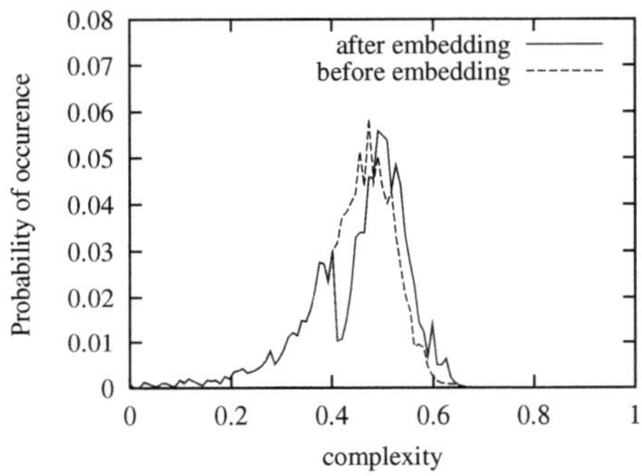

Fig. 8.6. Complexity histogram of 6th bitplane ($\alpha_{TH} = 0.41$).

We embedded pseudo random data into the gray scale image called Peppers (512×512, 8 bit/pixel) using BPCS with $\alpha_{\text{TH}} = 0.41$. Local regions on all bit-planes having more than the threshold in complexity were substituted with pseudo random data. Figs. 8.5 and 8.6 show complexity histograms of the 4th and 6th bit-planes using BPCS with $\alpha_{\text{TH}} = 0.41$. We can see an unusual shape in the form of a valley near the threshold. The distribution of the substituted pattern (complexities greater than the threshold) is a normal distribution. In the middle bit-planes, noise-like patterns and non noise-like patterns are mixed. In embedding in these planes, patterns that are above the threshold change to the normal distribution and a discontinuity in the complexity measure histogram around the threshold becomes noticeable.

8.3.2 Histogram Preserving Embedding

In BPCS, binary patterns for the replacement of noisy blocks are generated from only secret data. In the proposed method, on the other hand, binary patterns are generated both from secret data and the bits used to adjust the complexity.

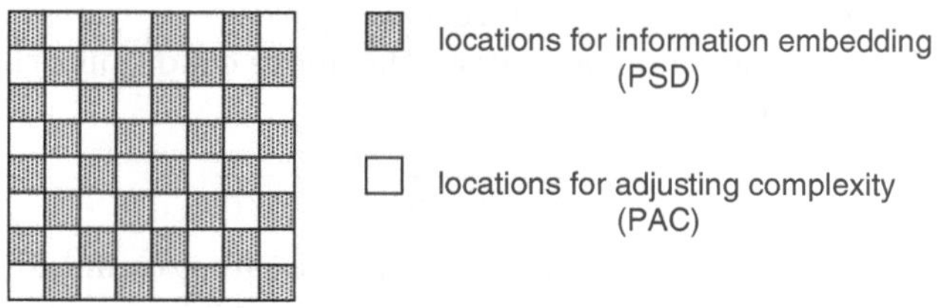

Fig. 8.7. Information assignment.

Approach to Adjust Complexity

In order to adjust the complexity of blocks in binary images, we use only half of the pixels in the image. The remaining half of the pixels are used for adjusting complexity. Pixels of the images are divided into two groups, *group A* and *group B*. Pixels in *group A* are used for secret information and pixels in *group B* are used for adjusting complexity. The pixels of group A are the pixels for secret data, and are termed *PSD*. The pixels of group B are the pixels for adjusting complexity, and are termed *PAC*. The locations of the PSD and PAC correspond to a checkerboard pattern. Fig. 8.7 shows the bit assignment of PSD and PAC in the images.

In the proposed method, we redefine noisy patterns as

$$0.5 - \delta \leq \alpha(P) \leq 0.5 + \delta. \tag{8.8}$$

where P is a binary image and δ is a constant coefficient satisfying $0 < \delta \leq 0.5$.

Next, to generate the binary patterns for embedding, we divide a bit-plane of the cover image into $m \times m$ size blocks. Let $P^i(i = 1, 2, \cdots, N)$ be the noise-like blocks and $C^i(= \alpha(P^i))$ be the complexity of P^i. The complexity histogram of blocks that are replaced with secret data is denoted by $h_{\mathrm{ORG}}(c), (0.5 - \delta \leq c \leq 0.5 + \delta)$. $h_{\mathrm{ORG}}(c)$ is the number of blocks of complexity c. In order to represent the complexity histogram of blocks that have been replaced with secret data, we define the another histogram denoted by $h_{\mathrm{EMB}}(c), (0.5 - \delta \leq k \leq 0.5 + \delta)$, and initialize $h_{\mathrm{EMB}}(c)$ to "0."

Firstly, we map a binary sequence having the size of $(m \times m)/2$ extracted from secret data on PSD in P^i. Then, we set the target complexity of P^i by the following steps.

a-1) C_{org} and e are initialized as C^i and 0 respectively.

a-2) Let k_c and k_s be $C_{\mathrm{org}} + e$ and $C_{\mathrm{org}} - e$. The k_c is the target complexity if the following condition is satisfied,

$$h_{\mathrm{ORG}}(k_c) > h_{\mathrm{EMB}}(k_c) \quad \text{and} \quad k_c \leq 0.5 + \delta. \tag{8.9}$$

The k_s is also the target complexity if the following condition is satisfied,

$$h_{\mathrm{ORG}}(k_s) > h_{\mathrm{EMB}}(k_s) \quad \text{and} \quad 0.5 - \delta \leq k_s. \tag{8.10}$$

If both k_c and k_s are the the target complexity, we choose one of them randomly. If k_c and k_s do not satisfy the above conditions, then the value of e is changed by

$$e \leftarrow e + \frac{1}{2 \times m \times (m-1)}, \tag{8.11}$$

and the above conditions are re-checked. The target complexity is denoted by C_t in the following.

The complexity of P^i is adjusted by the following steps using the target complexity and h_{EMB} and h_{ORG}. In PAC on P^i, there are pixels having the property that the complexity of P^i becomes larger by reversing its value. We denote the set of pixels having the property as B^+. There are also pixels having the property that the complexity of P^i becomes smaller by reversing its value. We denote the set of pixels having the property as B^-.

b-1) Go to the step **b-2** if P^i satisfies the following condition,

$$\alpha(P^i) < c. \tag{8.12}$$

Go to the step **b-3** if P^i satisfies the following condition,

$$\alpha(P^i) > c. \tag{8.13}$$

Go to the step **b-4** if the above conditions are not satisfied, this means $\alpha(P^i) = C_t$.

b-2) Choose a pixel from B^+, reverse the its value and remove it from B^+. Choose a pixel randomly if there are pixels having the same property. This step is repeated until $\alpha(P^i)$ is equal to C_t or greater, or B^+ is empty. In order for P^i to satisfy noisy pattern, the pixel value of the last pixel that has been reversed is reversed if the following condition is satisfied,

$$\alpha(P^i) > 0.5 + \delta. \tag{8.14}$$

Go to **b-4** if this step is finished.

b-3) Choose a pixel from B^-, reverse the its value and remove it from B^-. Choose a pixel randomly if there are pixels having the same property. This step is repeated until $\alpha(P^i)$ is equal to C_t or smaller, or B^- is empty. In oder for P^i to satisfy noisy pattern, the pixel value of the last pixel that has been reversed is reversed if the following condition is satisfied,

$$\alpha(P^i) < 0.5 - \delta. \tag{8.15}$$

Go to **b-4** if this step is finished.

b-4) $h_{\mathrm{EMB}}(c)$ is changed by the following equation,

$$h_{\mathrm{EMB}}(\alpha(P^i)) \leftarrow h_{\mathrm{EMB}}(\alpha(P^i)) + 1. \tag{8.16}$$

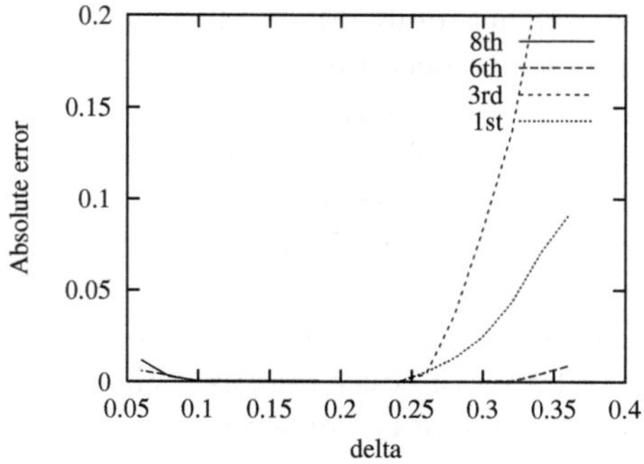

Fig. 8.8. Error of histogram adjustment.

8.3.3 Experiments and Discussions

We investigated the relation between δ and the accuracy of the adjusted complexity histogram. In the experiments, all of noise-like blocks in the cover image are replaced with random binary sequences representing secret data. In order to evaluate the accuracy in adjusting the shape of the complexity histogram, we defined the measure of the accuracy as follows,

$$\text{error} = \sum_i |h_o(i) - h_e(i)|, \tag{8.17}$$

where $h_o(i)$ and $h_e(i)$ represent the histograms of the cover image and the stego image, respectively.

The error was calculated from $\delta = 0.04$ to 0.36 with 0.02 increments. The result is shown in Fig. 8.8. As can be seen, the shape of the complexity histogram with $0.1 \leq \delta \leq 0.25$ is virtually identical before embedding and after embedding.

8.3.4 Conclusions

We have proposed an improved BPCS steganography technique that removes an identifying signature that can be found in conventional BPCS steganography. The improved BPCS is robust against attacks using complexity histogram because the complexity distribution is quasi-preserved by adjusting the complexity of the embedded patterns.

8.4 Visual Attack to BPCS Steganography and Countermeasure

BPCS replaces noisy blocks on bit-planes with the binary patterns mapped from secret data. The complexity is used to determine whether blocks are noise-like. BPCS can extract embedded information by using the simple thresholding in the complexity because secret data is replaced with only complex regions. To compensate the extraction, the logical operation called conjugate operation is used for the binary patterns look like informative regions. Therefore, we need to keep, for each block, the flag called conjugation flag representing whether the conjugate operation had been applied.

In the case where we build a secure system to exchange secret messages using BPCS, which is explained latter in detail, the conjugation flags must be embedded within a fixed area of cover images. When the conjugate flags are embedded in the manner, we can easily see unnatural patterns by observing the image visually. It can be used as a signature or a distinguishing mark between natural images and images with information embedded by BPCS, and it is regarded as a visual attack [10, 11, 12] to BPCS.

We propose a countermeasure to the visual attack of BPCS. The reason why BPCS is weak against the visual attack is to embed conjugation flags within a fixed area. The proposed method can embed the flags into each block by the thresholding in the complexity, as a result of the embedding, the distinguishing mark would be removed.

8.4.1 Finding Signature of Information Embedding by Visual Observation

In the secret key cryptosystem consisting of a sender and a receiver connected with an insecure channel, the important messages between them is encoded with a key at the sender and the encoded one is transmitted to the receiver over the insecure channel. At the receiver side, the received message is decoded with the key. It is possible to encode and decode with only one key. If we exchange somehow the key by using secure channel once, after that, we can keep exchanging encoded messages without exchanging the key again. If we require the convenience of the cryptosystem to BPCS, it is desirable to choose information which does not depend on image data and secret data as the key.

In order to extract the embedded information from stego-images with secret data embedded by BPCS, we need to know the information about the threshold and the block size used in embedding, and conjugation flags. Conjugation flags are not candidate for the key because those depend on image data, block size, secret data and the threshold. Therefore, conjugation flags must be embedded within cover images in the system.

The conjugation flags, however, are not embedded by the complexity thresholding because the additional conjugation flag is needed for the blocks in which the conjugation flags are embedded. Therefore the conjugation flags must be embedded into a fixed area of cover images.

There are several ways to embed conjugation flags within a fixed area on cover images. The simplest way to do that is to embed those information into a fixed area on LSB (Least Significant Bit) plane. We can embed it without degrading the quality of cover images because it is not noticeable

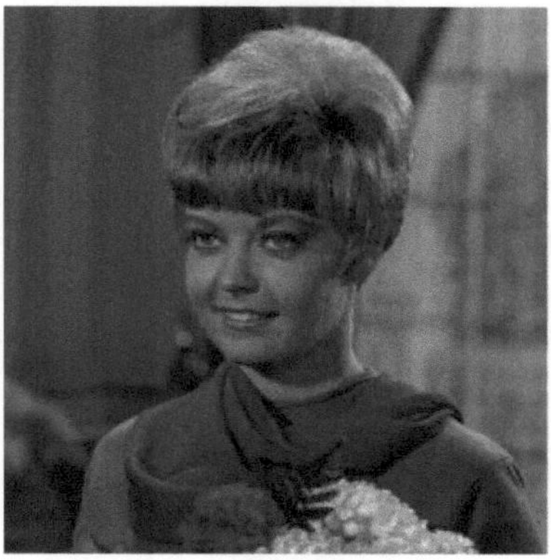

Fig. 8.9. Gray scale representation.

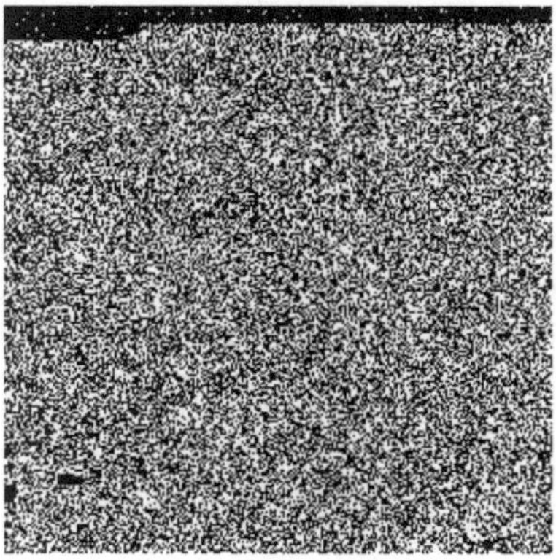

Fig. 8.10. LSB of Fig. 8.9 with Gray code.

intensity changes in the LSB plane for gray scale images. However, we can detect unnatural patterns by looking the LSB plane. For example, Fig. 8.9 shows the stego-image with secret data embedded by BPCS with $m = 8$ and $\alpha_{\mathrm{TH}} = 46/112$. The amount of the noisy region was about 31% of the original image. All of the regions are substituted with noisy patterns and the conjugation flags are embedded from the left upper block with raster scanning without checking whether blocks are noise-like. Fig. 8.10 shows the LSB plane of Fig. 8.9. We can easily see the unnatural pattern on upper part by comparing the image with the gray scale representation (Fig. 8.9). In general, the LSB plane for natural images looks like noisy patterns. Because we know such the characteristic of the LSB plane, it is easy to detect unnatural patterns from the stego-image, and it can be regarded as the signature of BPCS.

8.4.2 Robust Embedding against the Visual Attack

Outline

The reason why BPCS is weak against the visual attack is to embed conjugation flags without using the complexity thresholding. Therefore, if both secret data and the conjugation flags can be embedded by the complexity thresholding, BPCS would be robust against it. To realize this idea, we embed conjugation flags into each block.

Embedding

Let S be a $m \times m$ squared binary image mapped from the bit sequences of secret data. The conjugation flag, which takes on "0" or "1", of S can be embedded within S if we make the value of a pixel on S correspond to the flag. We call the pixel assigned the flag *a control pixel.* The value of the control pixel represents whether the conjugation operation had been applied. In this section we define that "1" of control pixel means the conjugate operation had been applied to S.

First, the proposed method initializes the control pixel as "0", then makes the bit sequences of secret data map on S except for the control pixel, next, calculates the complexity. By the complexity, the method determines whether the value of the control pixel should be changed form "0" to "1." In the following, $S_{\mathrm{CP}=0}$ and $S_{\mathrm{CP}=1}$ represent that the value of the control pixel is equal to "0" and "1."

We use one of the four corner of S as the control pixel. Because we consider 4 connectivity of pixels through this section, there are 2 adjacent pixels of the control pixel. Thus, we can categorize adjacent-pixel patterns into 3 patterns : the both values are 0, the both values are 1, and one is 0 and another is 1, and vice versa. Each pattern is denoted by BB, WW and BW in the following.

As mentioned earlier section, conjugation flags are not needed for the S whose complexity is within α_{TH} and $1 - \alpha_{\mathrm{TH}}$. In that case, it is better to embed secret data to the control pixel to increase data hiding capacity. In the extraction procedure, it is desirable that the meaning of the control pixel is determined by the complexity of a block in which the control pixel is, that is, when the complexity is greater than or equal to α_{TH} and less than or equal to $1 - \alpha_{\mathrm{TH}}$, the control pixel represents secret data and, otherwise, that represents conjugation flag. We can easily assign the meaning to the control pixel in embedding, however, in some case, the meaning may change in extraction because the complexity would be affected by changing the value of the control pixel.

We show here an example of that case. Let $\beta(S)$ be $\alpha(S) \times 2m(m-1)$, β_{TH} be $\alpha_{\mathrm{TH}} \times 2m(m-1)$, β^{*}_{TH} be $(1 - \alpha_{\mathrm{TH}}) \times 2m(m-1)$. We now consider the case where $\beta(S_{\mathrm{CP}=0}) = \beta_{\mathrm{TH}} - 2$ and the adjacent pixel pattern is BB. For the S, we need to apply the conjugate operation because the complexity of S

Table 8.1. Meaning of the control pixel and its value.

$\beta(S_{\mathrm{CP}=0})$	Adjacent pixel patterns	Control Pixel	
		Meaning	Value
$\lceil\beta_{\mathrm{TH}}\rceil - 2$ or $\lceil\beta_{\mathrm{TH}}\rceil - 1$	BB	CAB	1
	WW or BW	CF	1
$\lceil\beta_{\mathrm{TH}}\rceil$ or $\lceil\beta_{\mathrm{TH}}\rceil + 1$	BB or WW	SD	b_n
	BW	SD	0 (if b_n=0)
		CF	1 (if b_n=1)
$\lfloor\beta^*_{\mathrm{TH}}\rfloor - 1$ or $\lfloor\beta^*_{\mathrm{TH}}\rfloor$	BB	CAB	0
	WW or BW	SD	b_n
$\lfloor\beta^*_{\mathrm{TH}}\rfloor + 1$ or $\lfloor\beta^*_{\mathrm{TH}}\rfloor + 2$	BB or WW	CF	0
	BW	CF	0 (if b_n=0)
		SD	1 (if b_n=1)

is less than α_{TH}. If we make the value of the control pixel of S change to "1," then the maximum change in the border length is 2, thus the complexity of $S_{\mathrm{CP}=1}$ may become $\lceil\beta_{\mathrm{TH}}\rceil$. The control pixel of the $S_{\mathrm{CP}=1}$ can be extracted as the secret data because, after the conjugate operation, $\alpha(S_{\mathrm{CP}=1})$ falls within a range of α_{TH} and $1 - \alpha_{\mathrm{TH}}$. Thus, it would be impossible for this example to recover embedded information because the meaning of the control pixel is determined as not conjugation flag, but one bit of secret data.

To avoid this miss determination, we assign another function to adjust the complexity to the control pixel. Suppose that *CF*, *SD* and *CAB* represent conjugation flag, secret data and the complexity-adjustment bit, respectively. The control pixel holds one of CF, SD or CAB, and takes on one of 0 and 1 value. Those meaning and values depend on the complexity of S, one bit of the secret data which is embedded into the control pixel of S and the adjacent-pixel pattern of the control pixel.

The proposed method, which is robust against the visual attack, is given as the following.

Step 1) Choose a pixel from four corners of S as the control pixel, and initialize it as "0."

Step 2) Map the bit sequences of secret data to the pixels of S except for the control pixel.

Step 3) Calculate the complexity of $S_{\mathrm{CP}=0}$.

Step 4) By the calculated complexity, define the meaning and the value of the control pixel.

- If $\beta(S_{\mathrm{CP}=0}) < \beta_{\mathrm{TH}} - 2$, then the meaning of the control pixel of S is CF and its value is "1." Then the conjugate operation is applied to S.
- If $\beta_{\mathrm{TH}} + 2 \leq \beta(S_{\mathrm{CP}=0}) \leq \beta^*_{\mathrm{TH}} - 2$, then the meaning of the control pixel of S is SD and its value is one bit of the secret data.

- If $\beta(S_{\mathrm{CP}=0}) \geq \beta^*_{\mathrm{TH}} + 2$, the meaning of the control pixel of S is CF and its value is "0."
- Otherwise the meaning and the value of the control pixel depend on the complexity, the adjacent pixel patterns and a bit to be embedded into the control pixel. Table 8.1 shows the meaning and the value in each case. In the table, b_n means a bit of secret data which is embedded into the control pixel.

Step 5) Replace noisy blocks with S.

Extraction

Following BPCS extraction steps, we can extract the blocks, which are denoted by S', containing the secret data by the complexity thresholding. All of S' can be satisfied the following inequality about their complexity.

$$\alpha(S') \geq \alpha_{\mathrm{TH}} \tag{8.18}$$

Basically, the embedded secret data is recovered from S' by the simple rule described below.

- When the complexity of S' is less than or equal to $1 - \alpha_{\mathrm{TH}}$, then the control pixel means a bit of secret data. Thus all bits of S' are a part of secret data.
- When the complexity S' is greater than $1 - \alpha_{\mathrm{TH}}$, then the control pixel means a conjugation flag. If the conjugation flag is equal to "1," then we apply the conjugate operation to it. All the bits except for the control pixel of the S' applied the conjugate operation are a part of secret data.

In order to take account of Table 8.1 used in the embedding procedure, in addition, we need the exception rule described bellow.

- When the complexity of S' is equal to β_{TH} or $\beta_{\mathrm{TH}} + 1$, the control pixel means CAB if the its value is equal to "1" and the adjacent pixel pattern is BB.
- When the complexity of S' is equal to $\beta^*_{\mathrm{TH}} - 1$ or β^*_{TH}, the control pixel means CAB if the its value is equal to "0" and the adjacent pixel pattern is BB.

Embedded secret data can be recovered after the above steps are performed for all blocks containing secret data.

8.4.3 Experimental Result and Discussions

We used the GIRL (256 × 256, 8 bit/pixel) image as cover image. Noisy-regions determined with $m = 8$ and $\alpha_{\mathrm{TH}} = 46/112$ were replaced with another noisy pattern. We are unable to detect unnatural pattern from Fig. 8.11. in

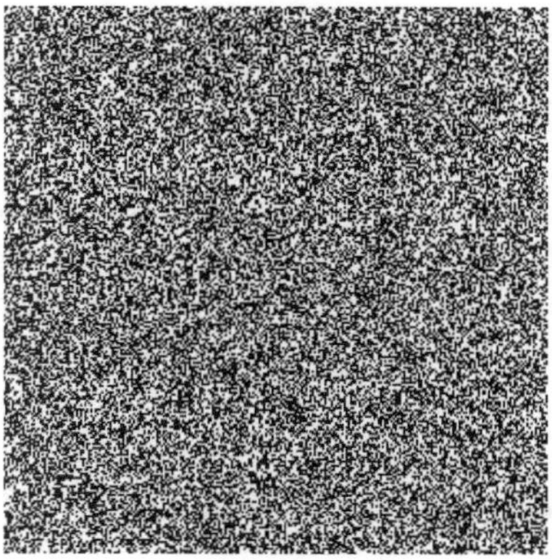

Fig. 8.11. LSB plane of the image with secret data embedded by the proposed method.

other words, we are unable to distinguish between the LSB of the cover image and that of the stego-image.

The proposed method decreases 1 bit of hiding data capacity for blocks whose complexity is less than α_{TH} or greater than $1 - \alpha_{\mathrm{TH}}$. If α_{TH} is getting close to 0, then the number of blocks we need to apply conjugate operation decreases. In such cases, the proposed method is useless because conjugation flags are not needed in extracting embedded information. However, image degradation will occur on the image data as detectable patterns. Moreover, by the comparison between bit-planes, one can easily recognize the existence of embedded information. Therefore, the proposed method is very effective, that is secure, when we embed secret data with keeping high image quality by using BPCS.

8.4.4 Conclusion

We have presented an improved BPCS steganography that removes an identifying signature that can be found in conventional BPCS steganography. The proposed method can embed both secret data and the conjugation flags into cover images with image segmentation using the complexity thresholding, therefore, unnatural patterns which can be used as the signature do not appear in the stego-images.

8.5 Application of BPCS Steganography to JPEG2000 Encoded Images

BPCS steganography is not robust with respect to lossy compression of dummy image, as are all other bit-plane-based steganography methods. To deploy the merits of BPCS steganography technique, in a practical scenario where the dummy image should be compressed before being transmitted, we propose a steganography technique based on JPEG2000 lossy compression scheme [13] and BPCS steganography. In JPEG2000 compression, wavelet coefficients of an image are quantized into a bit-plane structure and therefore BPCS steganography can be applied in the wavelet domain. The proposed JPEG2000-BPCS steganography provides a significant integration of JPEG2000 lossy compression scheme and BPCS steganography, and a solution to the aforementioned problem associated with bit-plane-based steganography methods.

8.5.1 JPEG2000 Compression Standard

JPEG2000 encoder consists of several fundamental components: pre-processing, discrete wavelet transform (DWT), quantization, arithmetic coding (tier-1 coding), and bit-stream organization (tier-2 coding) [13] (see the left part of Fig. 8.12). Pre-processing includes intercomponent transformation for multi-component images, typically color images. After the DWT is applied to each component, wavelet coefficients are quantized uniformly with deadzone. After the quantization step, an optional step to realize a functionality called region of interest (ROI) can be added. The ROI is realized by scaling up the wavelet coefficients in the relevant regions. The quantized wavelet coefficients are then bit-plane encoded by arithmetic coding.

In JPEG2000, each subband of the wavelet transformed image is encoded independently of the other subbands. Furthermore, each subband is partitioned into small blocks called codeblocks, and each codeblock is independently encoded by EBCOT algorithm [14]. This procedure is absolutely different from other well-known embedded wavelet coders such as EZW [15] and SPIHT [16]. The independent encoding of codeblocks provides many advantages such as localized random access into image, improved error resilience, efficient rate control, and flexible bit-stream ordering. The quantized wavelet coefficients in a codeblock are bit-plane encoded by three passes with arithmetic coding: significance propagation pass, refinement pass, and cleanup pass.

The compressed data from the codeblocks are organized into units called packets and layers in tier-2 coding. A precinct is a collection of spatially contiguous codeblocks from all subbands at a resolution level. The compressed data from the codeblocks in a precinct constitutes a packet. A collection of packets from all resolution levels constitutes a layer. Therefore a layer corresponds to one quality increment for the entire full resolution image. In JPEG2000, different types of progression orders are possible and a typical one is layer-resolution-component-position progression. Once the entire image has been compressed, a rate-distortion optimized bit-stream is generated for a target file size (bit rate).

8.5.2 JPEG2000-BPCS Steganography

Basically, secret data can be embedded in the bit-plane representation of the quantized wavelet coefficients after quantization step, provided that the rate-distortion optimization of JPEG2000 is bypassed. However, this procedure, which determines the optimal number of bit-planes for a given bit rate, is an essential part of the codec which contributes to its high compression efficiency. Thus, to avoid compromising the compression efficiency of JPEG2000, data embedding by BPCS is decided to be performed right after ROI descaling in decoding process where the optimal bit-plane structure for a given bit rate is available. The procedure for data embedding and extraction in JPEG2000-BPCS steganography is shown in Fig. 8.12.

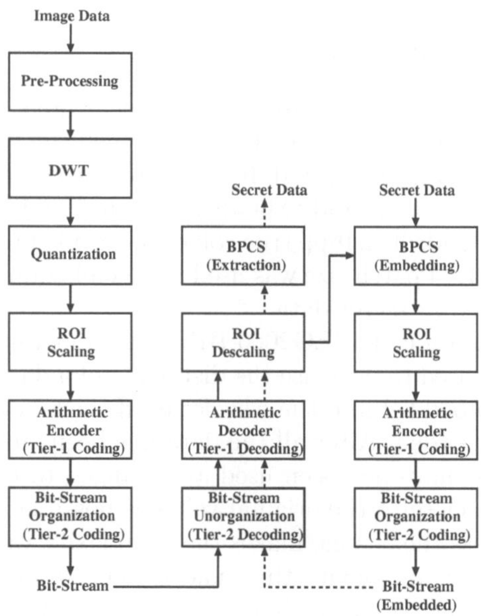

Fig. 8.12. A flowchart of data embedding and extraction in JPEG2000-BPCS steganography.

The entire process to embed data in JPEG2000-BPCS steganography follows the solid line arrows shown in Fig. 8.12. An image is encoded into JPEG2000 bit-stream, whose size can be met almost exactly to a target bit rate (bit per pixel; bpp). The encoding process is shown in the left part of Fig. 8.12; from pre-processing to bit-stream organization. The JPEG2000 bit-stream (compressed image file) is then decoded, but decoding is halted right after ROI descaling. The information at this point is used to construct the bit-planes of quantized wavelet coefficients and then used to embed secret data with BPCS steganography (see the top box of the right part in Fig. 8.12). The quantized wavelet coefficients modified by embedding are then subjected to JPEG2000 encoding again, which produces secret-data-embedded JPEG2000 bit-stream. Data embedding into an already compressed JPEG2000 file is also possible. In this case, the process starts with a JPEG2000 compressed image, i.e., a bit-stream from the bottom of the middle part in Fig. 8.12 and follows the same process as the aforementioned one.

The data extraction procedure follows the dashed arrows in the middle part of Fig. 8.12. JPEG2000 decoding of the secret-data-embedded bit-stream starts from bit-stream unorganization and is halted right after ROI descaling. At this point, extraction of secret data is carried out by the BPCS method using the bit-planes of quantized wavelet coefficients. We assume that the data extraction starts after the entire file of the bit-stream has been received.

8.5.3 Experimental Results

The JPEG2000-BPCS steganography was implemented using JJ2000 Java software of JPEG2000 compression [17], with which the program module for BPCS steganography was integrated. It was tested on several standard images including "Lena," "Barbara" and "Mandrill," "Lena" and "Barbara" are 8bpp gray images and "Mandrill" 24bpp true color image, all of which were 512×512 pixels in size. Here 4×4 patch size was used as an embedding unit and random binary data was used as secret data.

In the implementation of JPEG2000-BPCS steganography, an error correction scheme was devised to decrease the distortion of a data-embedded image. As data is being embedded into the wavelet coefficients, each bit that is used for embedding is recorded. After all the data has been embedded, the bits of each coefficient that have not been used are changed to bring the new value of the coefficient as close to the original value as possible. The change of bits is only allowed unless the change makes the complexity value for the relevant patch larger than the complexity threshold for embedding. The PSNR with the error correction increased by about 1.7 dB. In the following experiments, the error correction was always applied.

Results of embedding experiments are shown in Fig. 8.13. The least significant bit-plane and the two least significant bit-planes were used to embed data for 0.5bpp and 1.0bpp compressed image, respectively. 9 data points within each line in Fig. 8.13 were obtained by changing the complexity threshold α_0[3] from 2 to 10. In Fig. 8.13 data points for no data embedding are also included. Note that the compression rate for color "Mandrill" image is in fact three times less than those for the other gray images.

Generally, the JPEG2000-BPCS steganography was able to achieve embedding rates of around 9% of the final compressed image size for pre-embedding

[3] The complexity is hereinafter measured by k in Eq. (8.1), i.e., the total length of the black-and-white border without normalization by the maximum possible border length.

0.5bpp images, and 15% for pre-embedding 1.0bpp images with no noticeable degradation in image quality. These results were derived with the complexity threshold $\alpha_0 = 8$.

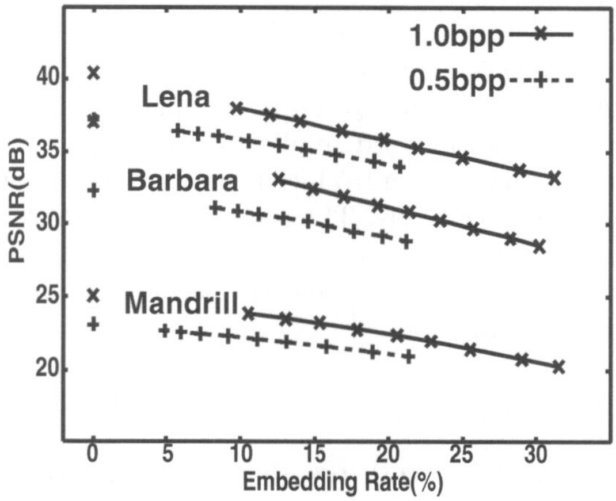

Fig. 8.13. Results of embedding experiments by JPEG2000-BPCS steganography.

8.5.4 Conclusions

This chapter presented a solution to the problem of hiding data into compressed image files in bit-plane-based steganography methods. The proposed scheme is based on a seamless integration of BPCS steganography with JPEG2000 image compression standard. Embedding rates of around 15% of the compressed image size were achieved for pre-embedding 1.0bpp compressed images with no noticeable degradation in image quality. The proposed JPEG2000-BPCS steganography will allow many more people access to the benefits of BPCS steganography due to many desirable features of JPEG2000 standard.

8.6 Histogram Preserving JPEG Steganography

The JPEG compression using the discrete cosine transform (DCT) is still the most common compression standard for still images, though the JPEG2000 standard has already been released. Getting less attention, JPEG images are therefore the most suitable dummy (cover) images for steganography using compressed images. Several steganographic techniques using JPEG images have already been proposed such as J-Steg [18] and F5 [19]. It is well known that embedding by J-Steg is detectable using the chi-square attack [19] since it is based on flipping the least significant bits (LSBs). F5 cannot be detected by the chi-square attack. However it can be detected by a specific technique [20] which exploits a significant change on the histogram of quantized DCT coefficients caused by embedding.

This section presents two histogram preserving JPEG steganographic methods. The first one is a histogram quasi-preserving method which uses quantization index modulation (QIM) [21] at quantization step of DCT coefficients. Since a straightforward application of QIM causes a significant histogram change, a device is introduced in order not to change the after-embedding histogram excessively. The second one is a histogram preserving method which uses a histogram matching technique. Here we call the first method QIM-JPEG steganography and the second one histogram matching JPEG (HM-JPEG) steganography.

8.6.1 QIM in DCT Domain

Consider applying QIM [21] with two different quantizers to embed binary data at the quantization step of DCT coefficients in JPEG compression. Each bit (zero or one) of binary data is embedded in such a way that one of two quantizers is used for quantization of a DCT coefficient, which corresponds to embed zero, and the other quantizer is used to embed one. Given a quantization table and a quality factor for JPEG compression, quantization step size $\Delta_k, 1 \leq k \leq 64$ for each frequency component is determined. Then, two codebooks, C^0 and C^1, for two quantizers are chosen as $C^0 = \{2j\Delta_k; j \in Z\}, C^1 = \{(2j+1)\Delta_k; j \in Z\}$ for k-th frequency. Given a k-th frequency DCT coefficient x, $2q$ with $q = \arg\min_j \parallel x - 2j\Delta_k \parallel$ becomes the quantized coefficient in case of embedding zero, for example, and $2q+1$ with $q = \arg\min_j \parallel x - (2j+1)\Delta_k \parallel$ in case of embedding one.

Assuming that the probabilities of zero and one are the same in binary data to be embedded, and considering how histograms of quantized DCT coefficients change after embedding. In the following, we assume that DCT coefficients belonging to k-th frequency are divided by its quantization step size Δ_k in advance and then two codebooks, C^0 and C^1 can be defined as $C^0 = \{2j; j \in Z\}, C^1 = \{2j+1; j \in Z\}$ for all frequency components. Let $h_i, i \in Z$ denote the number of DCT coefficients whose values x are in the interval $i - 0.5 < x < i + 0.5$, which is described as $h_i = N(i - 0.5 < x < i+0.5)$. Let h_i^- and h_i^+ denote the number of DCT coefficients in the interval $i - 0.5 < x < i$ and that in $i < x < i + 0.5$, respectively and therefore $h_i^- + h_i^+ = h_i$. After embedding by QIM, the histogram h_i is changed to $h_i^{'}$ as

$$h_i^{'} = \frac{1}{2}h_i + \frac{1}{2}(h_{i-1}^{+} + h_{i+1}^{-}). \tag{8.19}$$

The change in Eq. (8.19) can be understood as follows. If i is an even number, i.e., $i \in C^0$ and C^0 is used for embedding zero, half of DCT coefficients in the interval $i - 0.5 < x < i + 0.5$ are used for embedding zero and their quantized coefficients are unchanged after embedding. However, the other half, $(h_i^- + h_i^+)/2$ coefficients are used for embedding one, resulting in that $h_i^-/2$ coefficients are quantized to $i-1$ and $h_i^+/2$ coefficients to $i+1$. Alternatively, $h_{i-1}^+/2$ coefficients from the bin $i-1$ and $h_{i+1}^-/2$ coefficients from the bin $i+1$ are quantized to i for embedding zero. With similar consideration, it is easily understood that the change shown in Eq. (8.19) holds true for odd number i.

A typical example of before- and after-embedding histograms is shown in Fig. 8.14. These histograms are those of $(2,2)$ frequency component among 64 components $(k,l), 1 \leq k,l \leq 8$ for "Lena" image (512×512 pixels in size, 8 bit per pixel (bpp)) compressed with quality factor 80. It is seen that the numbers of quantized coefficients for low absolute values around zero change significantly after embedding. Eq. (8.19) indicates that if $h_i = h_{i-1}^+ + h_{i+1}^-$, then the number in the bin i does not change. In particular for $i = 0, \pm 1$, however, much difference between h_i and $h_{i-1}^+ + h_{i+1}^-$ causes the significant change on $h_i^{'}$ after embedding. Therefore a straightforward application of QIM in the DCT domain cannot be allowed for secure steganography against histogram-based attacks.

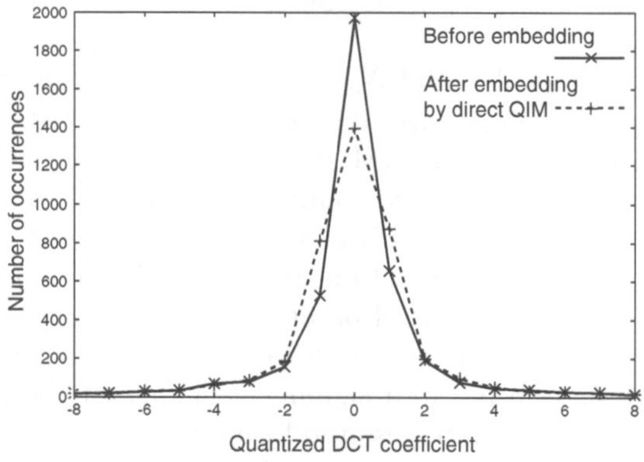

Fig. 8.14. Before- and after-embedding histograms of $(2,2)$ frequency component. Direct application of QIM causes a significant histogram change.

8.6.2 Histogram Quasi-Preserving QIM-JPEG Steganography

As shown in Fig. 8.14, the most significant changes caused by direct application of QIM are decrease of h_0 and increase of h_1 and h_{-1}. Let us try to preserve h_0, h_1 and h_{-1} after embedding. We introduce a dead zone for DCT coefficients x, $t_d^- < x < t_d^+$ $(-0.5 < t_d^- < 0 < t_d^+ < 0.5)$ where DCT coefficients are not used for embedding. The number of positive DCT coefficients

N_d^+ and that of negative coefficients N_d^- in the dead zone are described as $N_d^+ = N(0 < x < t_d^+)$ and $N_d^- = N(t_d^- < x < 0)$, respectively. t_d^+ and t_d^- are determined by optimum N_d^+ and N_d^- values which minimize the histogram changes for 0 and ± 1 bins.

After-embedding histogram $h_i^{'}$, shown in Eq. (8.19), it can be rewritten as

$$h_i^{'} = \frac{1}{2}(h_i^+ + h_{i+1}^-) + \frac{1}{2}(h_i^- + h_{i-1}^+), \tag{8.20}$$

where $(h_i^+ + h_{i+1}^-)/2$ and $(h_i^- + h_{i-1}^+)/2$ correspond to half of DCT coefficients in the interval $i < x < i+1$ and half in $i-1 < x < i$, respectively, and they are quantized to i. By introducing the aforementioned dead zone, part of h_0^+ and h_0^-, i.e., $h_0^+ - N_d^+$ and $h_0^- - N_d^-$ are used for embedding, and therefore $h_0^{'}$, $h_1^{'}$ and $h_{-1}^{'}$ become as follows,

$$h_0^{'} = N_d^+ + \frac{1}{2}\{(h_0^+ - N_d^+) + h_1^-\} + N_d^- + \frac{1}{2}\{(h_0^- - N_d^-) + h_{-1}^+\}, \tag{8.21}$$

$$h_1^{'} = \frac{1}{2}(h_1^+ + h_2^-) + \frac{1}{2}\{h_1^- + (h_0^+ - N_d^+)\}, \tag{8.22}$$

$$h_{-1}^{'} = \frac{1}{2}\{h_{-1}^+ + (h_0^- - N_d^-)\} + \frac{1}{2}(h_{-1}^- + h_{-2}^+). \tag{8.23}$$

The optimum values for N_d^+ and N_d^- can be derived by minimizing the sum of squared histogram changes over 0 and ± 1 bins, $\sum_{i=-1}^{1}(h_i - h_i^{'})^2$.

Note that in the proposed QIM-JPEG steganography, quantized coefficients 0's cannot be treated as zeroes embedded in them, because they cannot be discriminated from 0's in the dead zone. Therefore, if 0 coefficient is selected to embed a zero at quantization step, the embedding process to embed the zero should be continued until other even coefficient except 0 is chosen. This causes a serious problem on the histogram that a surplus of even coefficients is produced resulting in a significant change of the after-embedding histogram. This problem can be resolved by applying the exclusive OR (XOR) operation to a message bit with a random bit whenever embedding a message bit. That is, an embedding bit is the XOR-applied message bit. When 0 coefficient is selected to embed a zero of embedding bit, which means no message embedded, an embedding bit at subsequent embedding is not necessarily kept same though the message bit is same until non-0 coefficient is selected. The message bits can be recovered from the embedded XOR-applied message bits using the same random binary sequence as one used in embedding.

8.6.3 Histogram Preserving HM-JPEG Steganography

Consider histogram matching at quantization step of DCT coefficients, assuming that the probabilities of zero and one are same in binary data to be embedded. Histogram matching is here considered separately for positive coefficient part and negative one, since there sometimes exists asymmetry between both parts. In the following, the matching for positive part is only described (negative part can be treated in the same way).

Two quantizers, $Q^0(x)$ and $Q^1(x)$ are prepared: the former used to embed zero and the latter to embed one,

$$Q^0(x) = 2j,\ t_j^0 < x < t_{j+1}^0,\ j \in \{0, 1, 2, \ldots\}, \tag{8.24}$$

$$Q^1(x) = 2j + 1,\ t_j^1 < x < t_{j+1}^1,\ j \in \{0, 1, 2, \ldots\}, \tag{8.25}$$

where x is a positive DCT coefficient and $t_0^0 = t_0^1 = 0$. The decision threshold values $t_j^0, j \in \{1, 2, \ldots\}$ for $Q^0(x)$ are set so that they satisfy

$$\frac{1}{2}N(t_j^0 < x < t_{j+1}^0) = \begin{cases} h_0^+ & \text{for } j = 0, \\ h_{2j} & \text{for } j \in \{1, 2, \ldots\}, \end{cases} \tag{8.26}$$

where $N(t_j^0 < x < t_{j+1}^0)$ depicts the number of coefficients in the interval $t_j^0 < x < t_{j+1}^0$. Note that 1/2 in Eq. (8.26) means that half of relevant coefficients are used for embedding zero and its number is adjusted to h_0^+ or h_{2j} of cover image to preserve the histogram of cover image. The decision threshold values $t_j^1, j \in \{1, 2, \ldots\}$ for $Q^1(x)$ are similarly set as they satisfy

$$\frac{1}{2}N(t_j^1 < x < t_{j+1}^1) = h_{2j+1},\ j \in \{0, 1, 2, \ldots\}. \tag{8.27}$$

From Eqs. (8.26) and (8.27), it is found that the histogram preservation can be realized if $h_0^+ + \sum_{j=1}^{\infty} h_{2j} = \sum_{j=0}^{\infty} h_{2j+1} = N(0 < x < \infty)/2$. The condition $h_0^+ + \sum_{j=1}^{\infty} h_{2j} = \sum_{j=0}^{\infty} h_{2j+1}$, i.e., $\sharp even = \sharp odd$ is infrequently approximately satisfied in histograms for very low frequency components, but never hold true in general. The relation $\sharp even > \sharp odd$ generally holds true, and in high frequency components, $\sharp even \gg \sharp odd$ because h_0^+ is much larger than others.

Consider how to match after-embedding histogram with before-embedding one under the relation of $\sharp even > \sharp odd$. We introduce a dead zone, $0 < x < t_d$ ($t_d < 0.5$) in which DCT coefficients are not used for embedding[4]. t_d is determined as it fulfills

$$N_d = N(0 < x < t_d) = \sharp even - \sharp odd. \tag{8.28}$$

Eq. (8.28) means that $\sharp odd$ is equal to $\sharp even$ with least N_d coefficients removed. Then using t_d and N_d, the decision threshold values $t_j^0, t_j^1, j \in \{1, 2, \ldots\}$ for $Q^0(x)$ and $Q^1(x)$ are set so that they satisfy Eqs. (8.29)–(8.32),

[4] In case that $\sharp even < \sharp odd$, we cannot introduce the dead zone, i.e., $t_d = 0$, and cannot fully match two histograms. Partial matching is however possible to match for smaller absolute value coefficients (bins). In practice, matching for larger absolute value bins is not needed since the number of samples in such a bin is small and mismatch in such a bin is not distinguishable by steganalysis.

$$\frac{1}{2}N(t_d < x < t_1^0) = h_0^+ - N_d, \tag{8.29}$$

$$\frac{1}{2}N(t_j^0 < x < t_{j+1}^0) = h_{2j}, \qquad j \in \{1, 2, \ldots\}, \tag{8.30}$$

$$\frac{1}{2}N(t_d < x < t_1^1) = h_1, \tag{8.31}$$

$$\frac{1}{2}N(t_j^1 < x < t_{j+1}^1) = h_{2j+1}, \qquad j \in \{1, 2, \ldots\}, \tag{8.32}$$

respectively. Eqs. (8.29) to (8.32) indicate that $\sharp odd$ and $\sharp even - N_d$ are equal to $N(t_d < x < \infty)/2$ and then histogram matching becomes possible. Note that in HM-JPEG steganography, the XOR operation should be applied to embedding message as applied in QIM-JPEG steganography.

The above-mentioned HM-JPEG steganography is a histogram matching method using two quantizers, where the representatives of each quantizer are given in advance and the intervals for each representative are set so as to preserve the histogram of cover image. Though the usage of two quantizers is common to HM-JPEG and QIM-JPEG, the histogram matching method is different from QIM in that the chosen representative of a relevant quantizer is not necessarily closest to a given input. Therefore stego images by HM-JPEG might be more distorted than those by QIM-JPEG.

8.6.4 Experimental Results

Embedding performance of the proposed methods were evaluated comparing with F5 using three standard images: "Lena," "Barbara" and "Mandrill." These images are 512 × 512 pixels in size, 8 bpp gray images, and were compressed with quality factor 80. The least 21 frequency components, including the DC component, in the zigzag scan of 64 components were used for embedding experiments. The histogram change can be measured by Kullback-Leibler divergence.

Experimental results are shown in Table 8.2. Fig. 8.15 shows four histograms of $(1, 1)$ frequency component for "Lena": histogram of cover image (before embedding) and after-embedding histograms by QIM-JPEG, HM-JPEG and F5. The KL divergence value shown in Table 8.2 is the mean for the least 21 frequency components except the DC component. The KL divergence value by F5 is much larger than those by QIM-JPEG and HM-JPEG. Smaller KL divergence values represent better histogram preservation. Furthermore, QIM-JPEG and HM-JPEG achieved higher embedding rates with less degradation of image quality (higher PSNR vales) than F5. Among the two proposed methods, QIM-JPEG produced a bit higher PSNR stego images than HM-JPEG, probably because in QIM-JPEG the closest representative of a relevant quantizer to a given DCT coefficient is chosen as a quantized coefficient.

Table 8.2. Results of embedding experiments.

image	method	embedded data size (bits)	compressed image (bpp)	embedding rate (%)	PSNR (dB)	KL divergence
Lena	(no embedding)	-	1.129	-	38.55	-
	QIM-JPEG	46318	1.163	15.2	37.60	0.00339
	HM-JPEG	45908	1.149	15.2	37.41	0.00138
	F5	35174	0.990	13.6	37.26	0.04783
Barbara	(no embedding)	-	1.517	-	36.92	-
	QIM-JPEG	54241	1.552	13.3	36.07	0.00285
	HM-JPEG	53645	1.543	13.3	35.91	0.00106
	F5	43555	1.392	11.9	35.69	0.04117
Mandrill	(no embedding)	-	2.364	-	32.63	-
	QIM-JPEG	71621	2.378	11.5	32.13	0.00293
	HM-JPEG	71234	2.369	11.5	32.04	0.00124
	F5	61481	2.258	10.4	31.89	0.04543

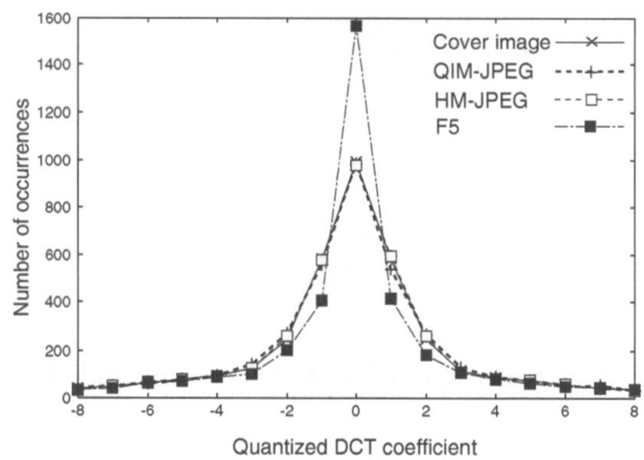

Fig. 8.15. Histograms of (1,1) frequency component for cover image and stego images by QIM-JPEG, HM-JPEG and F5.

8.6.5 Conclusions

We have realized two kinds of high performance JPEG steganography: QIM-JPEG steganography and HM-JPEG steganography. QIM-JPEG is a histogram quasi-preserving method using QIM with a dead zone at quantization step of DCT coefficients. HM-JPEG is a histogram preserving method based on histogram matching using two quantizers with a dead zone. In comparison with F5, the two methods show high performance with regard to embedding rate, PSNR of stego image, and particularly histogram preservation. The proposed methods are promising candidates for high performance as well as secure JPEG steganography against histogram-based steganalysis.

8.7 Experimental Program

We have developed an experimental program to embed and extract information data in/from BMP images according to BPCS method. We also developed another experimental program that was designed for embedding and extracting in/from JPEG images. The JPEG embedding method in this program is based on F5 embedding algorithm [19]. The two programs were put into one experimental system named "Qtech-Hide&View." This is a Windows-based system. All programs were developed under Visual C++ environment.

8.7.1 Components of the Experimental System

The system has two program components, i.e., information embedding and information extracting. Fig. 8.16 shows the menu window of the system.

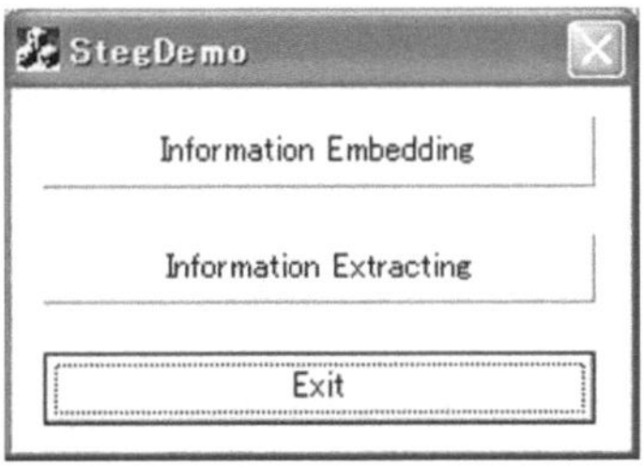

Fig. 8.16. Qtech-Hide&View menu window.

Information Embedding

Fig. 8.17 illustrates the Information Embedding component of Qtech-Hide & View. Embedding operation is executed by this component. The file types acceptable for vessel image are BMP, PNG, and JPG files. They must be in RGB-color format. The image size must be equal to or larger than 128×128, and less than or equal to $3,200 \times 3,200$ in pixel. The embedding data can be either one bare file (i.e., non-folder-covered file) or one folder having multiple of files and folders underneath. One special case is having an "index.html" file right under the top folder. In this case the extracting program will operate in a special manner.

The output image format, i.e., the stego image format, is selected from among BMP, PNG, and JPG files. The BMP and PNG embedding scheme is exactly the same. The only difference is that a BMP stego file is not compressed after embedding, while a PNG stego file is the compressed version of the BMP output in a lossless manner. Therefore, in case of BMP and PNG,

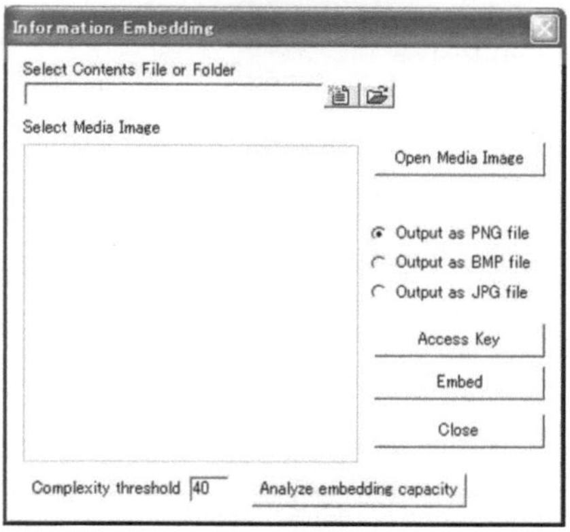

Fig. 8.17. Information embedding component.

the embedding capacity is always the same, and it is analyzable before actual embedding operation if a complexity threshold value is given. The threshold value can be formally set at any value ranging from 0 to 55. However, according to our experience, the best selection is to set it 40 or around. Therefore, the default complexity threshold was set 40. However, in JPG case the embedding capacity is not analyzable before embedding. If an access key is used in embedding, then it must be also used in the extracting operation. The length of the key was designed to have 4 to 16 bytes of alphanumeric characters. It is not an ordinary password, but is a set of special embedding parameters in the algorithm.

Information Extracting

The information extracting component of the system is illustrated in Fig. 8.18. This component extracts the embedded information data, i.e., files and folders, out of a stego image of BMP, PNG, and JPG file.

The Access Key must be provided in the same way as was given in embedding. Also, the complexity threshold value must be the same. The extraction mode is either "As it is" or "Link to Web." The As-it-is mode extracts the embedded data just as it was when embedding. Link-to-Web mode operates differently. In this mode, if the program finds an "index.html" file right under the top-folder, then after extracting, the program will start running the index.html file immediately. This operation can lead the system user (someone who runs the extracting program) to the WWW world instantly without starting a Web browser manually. This operation can seamlessly connect the users to a special information content space that is controlled by its owner, or by someone who embedded the content.

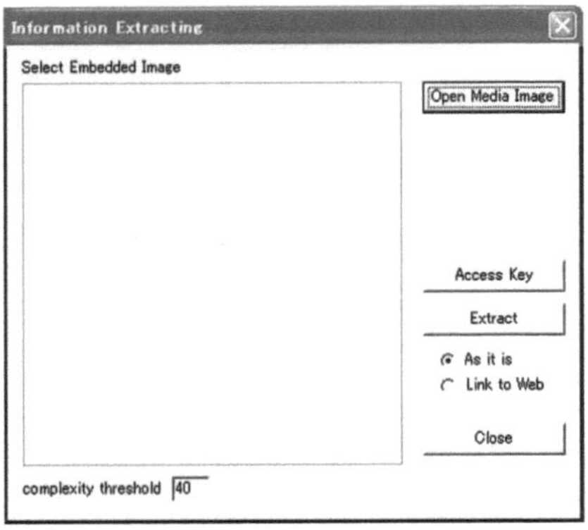

Fig. 8.18. Information extracting component.

8.7.2 Embedding and Extracting Experiments

We conducted a lot of embedding and extracting experiments using Qtech-Hide&View. We will show some of the results. Our major concerns are 1) embedding capacity, 2) before-and-after image difference, 3) embedding and extracting speed, etc.

BPCS Embedding and Extracting

Embedding and extracting by BPCS method is a standard operation of Qtech-Hide&View. We show our experiment using two vessel images (Image-1 and Image-2). As for the data to embed, we prepared two folders (Folder-1 and Folder-2) containing several files and folders underneath. Both folders included one index.html file right under their top folders. Folder-1 is for Image-1 embedding, and Folder-2 is for Image-2 embedding. Table 8.3 shows the properties of the two images before embedding. Image-1 and Image-2 are illustrated in Fig. 8.19 (A) and (B). Two folders for embedding are shown in Table 8.4 and Fig. 8.20. These two folders were the largest amount of data that Image-1-bef and Image-2-bef could embed, respectively. So, the compressed folder sizes in Table 8.4 were the maximum embedding capacities of the two vessel images. The folder compression was performed by a LHA compression program [22] which was incorporated in Qtech-Hide&View.

Table 8.3. Properties of the vessel images before embedding (RGB color).

Image name	Image size	BMP data size (KB)	PNG data size (KB)
Image-1-bef	950×713	1,986	1,492
Image-2-bef	600×465	818	575

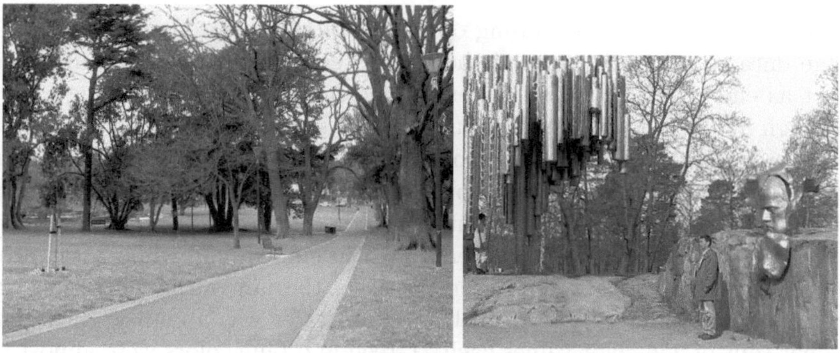

(A) Image-1-bef (950 × 713, BMP) (B) Image-2-bef (600 × 465, BMP)

Fig. 8.19. Vessel images.

Table 8.4. Folders for embedding.

Folder name	Original folder size (KB)	Compressed folder size (KB)
Folder-1	1,710	1,035
Folder-2	980	417

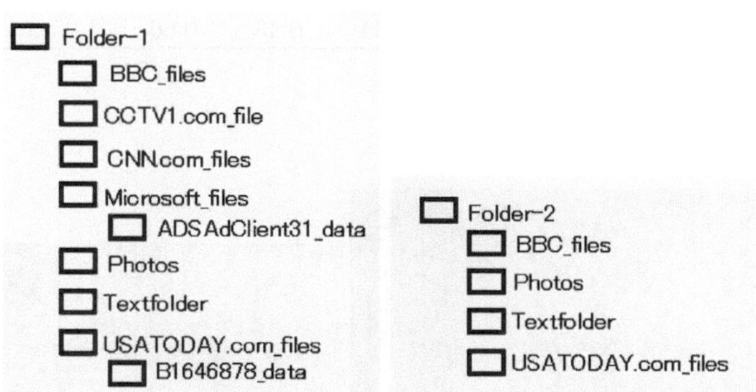

(A) Folder-1 (1,710KB) (B) Folder-1 (980KB)

Fig. 8.20. Folder structures to be embedded.

Embedding

We used the default complexity value 40. We did not use any Access Key in this experiment. The embedding operation starts by compressing the embedding data (actually, folders) in the embedding program. In each embedding, an image input in BMP was output in BMP, and in PNG then in PNG. Table 8.5 shows the properties of the two stego images after embedding. As we see in the table, the data sizes were unchanged after embedding in BMP, but increased a little in PNG. The reason why PNG embedding increases the file size is because the embedding operation increases the randomness of the image data to some degree, and the lossless compression by LHA algorithm is not as effective as it is for non-embedded images. The embedding ratio is very high in all embeddings. Especially, in PNG, we knew that the embedding ratio were almost always 0.65 or around. This is a very high score. Before and after embedding differences are shown in Fig. 8.21 (A) and (B) in black and white image patterns. This is about the Red color component. "Black area" in this pattern indicates the unaltered area in embedding, while "gray area" shows the altered area. The whiter the area, the larger the alteration was. The maximum difference between before and after was about 30 in decimal number (out of 256 color values each). Green and blue colors were almost the same as Red color. Embedding speed was quite high. In case of a notebook PC having a 1.4GH AMD Athlon CPU with 384MB memory, each embedding time in BMP image is shown in Table 8.5. PNG output took a little more time (0.2 second or less) in both cases.

Table 8.5. Properties of the stego images (RGB color).

Image name	Image size	BMP data size (KB)	PNG data size (KB)	Embedding ratio BMP	Embedding ratio PNG	Embedding time (BMP)
Image-1	950×713	1,986	1,584	0.52	0.65	2.0 sec (approx)
Image-2	600×465	818	634	0.43	0.66	1.0 sec (approx)

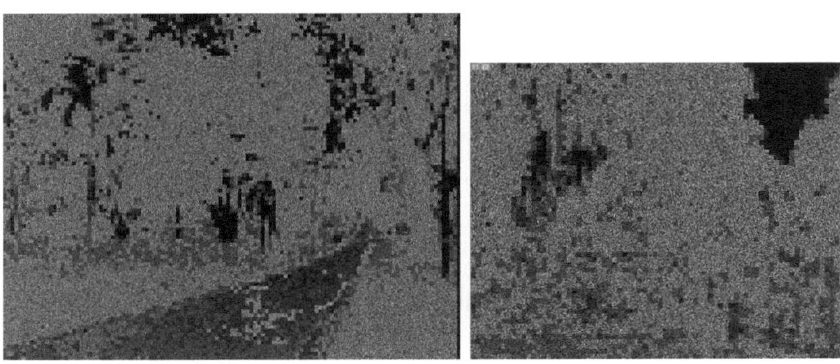

(A) Image difference in Red color (Image-1)

(B) Image difference in Red color (Image-2)

Fig. 8.21. Image difference patterns between before and after BPCS embedding in Red color component.

Extracting

The operation in the extracting program starts by checking the access key and the value of the complexity threshold value input by the operator. The default extraction mode is "As it is." It extracts the whole folder structure just as it was when embedding, and it is output in a temporary folder. "Link to Web" extraction mode extracts the whole folder structure first, and then searches for an "index.html" file directly under the top folder. If it is found, the program instantly starts running it, and No other folders and files are shown. Throughout all our experiments using variety of data, all embedded data (folders and files) were extracted exactly. In "As it is" mode the extracting times regarding the two BMP test images (Image-1 and Image-2) are listed in Table 8.6. Extractions from PNG images took a little more time (less then 0.2 sec). The PC we used for extracting was the same as we used for embedding. A "Link to Web" extracting mode took a longer time to go through all the extracting processes. Fig. 8.22 illustrates a "Link to Web" extraction from the stego Image-1 in PNG format.

Table 8.6. Extraction time (BMP stego image).

Image-1	Image-2
2.8 sec (approx)	1.5 sec (approx)

JPEG Embedding and Extracting

The vessel images for JPEG experiment were the same images that we used for BPCS experiments. Two BMP images (Image-1 and Image-2) were converted to JPEG images in two ways, i.e., high quality and low quality. "JPG-1-high.jpg" and "JPG-1-low.jpg" are high and low quality JPEG images, and "JPG-2-high.jpg" and "JPG-2-low.jpg" are the similar JPEG files converted from Image-2-bef. There was no obvious degradation in BMP to JPG conversion. The file sizes of these JPEG images are listed in Table 8.7.

Table 8.7. Size of the JPEG vessel image files.

JPG file name	JPG-1-high.jpg	JPG-1-low.jpg	JPG-2-high.jpg	JPG-2-low.jpg
File size (KB)	482	99	176	46

As for the data to embed, we prepared four bare text files (see Table 8.8). 1.highJPG.txt is for JPG-1-high.jpg, 1.lowJPG.txt is for JPG-1-low.jpg, and two other text files are for two other JPG-2 images. These files were the largest data amount that each JPEG image could embed. So, the compressed files sizes are the respective embedding capacities. The file compression was executed by a LHA program incorporated in the embedding program.

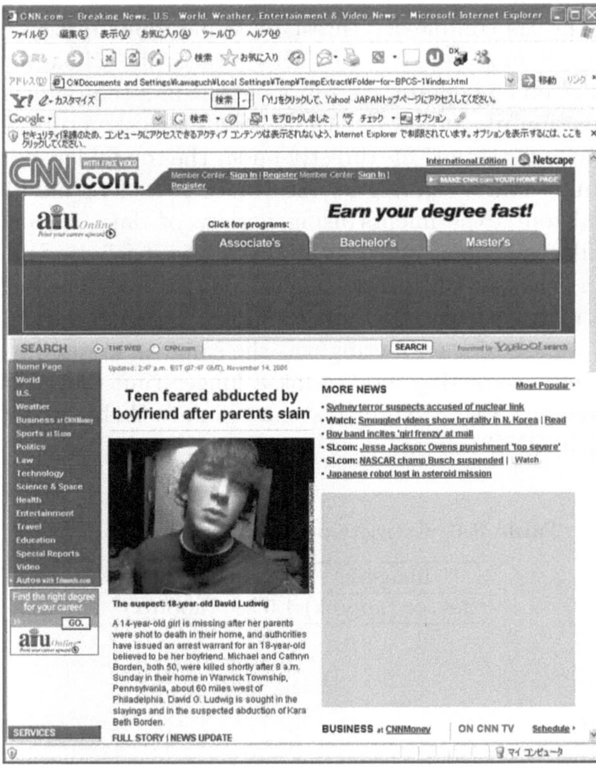

Fig. 8.22. An example of Link-to-Web extraction.

Table 8.8. Size of the text files for JPEG embedding.

File name	1.highJPG.txt	1.lowJPG.txt	2.highJPG.txt	2.lowJPG.txt
Original size (KB)	149	25	50	7
Compressed size (KB)	44	9	16	3

Embedding

We did not use any Access Key in the experiment. The result of the JPEG embedding is listed in Table 8.9. The file size of each JPEG output decreased a little. The embedding capacity was around 10% of each output JPG file (stego image) size. The reason why the JPG file decreases after embedding is as follows. The JPEG embedding operation increases the number of "0" elements of the quantized DCT coefficients and then the run-length-based data compression process in JPEG coding eventually decreases the file size. The embedding ratio was calculated as the ratio of the compressed text size vs the JPEG stego image size. The difference pattern between "before and after" embedding is shown in Fig. 8.23 (A) and (B). The largest differences in JPG-

1-high and low were 28 and 80 in Red color, respectively. Other colors were quite similar. It is obvious that JPG-1-high has a "finer" difference pattern than JPG-1-low case. The embedding times are shown in Table 8.9.

Table 8.9. Before and after embedding comparison.

JPG file name	JPG-1-high.jpg	JPG-1-low.jpg	JPG-2-high.jpg	JPG-2-low.jpg
File size (Before) (KB)	482	99	176	46
File size (After) (KB)	437	78	152	30
Embedding Ratio	0.10	0.12	0.11	0.10
Embedding time (approx)	0.4 sec	0.1 sec	0.1 sec	0.1 sec

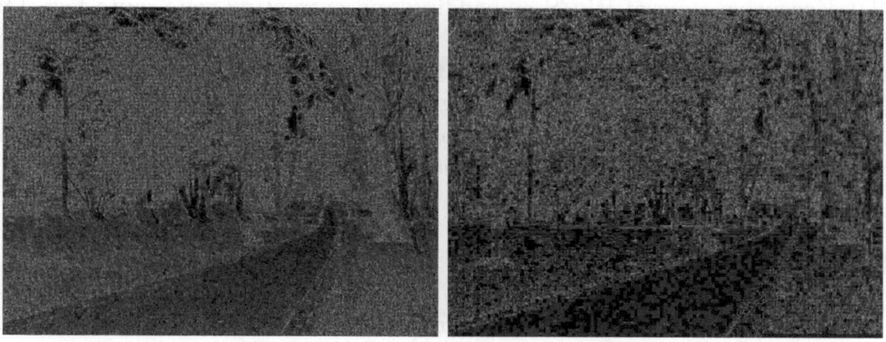

(A) Image difference in Red color (JPG-1-high)

(B) Image difference in Red color (JPG-1-lowf)

Fig. 8.23. Image difference patterns between before and after JPEG embedding in Red color component.

Extracting

The extracting operation was very smooth. All embedded data, i.e., bare text files, were extracted exactly. The extraction times are listed in Table 8.10.

Table 8.10. Extraction time.

JPG file name	JPG-1-high.jpg	JPG-1-low.jpg	JPG-2-high.jpg	JPG-2-low.jpg
Extraction time (approx)	0.6 sec	0.2 sec	0.3 sec	0.1 sec

Conclusions from the Experiments

Throughout varieties of embedding and extracting experiment using BMP, PNG, and JPEG, we confirmed the followings.

(A) BPCS-embedding method has a very large embedding capacity. Especially, in the case of PNG image, the capacity turned out to be 65% in most cases. When the embedded data are all text files, because the LHA compression program can reduce a text file into 1/3 of its original size, it is possible to embed almost 200% larger text data into one PNG image.
(B) Embedding capacity according to our JPEG embedding program was found to be 10% on average.
(C) Image quality after embedding did not change visually even in the case when we embedded the maximum capacity in both BPCS and JPEG method.
(D) Execution time of BPCS embedding and extracting were quite fast. Of course it depends on the size of the vessel image and the size of the embedding data. It was also true for JPEG embedding and extracting.
(E) The embedded data are very fragile in both BPCS and JPEG method. Changing color data by 1 bit on one single pixel of a stego image always hampered the extracting operation.

References

1. Hall, E.L. (1979): Computer image processing and recognition. Academic Press, New York
2. Jain, A.K. (1989): Fundamentals of digital image processing. Prentice Hall, Englewood Cliffs, NJ
3. Kawaguchi, E., Endo, T., Matsunaga, J. (1983): Depth-first picture expression viewed from digital picture processing. IEEE Trans. on PAMI **5** 373–384
4. Kawaguchi, E., Taniguchi, R.: Complexity of binary pictures and image thresholding — An application of DF-Expression to the thresholding problem. Proceedings of 8th ICPR, **2**, 1221–1225
5. Kawaguchi, E., Taniguchi, R. (1989): The DF-Expression as an image thresholding strategy. IEEE Trans. on SMC, **19**, 1321–1328
6. Kamata, S., Eason, R.O., Kawaguchi, E. (1995): Depth-first Coding for multivalued pictures using bit-plane decomposition. IEEE Trans. on Commun., **43**, 1961–1969
7. Kawaguchi, E., Niimi, M. (1988): Modeling digital image into informative and noise-like regions by complexity measure. Information Modelling and Knowledge Bases XV, IOS Press, 255–265
8. Nozaki, K., Noda, H., Kawaguchi, E., Eason, R. (2005): A model of unforgeable digital certificate document system. Information Modelling and Knowledge Bases XVI, IOS Press, 203–210
9. Niimi, M., Noda, H., Kawaguchi, E. (1999): Steganography based on region segmentation with a complexity measure. Systems and Computers in Japan, **30**, 1–9

10. Katzenbeisser, S., Petitcolas, F.A.P. (2000): Information hiding techniques for steganography and digital watermarking. Artech House, 79–93
11. Johnson, N.F., Duric, Z., Jajodia, S. (2001): information hiding: steganography and watermarking — attacks and countermeasures. Kluwer Academic Publishers, 47–76
12. Wayner, P. (2002): Disappearing cryptography: information hiding: steganography & watermarking. Morgan Kaufmann Publishers, 303–314
13. Rabbani, M., Joshi R. (2002): An overview of JPEG 2000 still image compression standard. Signal Processing: Image Communication, **17**, 3–48
14. Taubman, D. (2000): High performance scalable image compression with EBCOT. IEEE Trans. Image Process., **9**, 1158–1170
15. Shapiro, J.M. (1993): Embedded image coding using zerotrees of wavelet coefficients. IEEE Trans. Signal Process., **41**, 3445–3462
16. Said, A., Pearlman, W.A. (1996): A new, fast, and efficient image codec based on set partitioning in hierarchical trees. IEEE Trans. Circuits and Systems for Video Technology, **6**, 243–250
17. `http://jj2000.epfl.ch/index.html`
18. Upham, D. (1997): `http://ftp.funet.fi/pub/crypt/cypherpunks/steganography/jsteg/`
19. Westfeld, A. (2001): F5 – A steganographic algorithm: high capacity despite better steganalysis. Lecture Notes in Computer Science, **2137**, 289–302
20. Fridrich, J., Goljan M., Hogea, D. (2003): New methodology for breaking steganographic techniques for JPEGs. Proc. of SPIE, **5020**, 143–155
21. Chen, B., Wornell, G.W. (2001): Quantization index modulation: A class of provably good methods for digital watermarking and information embedding. IEEE Trans. on Information Theory, **47**, 1423–1443
22. `http://www.csdinc.co.jp/archiver/lib/main-e.html`
`http://www2.nsknet.or.jp/~micco/english/unlha32_e.htm`

Part IV

Practical Applications of Intelligent Multimedia Signal Processing and Data Hiding Systems

9

Intelligent Video Event Detection for Surveillance Systems

Hong-Yuan Mark Liao[1], Duan-Yu Chen[1], Chih-Wen Su[1], and Hsiao-Rong Tyan[2]

[1] 128, Section 2, Academy Road, Institute of Information Science, Academia Sinica, Nankang, Taipei, Taiwan
{liao, dychen, lucas}@iis.sinica.edu.tw
[2] 200, Chung Pei Rd., Chung Li, Department of Information and Computer Engineering, Chung-Yuan Christian University, Taiwan
tyan@ice.cycu.edu.tw

Summary. In recent years, real-time direct detection of events by surveillance systems has attracted a great deal of attention. In this chapter, we present solutions for video-based surveillance systems in the spatial domain and in the compressed domain, respectively. In spatial domain, we propose a new video-based surveillance system that can perform real-time event detection. In the background modelling phase, we adopt a mixture of Gaussian approach to determine the background. Meanwhile, we use color blob-based tracking to track foreground objects. Due to the self-occlusion problem, the tracking module is designed as a multi-blob tracking process to obtain similar multiple trajectories. We devise an algorithm to merge these trajectories into a representative one. After applying the Douglas-Peucker algorithm to approximate a trajectory, we can compare two arbitrary trajectories. The above mechanism enables us to conduct real-time event detection if a number of wanted trajectories are pre-stored in a video surveillance system. In compressed domain, we propose the use of motion vectors embedded in MPEG bitstreams to generate so called motion-flows, which are applied to perform quick video retrieval. By using the motion vectors directly, we do not need to consider the shape of a moving object and its corresponding trajectory. Instead, we simply link the local motion vectors across consecutive video frames to form motion flows, which are then annotated and stored in a video database. In the video retrieval phase, we propose a new matching strategy to execute the video retrieval task. Motions that do not belong to the mainstream motion flows are filtered out by our proposed algorithm. The retrieval process can be triggered by a query-by-sketch (QBS) or a query-by-example (QBE). The experimental results show that our method is efficient and accurate in the video retrieval process.

H.-Y.M. Liao et al.: *Intelligent Video Event Detection for Surveillance Systems*, Studies in Computational Intelligence (SCI) **58**, 233–259 (2007)
www.springerlink.com

9.1 Introduction

Intelligent video-based surveillance has become a very popular research topic in recent years due to increasing crime. In the past, video-based surveillance systems relied primarily on human operators to observe several, or dozens, of monitors simultaneously. However, this kind of monitoring is not practical, because a human operator cannot watch so many TV screens simultaneously and observe everything that happens. Furthermore, unlike machines, human operators become tired, especially after working long hours. Therefore, it is essential to develop a smart real-time video-based surveillance system. Some difficult design issues must be taken into account. Firstly, the motion of a human being is highly articulated, which makes the task of description very difficult. Secondly, in order to correctly identify an event, comparison of two arbitrary motion sequences is indispensable.

In the past decade, extensive research have been conducted into surveillance-related issues [1]–[16]. In [1], Wren et al. proposed a statistical background model to locate people and utilized 2D image analysis to track a single person in complex scenes with a fixed camera. Lipton et al. [2] proposed the use of a human operator to monitor activities over a large area using multiple cameras. Their system can detect and track multiple people and vehicles in crowded scenes for long periods. Grimson et al. [3] established a multiple-camera environment to learn patterns common to different object classes and detect unusual activities. Bobick et al. [4] proposed a combination of a Hidden Markov Model and stochastic grammar to recognize activities and identify different behavior based on contextual information acquired by a static camcorder. Kanade et al. [5] proposed the use of multiple sensors to detect and track moving objects. Haritaoglu et al. [6] proposed a method for the detection and tracking of multiple people and monitoring of their activities in an outdoor environment. Stauffer and Grimson [7] focused on motion tracking in outdoor environment. They used observed motions to learn patterns from different kinds of activities. In [8], Zelnik and Irani proposed a non-parametric approach to characterize video events by Spatio-Temporal Intensity Gradients calculated at multiple temporal scales. Medioni et al. [9] used a set of features derived from multiple scales to stabilize an image sequence. They proposed the extraction of the trajectories of moving objects using an attribute graph representation. Davis and Bobick [10] proposed an activity recognition method based on view-dependent template matching. In [11], Davis et al. proposed the representation of simple periodic events, such as walking, by constructing dynamic models based on computing periodic patterns in people's movements. Makris and Ellis [14] proposed to automatically learn an activity-based semantic scene model based on motion trajectories from video streams. In [15], Su et al. proposed the concept of motion flow and used it to represent an event directly in a compressed domain. They also proposed a scale and translation invariant matching algorithm to compare an unknown event with database events.

In this chapter, we present solutions for video-based event detection system in the spatial domain and the compressed domain, respectively. In the spatial domain, we first adopt a mixture of Gaussian approach to determine the background. Through this simple modelling, we can separate foreground objects from the background efficiently and accurately. To track foreground objects, we use color blob-based tracking. However, the method is not perfect due to the effect of self-occlusion or mutual occlusion among various body parts [12, 13, 17]. Therefore, the tracking process is designed as a multi-blob tracking process that generates multiple similar trajectories. We have also designed an algorithm that merges these trajectories into one representative trajectory and then apply the Douglas-Peucker algorithm to approximate it. To compare a trajectory extracted from a real-time environment with those stored in the database, we propose a translation and scaling invariant metric to execute the matching task. Using the above procedure, we can detect abnormal intrusion events in real time by pre-storing a number of possible intrusion trajectories in a local computer linked to a camcorder monitor. If the path of an intruder is close to one of the pre-stored trajectories, the system sends a signal directly to the control center. The contribution of this work is twofold. First, it simplifies the real-time event detection problem by comparing the degree of similarity between two arbitrary trajectories. Second, the proposed method is translation and scaling invariant. It can therefore be applied to different application domains, such as home security systems, complex surveillance systems, or parking lot management systems.

In the compressed domain, since stored surveillance videos are compressed, we directly utilize the motion vectors embedded in MPEG bitstreams to develop a motion descriptor. It is known that motion vectors only record the direction and magnitude of movement between corresponding macroblocks of two consecutive anchor frames, as they are only comprised of local data that do not have much semantic meaning. In this study, we utilize the consistency of motion direction, the color distribution, and the overlapping area between macroblocks of two consecutive frames to link all neighboring motion vectors. These linked motion vectors form so-called motion-flows, which contain more semantic meaning than the original motion vector data. Since a large moving object may occupy several macroblocks and produce multiple motion flows, we also propose an algorithm to reduce motion flows that are similar in shape to one or more representative motion flows. We approximate these representative motion flows by generating control points and storing them in a database as models. When a user wants to query a specific motion, he/she can draw a trajectory on a sketch-based interface, and the system will retrieve a set of shots that contain similar motion content. Since the temporal information of a trajectory is hard to express precisely, we only consider the spatial information in a QBS (Query-By-Sketch) process. Initially, a user executes the process to retrieve some candidate shots from the database. Then, he/she can choose one of candidate shots and execute a QBE (Query-By-Example) process to extract the video clips that are most similar to the query.

The remainder of this chapter is organized as follows. In Section 9.2, we describe how to detect video events in spatial domain for real-time applications. In Section 9.3, we introduce novel motion-flow based event detections in compressed domain for off-line usage. Conclusions are given in Section 9.4.

9.2 Real-Time Video Event Detections

9.2.1 Foreground and Background Estimation

Even though there are numerous background estimation algorithms existing in the literature, most of them follow a simple flow diagram shown in Fig. 9.1. The four major steps in a background estimation algorithm are preprocessing, background modelling, foreground detection, and data validation [18]. Preprocessing consists of a collection of simple image processing tasks that change the input video frames into a format that can be used in the subsequent processes. Background modelling uses the preprocessed video frame to calculate and update a background model, and provides a statistical description of the background scene. Foreground detection identifies pixels in the video frame that cannot well be explained by the background model, and outputs them as a binary candidate foreground mask. Finally, data validation analyzes the candidate mask, eliminates those pixels that do not correspond to actual moving objects, and outputs the final foreground mask. The most common approach is to combine morphological filtering and connected component grouping to eliminate noises.

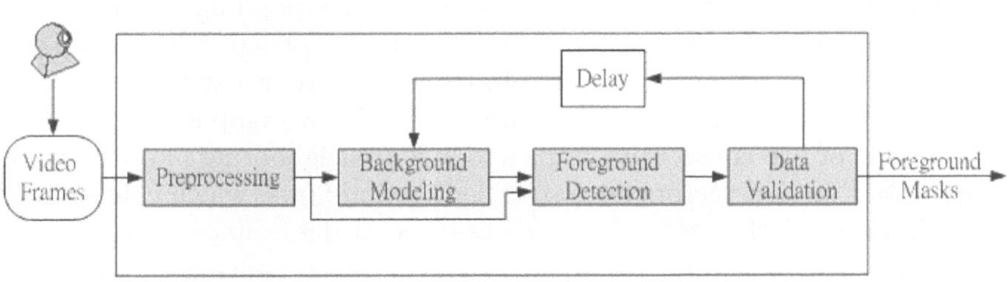

Fig. 9.1. Flow diagram of a typical foreground and background estimation algorithm.

Since our objective is real-time event detection using a stationary camera, distinguishing foreground objects from the background is an important step. Foreground estimation is relatively easy in an indoor environment, because the illumination conditions do not change significantly. An outdoor environment, on the other hand, is much more complicated, as varying weather and sunlight affect the correct detection of foreground. Some researchers have adopted an adaptive Gaussian approach to model the behavior of a pixel. However, the background region of a video sequence often contains several moving objects. Therefore, rather than explicitly estimating the values of all pixels as one distribution, we prefer to estimate the value of a pixel as a mixture of Gaussians [19, 20, 21]. In [19], the probability that an observed pixel will have an intensity value x_t at time t is estimated by K Gaussian distributions defined as follows:

$$P(x_t) = \sum_{l=1}^{K} \frac{\omega_{l,t}}{(2\pi)^{1/2}} e^{-\frac{1}{2}(x_t-\mu_l)^T \Sigma_l^{-1}(x_t-\mu_l)}, \tag{9.1}$$

where $\omega_{l,t}$ is the weight of the lth distribution of pixel x_t's mixture model; μ_l is the mean of the lth distribution; and Σ_l is its covariance matrix, where $\Sigma_l = \sigma_l^2 I$, σ_l is the standard deviation of the lth distribution, and I is an identity matrix. To update the model, each new pixel is checked to see it matches the existing Gaussian distributions. To adjust the weight of each distribution, the weight $\omega_{l,t}$ is updated by:

$$\omega_{l,t} = (1-\alpha) + \alpha(M_{l,t}), \tag{9.2}$$

where α is the learning rate that controls the speed of the learning; M is a Boolean value indicating whether or not a match is found. The definition of M is as follows: $M_{l,t} = 1$ when a match is confirmed on the lth distribution at time t; otherwise, $M_{l,t} = 0$.

The parameters μ and σ can be updated as follows:

$$\mu_{l,t} = (1-\beta)\mu_{l,t-1} + \beta x_t, \tag{9.3}$$

$$\sigma_{l,t}^2 = (1-\beta)\sigma_{l,t-1}^2 + \beta(x_t - \mu_{l,t})^T(x_t - \mu_{l,t}), \tag{9.4}$$

where $\beta = \alpha P(x_t \mid \mu_{l,t-1}, \sigma_{l,t-1})$. In each frame, pixels far away from the background distributions are recognized as foreground. A connectivity algorithm is then applied to identify possible objects in motion. It is widely recognized that an overly segmented result may break the detected objects into pieces. Therefore, morphological operations must be applied to fix the completeness of foreground objects. A detected foreground object is considered as a blob and characterized by its position and color distribution to support the subsequent tracking process. Fig. 9.2 illustrates the process of background estimation and foreground segmentation. Fig. 9.2(a) is the original video frame with a moving subject. After background estimation, an estimated background is shown in Fig. 9.2(b). The foreground pixels obtained after applying background subtraction are shown in Fig. 9.2(c), in which noise, caused by wavering tree branches, for example, can be filtered out by morphological operations. In the meantime, blobs with high connectivity can be separated from the background and detected as foreground objects as shown in Fig. 9.2(d).

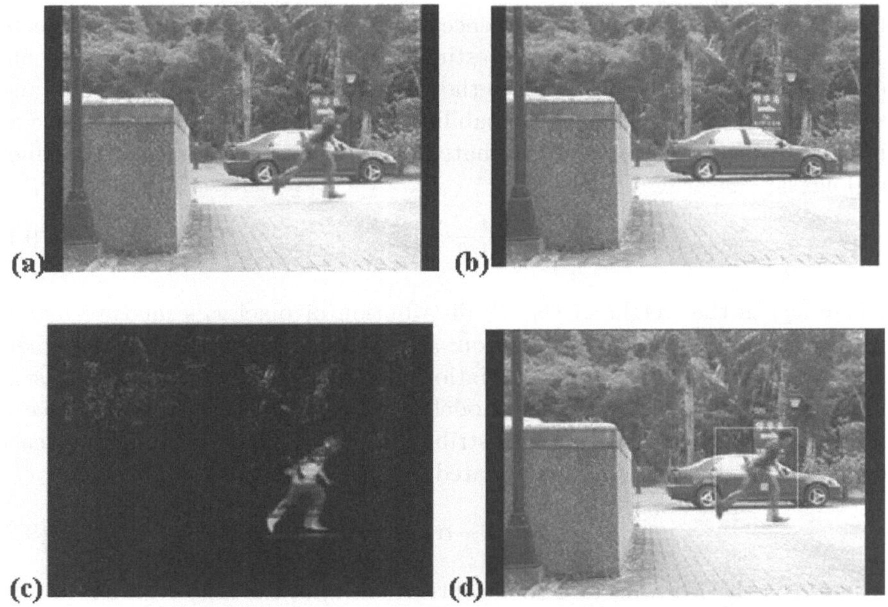

Fig. 9.2. Background estimation and foreground segmentation. (a) Original frame. (b) Background model. (c) Foreground pixels. (d) Detected moving subject.

9.2.2 Color-Based Blob Tracking

In this section, we propose a hybrid blob tracker that is comprised of two stages. The first stage is executed by a color-based blob tracker, which provides reliable and fast tracking results if the moving blobs are pre-segmented.

Color-Based Blob Tracker

After background estimation, an estimated foreground can be derived. Ideally, residual pixels obtained after applying background subtraction should represent foreground objects. However, noise, such as that caused by wavering tree branches, needs to be filtered out. Therefore, morphological operations are performed to remove noise. In the meantime, blobs with high connectivity can be separated from residual pixels and detected as foreground objects. In order to satisfy the real-time constraint, we employ color histograms to characterize the extracted blobs. Although a color histogram is not the best nonparametric estimator [22], it is a good target tracker due to its low computation cost. Moreover, since it disregards all geometric information, it is robust against complicated non-rigid motions. Using a color histogram, a target R and its corresponding candidates P can be modelled as

$$\text{Target:} \quad R_t = \{r_{i,t}\}_{i=1,\cdots,n}, \quad \text{where} \sum_{i=1}^{n} r_{l,t} = 1, \tag{9.5}$$

$$\text{Corresponding candidates:} \quad P_t(x,y) = \{p_{i,t}(x,y)\}_{i=1,\cdots,n}, \quad \text{where} \sum_{i=1}^{n} p_{i,t} = 1. \tag{9.6}$$

$P_t(x, y)$ and $p_{i,t}(x, y)$ denote a candidate located at (x, y) and the value of its ith bin at time t, respectively; and $r_{i,t}$ represents the value of the ith bin at time t. The histogram with n bins of R and P are normalized by their own total pixel numbers. Next, we employ a similarity function, called the Bhattacharyya coefficient [23], to calculate the degree of similarity between the target and a candidate in the database. A Bhattacharyya coefficient is a divergence-type measure with a straightforward geometric interpretation. It is defined as the cosine of an angle measured between two n-dimensional unit vectors, $(\sqrt{p_1}, \sqrt{p_2}, \cdots, \sqrt{p_n})^T$ and $(\sqrt{r_1}, \sqrt{r_2}, \cdots, \sqrt{r_n})^T$. Detailed definitions of the Bhattacharyya coefficient can be found in [24]. The formal definition of the distance between a target at time t and a candidate at time $t + 1$ is

$$d(x, y) = \sqrt{1 - \sum_{i=1}^{n} \sqrt{p_{i,t+1}(x, y) r_{i,t}}}\,. \tag{9.7}$$

Therefore, to find the best match among a set of candidates located in the subsequent frame, the candidate that has the smallest distance with the target is chosen. We then use the color distribution of this chosen candidate to update the color distribution of the target. The tracking procedure is iterated until the target cannot find any further match. Since a color-based blob tracker may generate more than one trajectory due to occlusion or the distinct movements of different body parts, we now discuss how to merge these trajectories into one representative trajectory.

Single out a Representative Trajectory from a Group of Trajectories

Since the movement of an articulated object like a human being may cover more than one trajectory due to occlusion or the movements of different body parts, it is possible to derive more than one trajectory from a moving person. Therefore, we adopt an algorithm proposed in our previous work [15] to single out one representative trajectory from a set of derived trajectories. Initially, we select a trajectory, a, that has the longest duration in a tracking sequence. Suppose a starts from time t_i and ends at time t_j is the set of trajectories whose start or end times are within the duration. We merge b (b is a member of $\{B\}$) with a, if it satisfies the following condition:

$$\sum_{t\in[t_s,t_e]} \frac{\| (a(t) - a(t_s)) - (b(t) - b(t_s)) \|}{t_e - t_s} < \epsilon, \tag{9.8}$$

where t_s and t_e are respectively the start and end times of trajectory b. Let $a(t)$ and $b(t)$ be the spatial positions of a and b at time t, respectively; and let $a(t_s)$ and $b(t_s)$ be the spatial position of a and b at time t_s, respectively. If the average of the relative spatial distances between a and b is smaller than a threshold, ϵ, we consider b a highly correlated trajectory of a. Therefore, the trajectory a is updated by the average position of trajectories a and b using Eq. (9.9),

$$a(t) = \begin{cases} b(t), & \text{if } a(t) \cap b(t) \in \phi \\ \frac{1}{2}(a(t) + b(t)), & \text{otherwise} \end{cases}, \quad t \in [t_s, t_e], \tag{9.9}$$

where ϕ represents an empty set. We consider a as the representative trajectory of $\{B\}$ and store it temporally. Next, we select the longest trajectory from the remaining trajectories, and repeat the above process. If the trajectory under consideration is longer than the temporary one, we replace it; otherwise, it is removed. This process continues until all trajectories in $\{B\}$ are processed. Here, we only consider trajectories with duration longer than three seconds in order to avoid the effects of noise. The trajectory that survives until the last moment is chosen as the representative trajectory.

Fig. 9.3 explains how the above algorithm works. Figs. 9.3(a)–9.3(c) show three discontinuous frames indicating a man climbing a stairway. Due to the occlusion of the handrail, the person is split into three blobs in Figs. 9.3(a) and 9.3(b), and two blobs in Fig. 9.3(c). From the blob-moving sequence, our algorithm detects several trajectories, as illustrated in Fig. 9.3(d), and singles out a representative trajectory as shown in Fig. 9.3(e).

9.2.3 Representing a Trajectory and Matching

After obtaining a trajectory calculated by a real-time tracking process, we need an efficient algorithm that can compare the degree of similarity between this trajectory and the trajectories stored in the local database.

We adopt the Douglas-Peucker algorithm [25] to select the necessary control points from a trajectory. The algorithm starts by using a straight line segment to connect the start and end points of the trajectory. If the perpendicular distance between any intermediate point to the anchor line is larger than a threshold, we split the trajectory into two segments via the farthest intermediate point. This process continues until all perpendicular distances are smaller than the preset threshold. The selected points and the two end points form the set of control points of the trajectory.

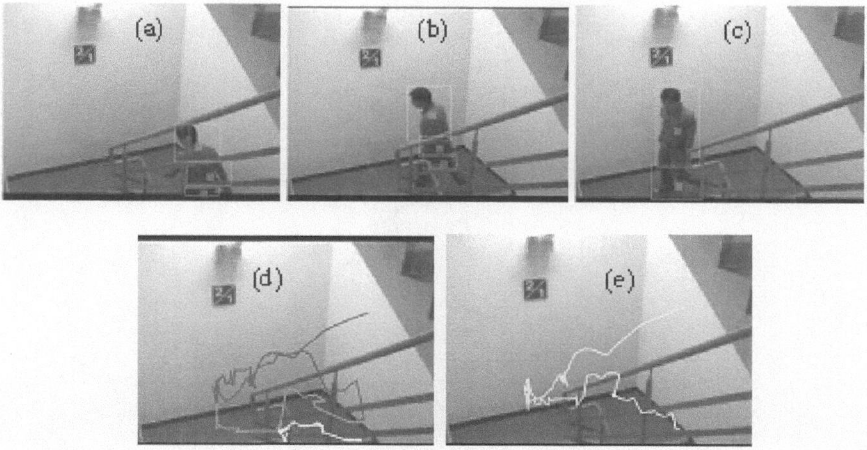

Fig. 9.3. An example showing a representative trajectory is singled out from a group of trajectories. (a)-(c): tracking of a person whose body is split into three parts due to occlusion of the handrail; (d) the group of calculated trajectories; and (e) the representative trajectory derived by applying the proposed algorithm.

Conventionally, (x, y) is used to denote the position of a point in the spatial domain. In contrast, we use five positive real numbers (x^+, x^-, y^+, y^-, d) to represent the position of a control point. Here, d denotes the cumulative length of the trajectory from the first control point to the current control point, and $+/-$ denotes the cumulative positive/negative movement along the x- or y-axis from the first control point. Now, let Q and D be the trajectories of the query and a model in the database, respectively. We normalize the length of both trajectories into a unit length before making a comparison. This technique guarantees the requirement of scale invariance. Therefore, the parameters d, $x+$, $x-$, $y+$, and $y-$ of each control point on the two trajectories must be normalized by dividing them by the length of Q and D, respectively.

We align both Q and D by calculating the length d from the first control point. For each control point on $Q(D)$, we interpolate a corresponding point that has the same cumulative length onto $D(Q)$. The d value is used as the basis of the alignment task, because we only consider the similarity between Q and D in the spatial domain. The control points and the corresponding points are labelled by circles and triangles, respectively (Fig. 9.4). The insertion of the corresponding points on Q and D is dependent of d. Now, for each control point on the trajectory $Q(D)$, we can interpolate a corresponding point located on $D(Q)$. Assume the total number of control points and their corresponding points located on Q and D are both N. Let $Q' : \{Q'_1, Q'_2, \cdots, Q'_N\}$ and $D' : \{D'_1, D'_2, \cdots, D'_N\}$ be the set of points including the control points and the

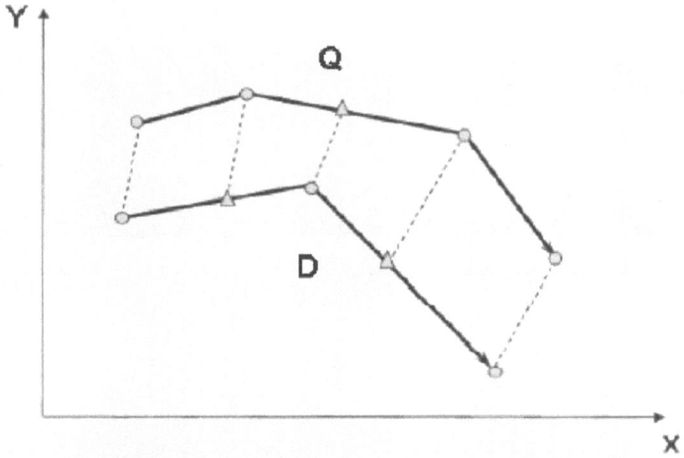

Fig. 9.4. The alignment task between two trajectories.

inserted corresponding points located on Q and D, respectively. The set of points Q' and D' can be called check-points, each of which can be represented by $(x+, x-, y+, y-)$ in the spatial domain. In order to compare two arbitrary trajectories, we define a metric as follows:

$$\text{Dist}_{i,j}^{Q',D'} = \left|(Q'_j - Q'_i) - (D'_j - D'_i)\right| \bullet \begin{pmatrix} 1 & 0 \\ 1 & 0 \\ 0 & 1 \\ 0 & 1 \end{pmatrix}, \tag{9.10}$$

where i and j $(i < j)$ denote the i-th and j-th check points of two partial trajectories of Q' and D', respectively; $Q'_j - Q'_i$ and $D'_j - D'_i$ represent the difference between the i-th and j-th check points of Q' and D', respectively; and $(Q'_j - Q'_i) - (D'_j - D'_i)$ is a 1×4 vector, and its subsequent term in Eq. (9.10) is a 4×2 matrix. Before executing the matrix operation, the absolute value of each element of $(Q'_j - Q'_i) - (D'_j - D'_i)$ must be taken. The operation on the right-hand side of Eq. (9.10) will result in a 1×2 vector. In addition, $\left\|\text{Dist}_{i,j}^{Q',D'}\right\|$ is basically an estimation of the distance between two partial trajectories on Q' and D', respectively. With the above distance metric, we can define the total distance between Q and D as follows:

$$\text{TDist}(Q, D) = \sum_{i=1}^{N-1} \left\|\text{Dist}_{i,i+1}^{Q',D'}\right\|. \tag{9.11}$$

The norm defined in Eq. (9.11) is an $l2$-norm.

The advantage of the proposed representation scheme is that we do not really need to compare the check points pair by pair. It should be noted, however, that all the elements that form the vector of a check-point on a trajectory are positive and their magnitudes are accumulated from the beginning. Therefore, if we choose an intermediate check point, Q'_k, in Q' and its corresponding check point, D'_k, in D', we can be sure that

$$\left\|\mathrm{Dist}_{i,j}^{Q',D'}\right\| \leq \left\|\mathrm{Dist}_{i,k}^{Q',D'}\right\| + \left\|\mathrm{Dist}_{k,j}^{Q',D'}\right\|. \tag{9.12}$$

Eq. (9.12) shows that a coarse-to-fine search strategy is appropriate for a trajectory-based query. In the first step of the comparison between Q' and D', we simply check the value of $\left\|\mathrm{Dist}_{1,N}^{Q',D'}\right\|$. This step only needs to consider four check points Q'_1, D'_1, Q'_N, and D'_N. Since the value of $\mathrm{TDist}(Q, D)$ must be equal to or larger than that of, we can quickly determine that trajectory D is not similar to Q if the returned value of $\left\|\mathrm{Dist}_{1,N}^{Q',D'}\right\|$ is greater than a predefined threshold δ.

Once the value of $\left\|\mathrm{Dist}_{1,N}^{Q',D'}\right\| < \delta$, we seek the second check points on Q' and D', respectively, by checking Q_2 and D_2. If Q_2 is chosen as Q'_2, we can insert D'_2 into the right position between D_1 and D_2 and vice versa. Furthermore, Q' and D' can be divided into four sub-trajectories by Q'_2 and D'_2. Under these circumstances, we only compute the sum of $\left\|\mathrm{Dist}_{1,2}^{Q',D'}\right\|$ and $\left\|\mathrm{Dist}_{2,N}^{Q',D'}\right\|$ as the distance between the sub-trajectories. If the distance between two distinct sub-trajectories is still larger than a predefined threshold δ, D will be filtered out. Otherwise, we insert Q'_3 and D'_3 to further compute $\left\|\mathrm{Dist}_{2,3}^{Q',D'}\right\|$ and $\left\|\mathrm{Dist}_{3,N}^{Q',D'}\right\|$. The above newly computed distances replace the value of $\left\|\mathrm{Dist}_{2,N}^{Q',D'}\right\|$, and the process is executed repeatedly until the computed distance is larger than δ, or there are no more intermediate check points within each sub-trajectory. Since most of the trajectories would be filtered out by checking the first few control points, our proposed algorithm is very efficient.

9.2.4 Experiment Results

In order to test the effectiveness and efficiency of our real-time event detection method, we tested our algorithm on the proposed surveillance systems with monitors placed at eight different locations. These indoor/outdoor environments included a parking lot, the area in front of an elevator, and a stairway. The corresponding background views taken at these locations are shown in Fig. 9.5. To demonstrate the performance of the proposed color-based blob tracking algorithm, the tracking results of the outdoor and indoor environments are demonstrated in Figs. 9.6(a)–(b) and Fig. 9.6(c), respectively. Moving objects in Figs. 9.6(a)–(b) were successfully tracked because adaptive mixture Gaussian model is advantageous under changing illuminations. In addition, the color histograms provide efficient computation and

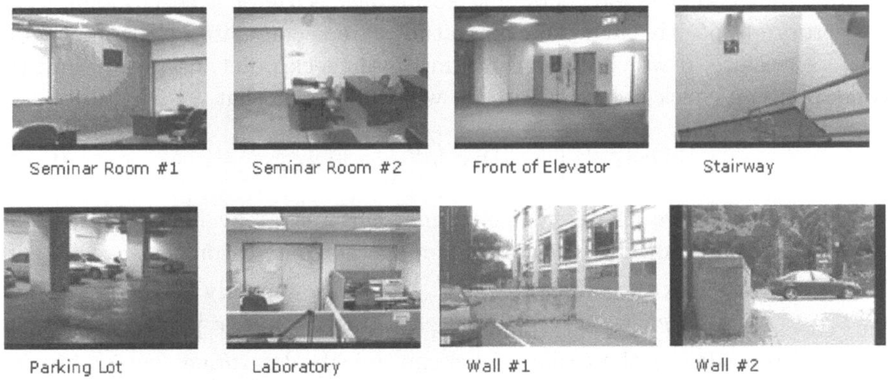

Fig. 9.5. Surveillance systems placed at eight different locations.

robustness against the occlusion problem. From Fig. 9.6(c), we can see that a moving person is occluded by the handrail and separated into two parts. Due to the superior characteristics of our color-based blob tracking algorithm, the moving person can be successfully tracked from two parts (Frame 2210 and Frame 2230) to only one part (Frame 2300). Finally, the representative trajectory was singled out by merging two distinct trajectories into one.

In the second set of experiments, we conducted a robustness test on our proposed system. The purpose of this set of experiments was to analyze the effect of false alarms. The ultimate goal of our system is to detect the movement of human beings and to ignore the movement of other moving objects. In order to perform real-time anomalous event detection, we pre-stored a set of trained trajectories to support real-time event detection. The pre-stored trajectories are shown in Fig. 9.7(a). The left-hand side of Fig. 9.7(a) shows the five derived trajectories corresponding to the five climbing-wall sequences shown on the right-hand side. Fig. 9.7(b) shows the merged trajectories of Fig. 9.7(a). As one can see from Fig. 9.7(b), the five trajectories are very similar. Fig. 9.8(a) shows the trajectories detected in real-time when an intruder tried to climb the wall. Since the detected trajectories (the black curve shown in Fig. 9.8(b)) was very close to the trained set of trajectories, the proposed surveillance system triggered an alarm to alert the human operator working in the control center. To test the robustness of the system, we conducted another experiment. Fig. 9.9(a) shows the detected path of a moving basketball. The corresponding trajectory of the path shown in Fig. 9.9(a) is illustrated by the black curve and shown in Fig. 9.9(b). As one can see from Fig. 9.9(b), the detected trajectory was very different from the pre-trained trajectories. Therefore, our system did not detect it as an intrusion event, because our algorithm could measure the difference between this trajectory and the database

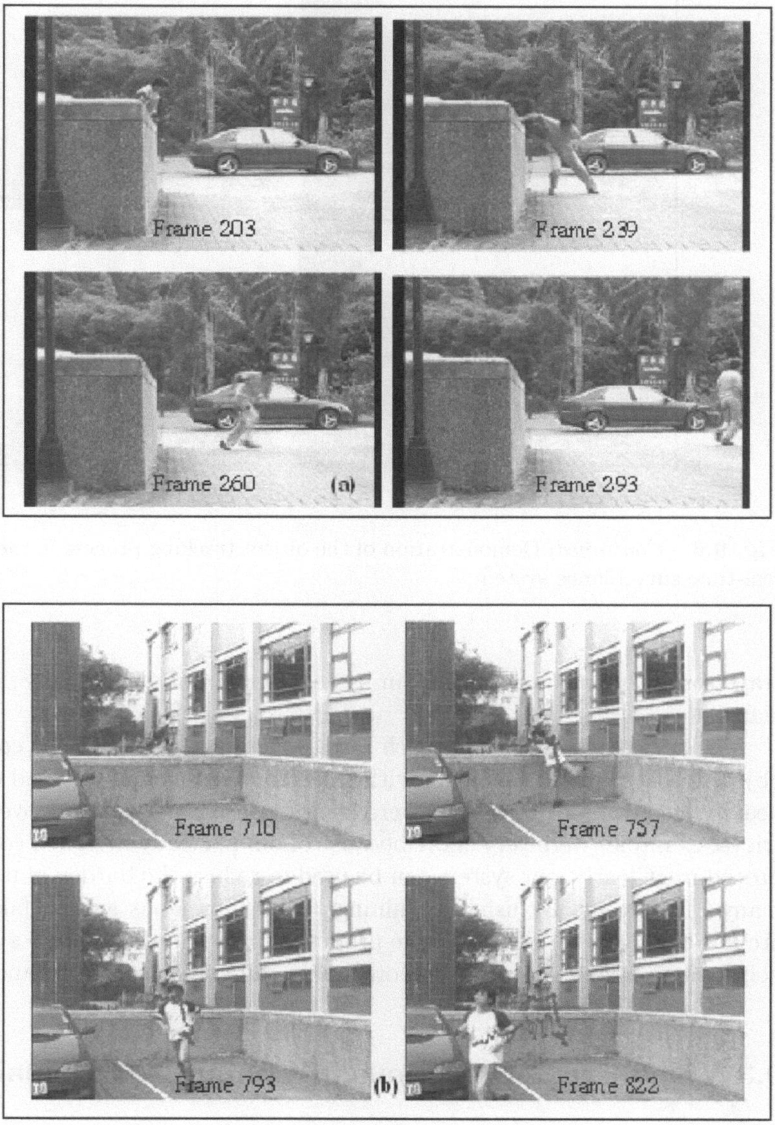

Fig. 9.6. Demonstration of the object tracking process in the proposed real-time surveillance system.

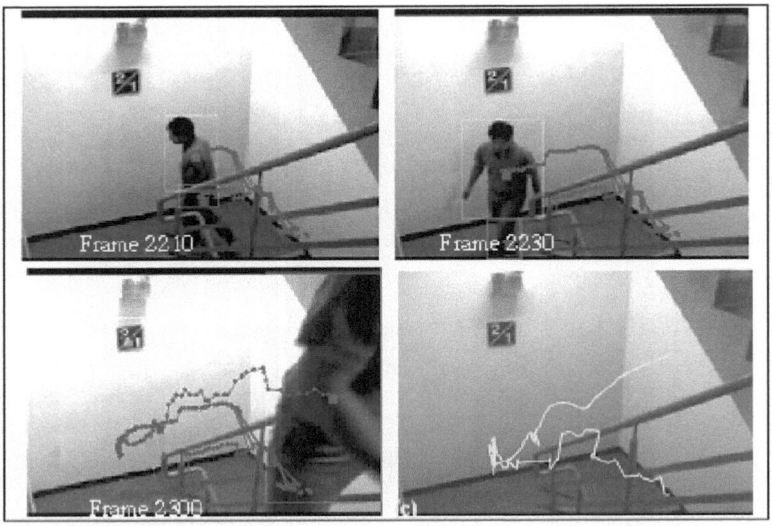

Fig. 9.6. (*Continued*) Demonstration of the object tracking process in the proposed real-time surveillance system.

trajectories. In such a scenario, our system would not usually generate a false alarm.

The advantage of our approach is that a simple, but efficient, color-based object tracker is used following with trajectory refinement, instead of relying heavily on a complex object tracker. The response times of the above video retrieval examples were very short because of our specially designed comparison procedure. Clearly, our system can be used to reduce the burden of monitoring many TV screens. By using a training set of anomalous events, false alarms are not be triggered; and thus, the proposed real-time surveillance system can help human operators conduct more precise and efficient surveillance tasks.

9.3 Video Event Detections in Compressed Domain

9.3.1 Constructing Motion Flows from MPEG Bitstreams

In this section, we introduce the method for constructing motion flows from an MPEG bitstream. Some methods [26, 27, 28] have been proposed for annotating motion information in a video. Among them, the trajectory-based approach is probably the most popular. However, its unstable nature and high computation cost have discouraged its use as a representation/annotation tool. Furthermore, such schemes take the path formed by linking the centroids of a video object that appears across consecutive anchor frames. Therefore, if a

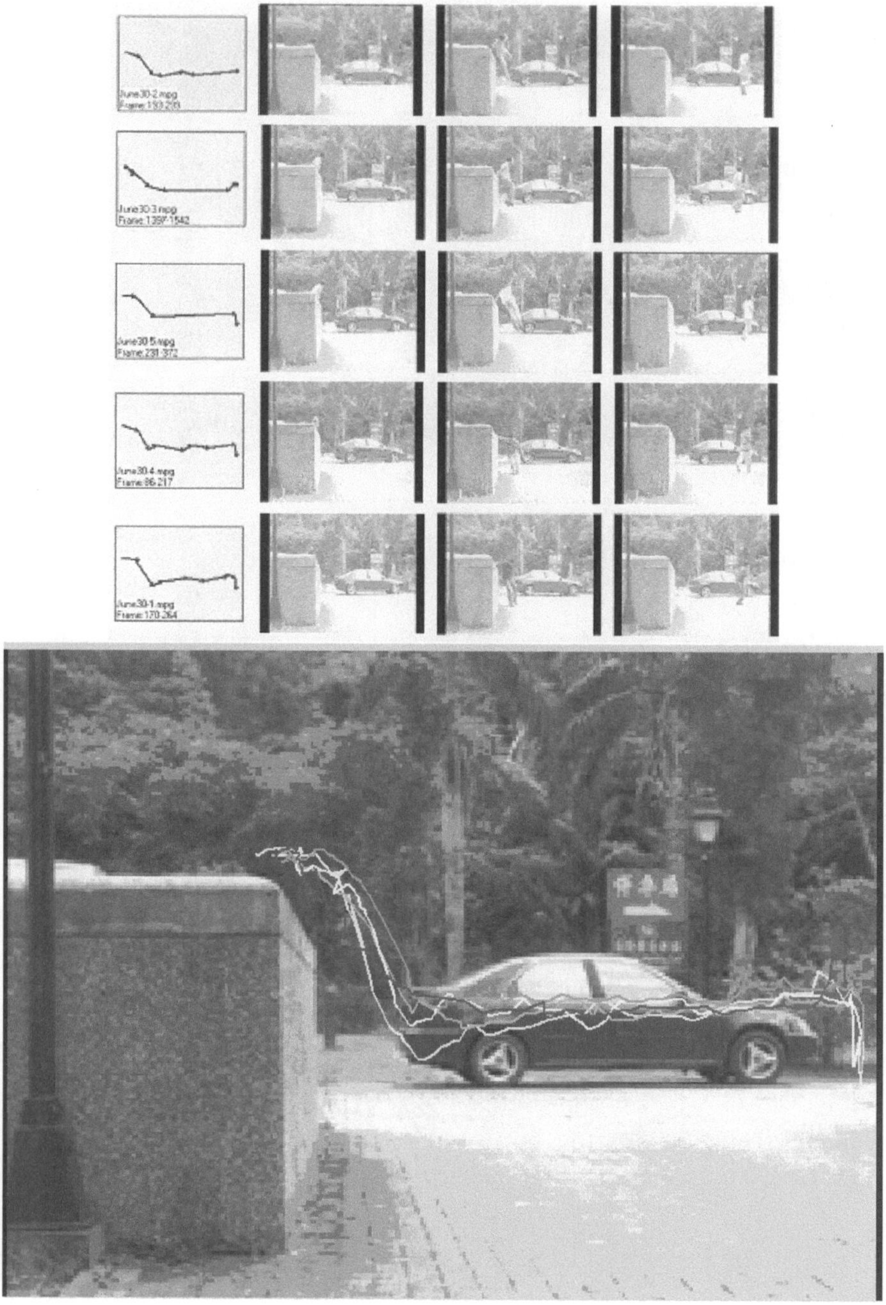

Fig. 9.7. A training set of pre-stored trajectories derived from the climbing-wall movements of five different human subjects.

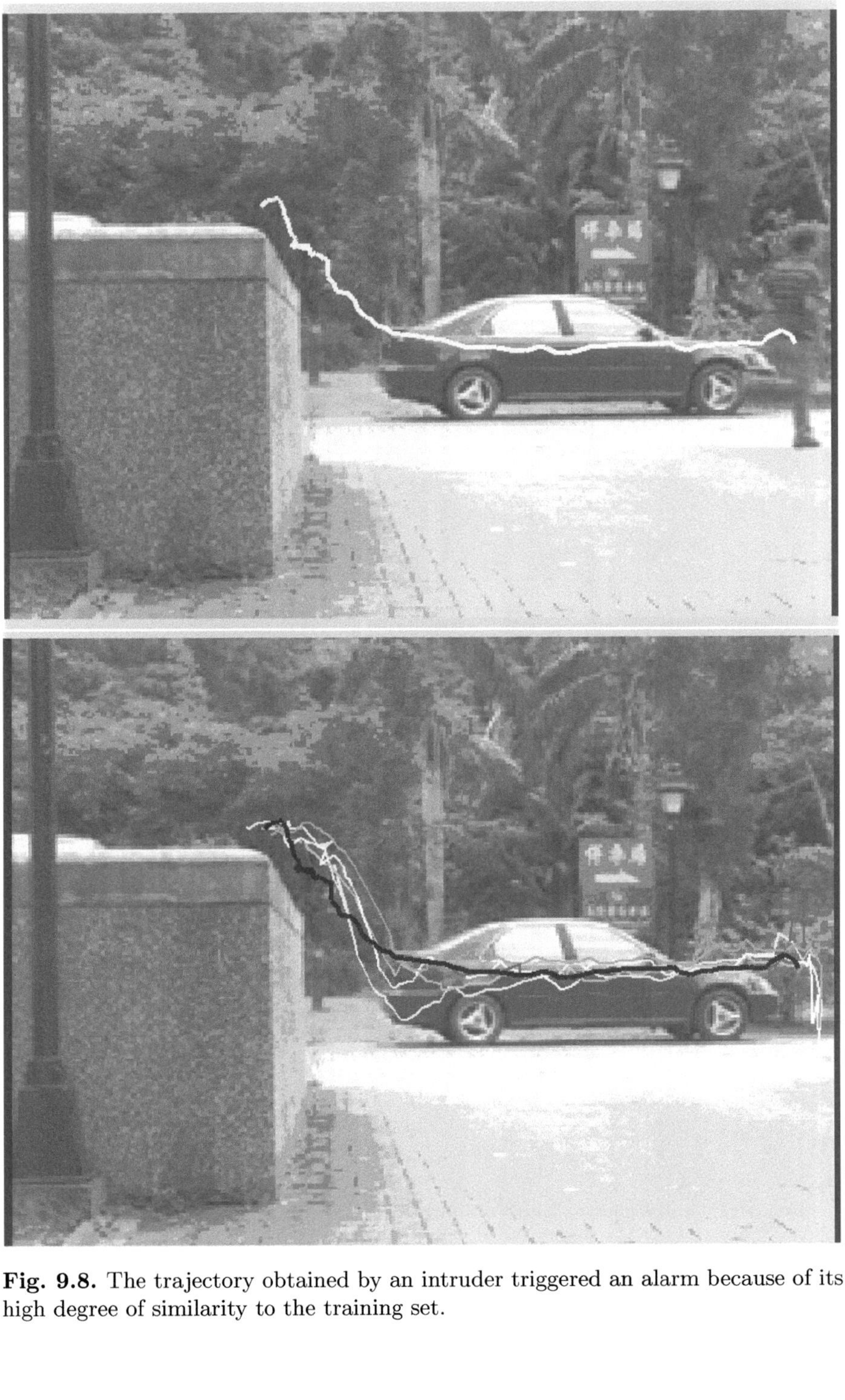

Fig. 9.8. The trajectory obtained by an intruder triggered an alarm because of its high degree of similarity to the training set.

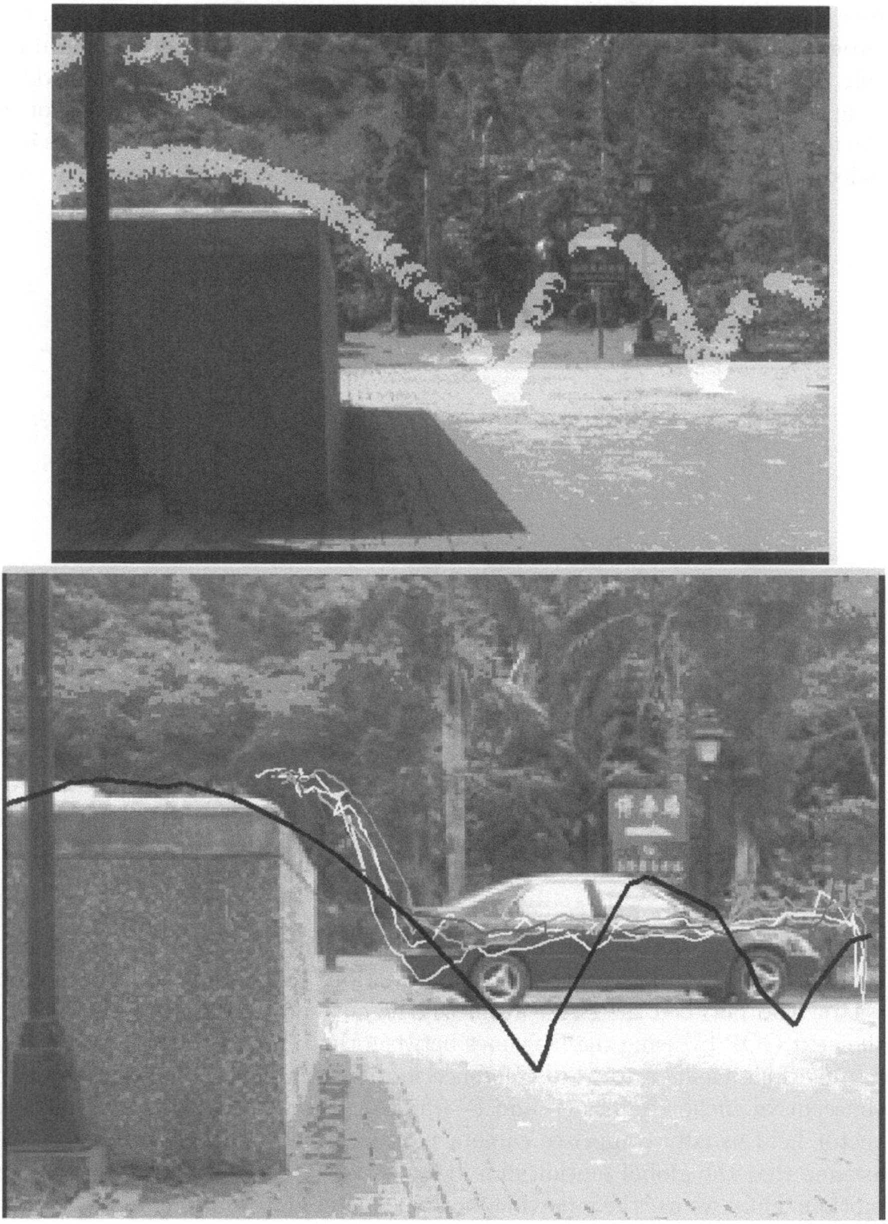

Fig. 9.9. The trajectory of a basketball does not trigger an alarm, since it is very different to the pre-stored trajectories.

user wants to retrieve the motion contributed by part of a video object, the trajectory-based representation scheme can not provide a correct retrieval result. We therefore propose the use of the motion vectors originally embedded in an MPEG bitstream to construct motion flows in a single shot. Although the motion vectors do not always correspond to the real motion of objects in a video when compared with the optical flow, they are relatively easy to derive.

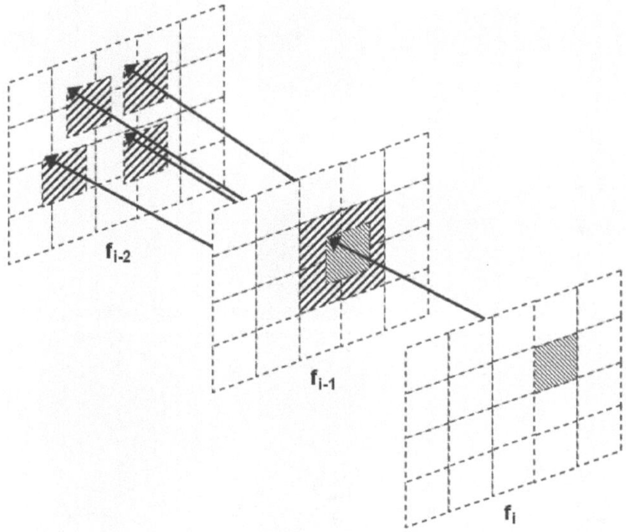

Fig. 9.10. A current motion vector and the four possible previous motion vectors that could be linked to it.

Before constructing the motion flows, we must do some pre-processing steps in order to compensate for camera motion. First, we produce a motion vector field between the last P-frame in the current GOP and the I-frame in the next GOP by using the B-frames between the P- and I-frame, as proposed in [26]. This yields a forward reference motion vector field between any two consecutive anchor-frames (I- and P- frames). It is well known that a motion vector field usually comprises camera motion, object motion, and noise. We assume that the global motion in a video is contributed primarily by camera motion. Thus, we use the following four-parameter global motion model, which is fast and valid for most videos [26], to estimate the camera motion from the motion vector field,

$$\overrightarrow{MV_{\text{cam}}} = \begin{pmatrix} \text{zoom} & \text{rotate} \\ -\text{rotate} & \text{zoom} \end{pmatrix} \bullet \begin{pmatrix} x \\ y \end{pmatrix} + \begin{pmatrix} \text{pan} \\ \text{tilt} \end{pmatrix} . \tag{9.13}$$

Once the four parameters have been estimated, we can find the degree of correspondence between each pixel in the current frame and its counterpart in the previous frame. The foreground pixels in the current frame can be identified if their color changes significantly after the camera motion. In addition, information about local motion can also be derived if one subtracts the estimated camera motion from the original motion vector field. If several foreground pixels within a macroblock survive the erosion process, the local motion corresponding to the macroblock can be regarded as robust. Otherwise, we ignore the local motion, because it probably arises from the background.

After the camera motion has been compensated for, we can extract the local motion fields from the bitstreams. Each field represents the movement of a macroblock between two consecutive anchor frames. However, a field is not usually continuous in the spatio-temporal domain, since motion vectors always start at regular places, but could end anywhere. Thus, when we try to make the necessary connections between two local motion fields, each macroblock in the current frame may overlap with four macroblocks in the previous frame, as shown in Fig. 9.10. In other words, it is possible that several candidate local motions located in the previous frame could be connected to a local motion in the current frame. Therefore, we use the following three criteria to choose the most reliable candidate for the current local motion: (1) the consistency of motion direction, (2) the color distribution, and (3) the overlapping area between macroblocks in the previous and the current frames. Suppose $\mathrm{LM}_{\mathrm{Cur}}$ is a local motion and C denotes the set of candidates of $\mathrm{LM}_{\mathrm{Cur}}$ in the previous anchor frame. The most reliable candidate, $\mathrm{LM}_{\mathrm{ancestor}}$, is chosen according to the following rule:

$$\mathrm{LM}_{\mathrm{ancestor}} = \arg\min_{m \in C} \left\| (\theta_m, \alpha\phi_m, \beta\varphi_m) \right\| , \tag{9.14}$$

where θ, ϕ, and φ denote the angle formed by $\mathrm{LM}_{\mathrm{Cur}}$ and a possible candidate m, the color histogram difference between macroblocks, and the overlapping area between macroblocks, respectively. Furthermore, all the parameters are normalized so that all values fall within the range [0,1], and α and β are weighted values that balance the influence of the three factors. Once the most reliable candidate of $\mathrm{LM}_{\mathrm{Cur}}$ has been determined, we link the local motions acquired at different time spots to form a single motion flow for each macroblock. Since a large moving object may cover several similar motion flows, we remove redundant flows and preserve one or more representative motion flows from all the similar motion flows. Initially, we select a motion flow, a, that has the longest duration in a shot. Suppose a starts from time t_i and ends at time t_j , and let $\{B\}$ be a set of motion flows whose start and end times are both within the duration of t_i and t_j . We remove a motion flow b, belonging to $\{B\}$, if it satisfies the following condition:

$$\frac{\sum_{t \in [t_s, t_e]} \left\| (a_t - a_{t_s}) - (b_t - b_{t_s}) \right\|}{t_e - t_s} < \epsilon, \tag{9.15}$$

where t_s and t_e are respectively the start and end times of motion flow b; a_t and b_t denote the spatial position of a and b at time t respectively; and a_{t_s}

and b_{t_s} denote the spatial position of a and b at time t_s respectively. If the average of the relative spatial distance between a and b is lower than a given threshold ϵ, we consider b to be a sub-segment of a. As b can be retrieved from a by a partial matching process, it is redundant and can be removed.

We then consider a as the representative of the motion flow removed from $\{B\}$ and store it in the database. Next, we again select the motion flow with the longest duration from the remaining motion flows, and repeat the above process until all motion flows are either stored or removed. Here, we only consider motion flows longer than 3 seconds in order to avoid the effects of noise and reduce the size of the database.

Fig. 9.11(b) shows different representative motion flows of the video clip shown in Fig. 9.11(a). The original motion flows (with $\epsilon = 0$) are shown on the left-hand side, and the motion flows after applying the removal process using different thresholds are shown in the middle and on the right-hand side, respectively. It is obvious that the redundant motion flows have been successfully removed, and that the number of representative motion flows is controlled by the value of ϵ. Fig. 9.12 shows another example of representative motion flows derived from a video sequence containing multiple moving objects and global camera motion. Since the movement of each object is different, several representative motion flows are generated concurrently to represent the way the objects move. The extraction of motion flows is therefore much faster and easier than deriving a trajectory, but there still exist two problems when we construct motion flows from motion vectors. First, the occlusion of multiple moving objects can cause a macroblock to be intra-coded, which means we could miss motion information. Thus, a complete motion flow for each moving object may not be derived. The region surrounded by dotted lines in Fig. 9.12 illustrates the above situation. The sudden termination of motion flows is apparently caused by the occlusion of two of the football players. Second, since we remove the camera motion before extracting the local motion from a video, the motion flow will break off if a moving object stops temporarily.

9.3.2 Coarse-to-Fine Trajectory Comparison

Having constructed the motion flows from each shot, we propose a new algorithm that compares the degree of similarity between a query trajectory and the trajectories formed by the motion flows in a database. Since we are looking for similar clips in the database, some geometric transformation, such as scaling or translation, should be handled. Here, we do not consider rotation invariance because the direction, that is, up-and-down or left-and-right, usually has semantic meaning in a video. For example, if one wants to query a jump motion, the trajectory should start from a lower position, pass through a higher position and then return to the lower position. Also, the issue of partial matching must be handled if a user provides an incomplete query. In the following, we propose a simple, but fast, algorithm for comparing two distinct trajectories (motion flows). To reduce the time complexity and minimize the

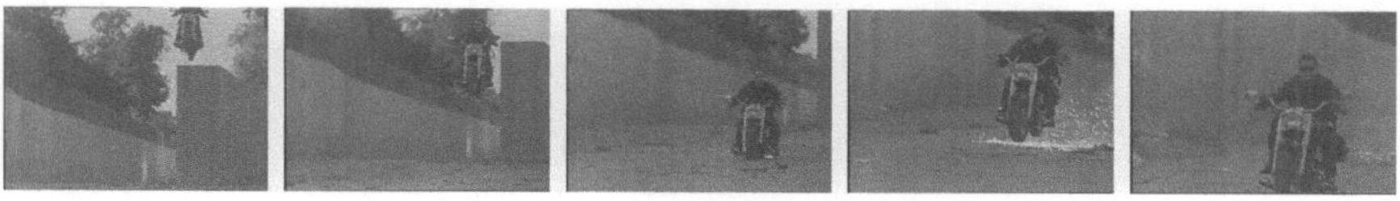

(a)

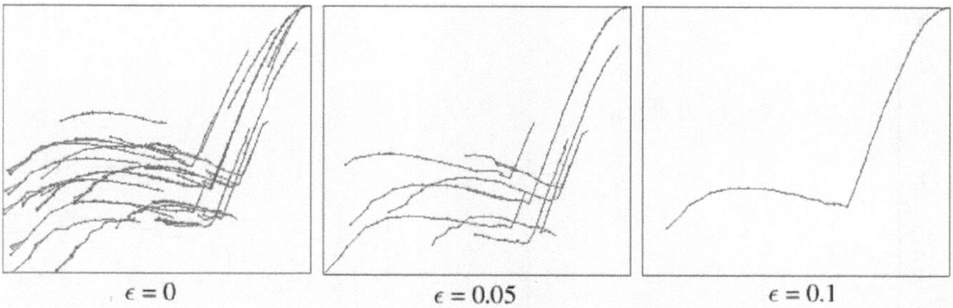

(b.1) (b.2) (b.3)

Fig. 9.11. (a) Original video clip. (b.1)–(b.3) The representative motion flows selected with threshold $\epsilon = 0$, 0.05, and 0.1.

storage space required, we remove redundant points from a trajectory, leaving only a few necessary points to represent it. We then use the Douglas-Peucker algorithm introduced in Section 9.2.3 to select the necessary control points from the trajectory. The algorithm starts by using a straight line which is called the anchor line to connect the start and end points of the trajectory. Once the perpendicular distance between any intermediate point and the anchor line is larger than a given threshold, the trajectory is split into two segments via the farthest intermediate point. The process continues until all the perpendicular distances are smaller than a pre-set threshold. Finally, the chosen intermediate points and the two end points are reserved as the control points of the trajectory.

We use six positive real numbers $(x+, x-, y+, y-, d, t)$ to represent a control point on a trajectory, where d denotes the cumulative length of the trajectory from the first control point to the current control point. Here $+/-$ denotes the cumulative positive/negative movement along the $x-$ or $y-$axis from the first control point to the current control point. Now, let Q and D be the trajectories of the query and a model in the database, respectively. In a QBS case, we normalize the length of both trajectories into a unit length before comparing them. This guarantees the requirement of scale invariance. Therefore, the parameters d, $x+$, $x-$, $y+$ and $y-$ of each control point on the two trajectories have to be normalized by dividing them by the length of Q and D, respectively.

According to the six parameters of a control point, d and t are utilized to make a fair comparison. We align both Q and D by calculating the length d

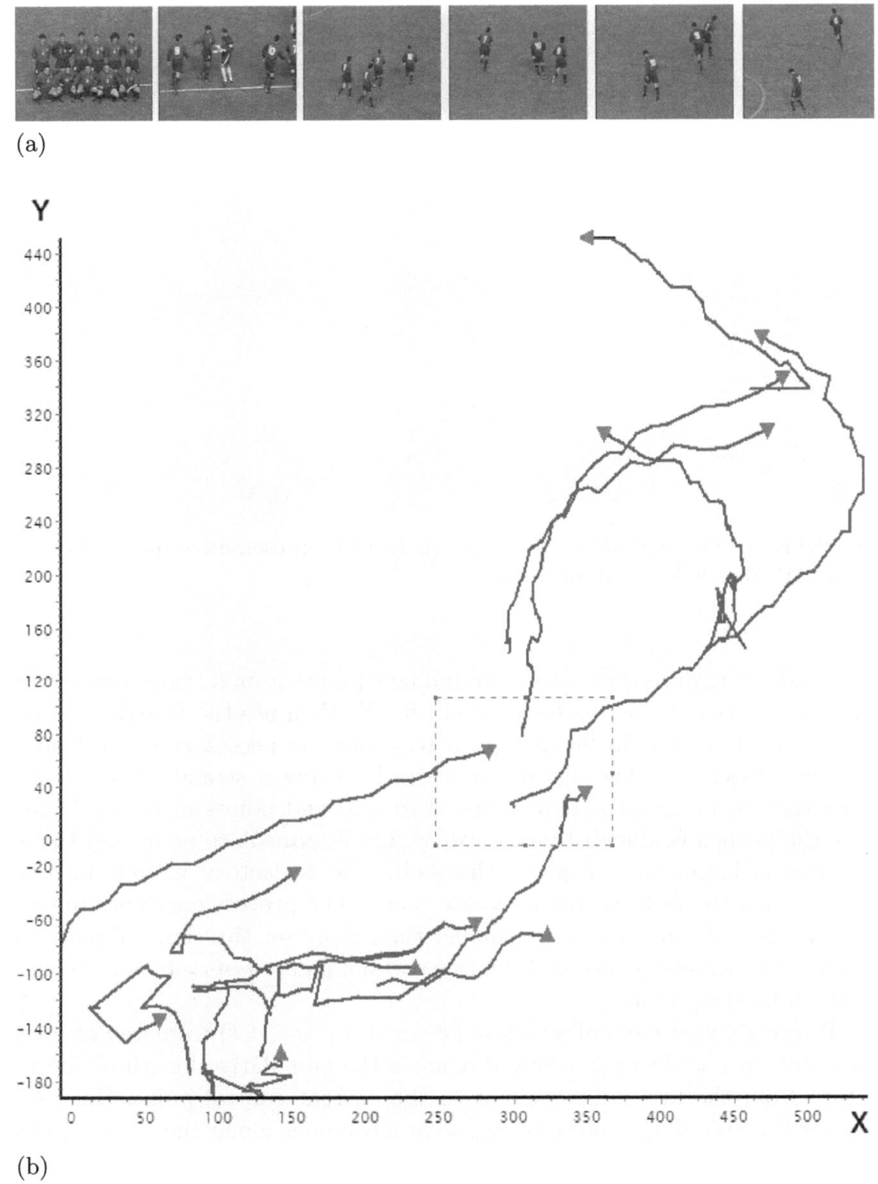

Fig. 9.12. (a) An original video clip. (b) The representative motion flows derived from the video sequence in (a).

or duration t from the first control point. For each control point on $Q(D)$, we interpolate a corresponding point that has the same cumulative length onto $D(Q)$. In a Query-By-Sketch (QBS) video retrieval system, the d value is used as the basis to conduct the alignment task, because we only consider the similarity between Q and D in the spatial domain, as shown in Fig. 9.4. On the other hand, the t value plays a crucial role when a video retrieval system incorporates the Query-By-Example (QBE) approach, as shown in Fig. 9.13. The control points and the corresponding points are labelled by circles and triangles, respectively. In this scenario, the insertion of corresponding points on Q and D is dependent on either d or t. Now, for each control point on the trajectory $Q(D)$, we can interpolate a corresponding point located on $D(Q)$. Assume the total number of control points and their corresponding points located on Q and D are both N. Let $Q' : \{Q'_1, Q'_2, \cdots, Q'_N\}$ and $D' : \{D'_1, D'_2, \cdots, D'_N\}$ be the set of points (including the control points and inserted corresponding points) located on Q and D, respectively. We call the points in set Q' and D' check-points, each of which can be represented by $(x+, x-, y+, y-)$ in the spatial domain. To compare two arbitrary trajectories, we use the matching process described in Section 9.2.3. The process is executed repeatedly until the computed distance is larger than δ, or there are no more intermediate check points within each sub-trajectory. Since most of the trajectories are filtered out by checking the first few control points, our proposed algorithm is very efficient. Furthermore, the partial matching problem can be solved by choosing two distinct control points on D as the new start and end points of D.

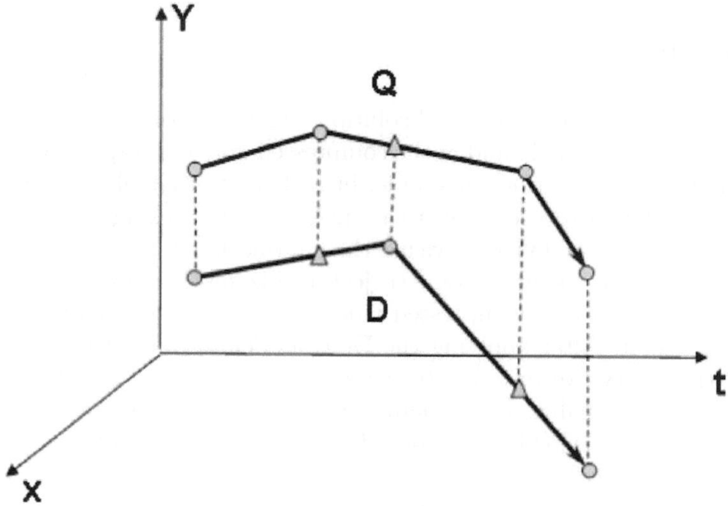

Fig. 9.13. The alignment task in QBE.

9.3.3 Experiment Results

To test the effectiveness and efficiency of our method, we took a compressed four-hour MPEG-2 test video from eight different locations as shown in Fig. 9.6. From the four-hour video, we extracted 108 video clips that contained motion. We call these clips with motion events. To simplify the QBS process, we used one of the eight locations as the background to assist in drawing a query sketch. The left-hand side of Fig. 9.14 shows a query sketch of a man climbing a stairway. Among the 108 events, the top three retrieved events were all of the man climbing the stairway at different times in the sequence. The 4th retrieved sequence was a descending the stairway event, which was retrieved because of its high degree of similarity to the top three retrieved events. In another experiment, we drew a climbing-wall trajectory with the help of the user interface (as shown in Fig. 9.15). From the top six retrieved events, it is obvious that the 1st, 3rd, 4th, 5th, and 6th all relate to the query. The 2nd retrieved event happened at another location; however, its corresponding trajectory was very close to the query sketch. In sum, we consider that the proposed method is especially useful in surveillance-related systems. It is also useful for a general coarse search. Since the approach can retrieve video clips from a large database in a very efficient manner and most of the retrieved results are close to the input query, we can use the approach as a coarse search engine. It is obvious that video databases of the future will be very large indeed. If we do not manage this kind of database efficiently, it will not be possible to enjoy to the full extent of the multimedia world of the future.

9.4 Conclusion

In this chapter, we have presented solutions for video-based surveillance systems in the spatial domain and in the compressed domain, respectively. In spatial domain event detections, a simple, but efficient, color blob-based tracker has been developed to accomplish the multi-object tracking task. For event detection in compressed videos, we use the information of motion vectors in an MPEG bitstream to generate some trajectory-like motion flows. Since motion vectors are embedded in compressed videos, we can process multiple moving objects in a shot. After applying the Douglas-Peucker algorithm to approximate a trajectory, we are able to compare two arbitrary trajectories. The above mechanism enables us to conduct both spatial domain and compressed domain event detections if a number of wanted trajectories are pre-stored in a video-based surveillance system.

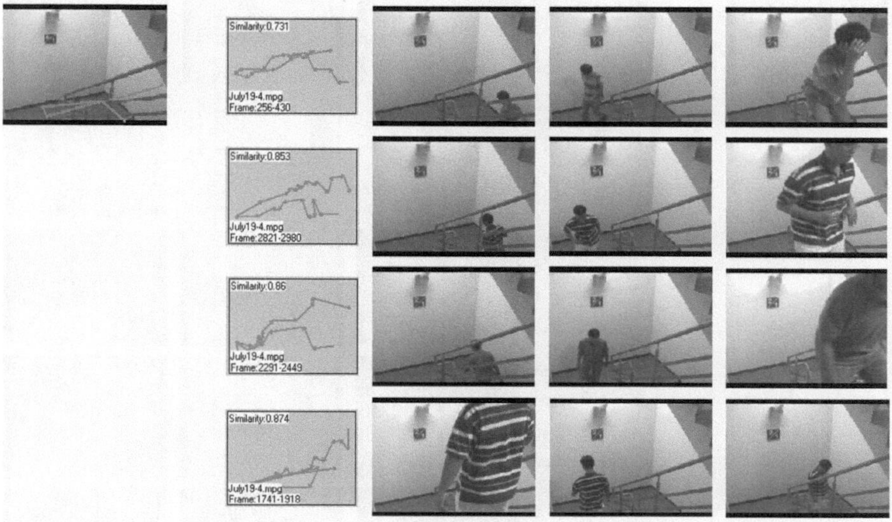

Fig. 9.14. An example of the retrieval result using query-by-sketch in a stairway scenario. The top four retrieved results (out of 108 video clips) are all related video clips.

References

1. Wren, C., Azarbayejani, A., Darrell, T., and Pentland, A. (1997): Pfinder: Real-time tracking of the human body. IEEE Trans. Pattern Analysis and Machine Intelligence, **19**, 780–785
2. Lipton, A., Fujiyoshi, F., and Patil, R. (1998): Moving target detection and classification from real-time video. Proc. IEEE Workshop Application of Computer Vision, 8–14
3. Grimson, E., Stauffer, C., Romano, R., and Lee, L. (1998): Using adaptive tracking to classify and monitoring activities in a site. Proc. Computer Vision and Pattern Recognition Conf., 22–29
4. Bobick A. and Ivanov, Y.A. (1998): Action recognition using probabilistic parsing. Proc. IEEE Conf. Computer Vision and Pattern Recognition, 196–202
5. Kanade, T., Collins, R.T., Lipton, A.J., Burt, P., and Wixon, L. (1998): Advances in cooperative multi-sensor video surveillance. Proc. DARPA Image Understanding Workshop, 3–24
6. Haritaoglu, I., Harwood, D., and David, L.S. (2000): W4: Real-time surveillance of people and their activities. IEEE Trans. Pattern Analysis and Machine Intelligence, **22**, 809–830
7. Stauffer, C. and Grimson, W.E. (1999): Learning patterns of activity using real-time tracking. IEEE Trans. Pattern Analysis and Machine Intelligence, **22**, 747–757
8. Zelnik-Manor, L. and Irani, M. (2001): Event-based video analysis. Proc. IEEE Conf. Computer Vision and Pattern Recognition, 123–130

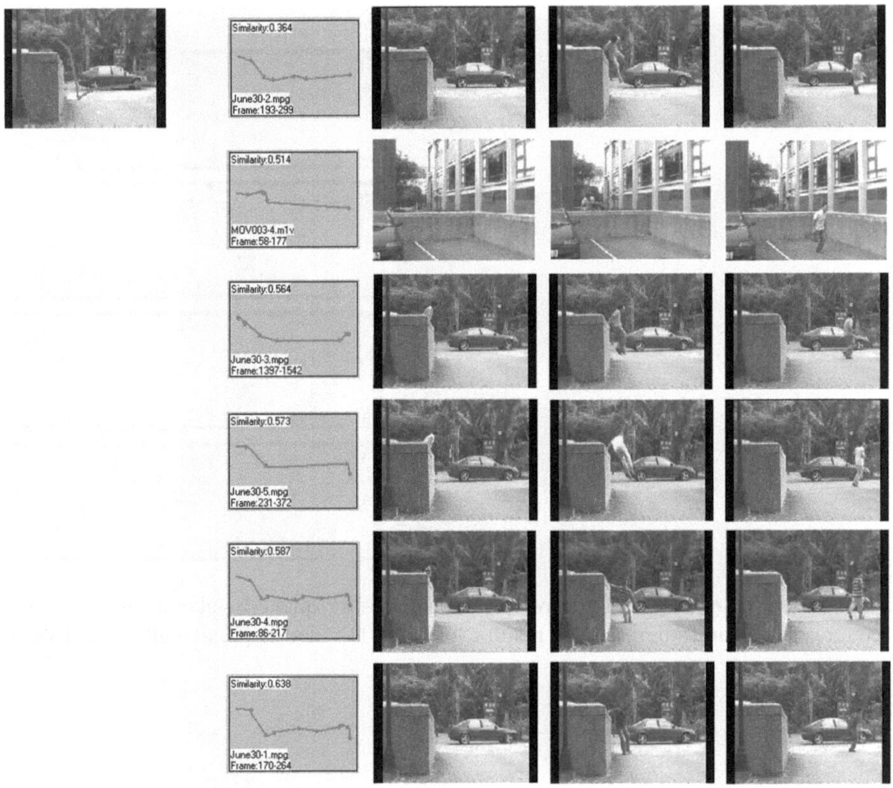

Fig. 9.15. An example of retrieval results using query-by-sketch on frames from an in-house video surveillance system. Except for the frames in the second row, all the retrieved results (out of 108 video clips) are related to the query trajectory. The trajectory of the clips in the second row is included because it has a very similar shape to those of the other retrieved results.

9. Medioni, C., Cohen, I., Bremond, F., Hongeng, S., and Nevatia, R. (2001): Event detection and analysis from video streams. IEEE Trans. Pattern Analysis and Machine Intelligence, **23**, 873–889
10. Davis, J. and Bobick, A. (1997): Representation and recognition of human movement using temporal templates. Proc. IEEE Conf. Computer Vision and Pattern Recognition, 928–934
11. Davis, L., Chelappa, R., Rosenfeld, A., Harwood, D., Haritaoglu, I., and Cutler, R. (1998): Visual surveillance and monitoring. Proc. DARPA Image Understanding Workshop, 73–76
12. McKenna, S.J., Jabri, S., Duric, Z., Rosenfeld, A., and Wechsler, H. (2000): Tracking groups of people. Computer Vision and Image Understanding, **80**, 42–56
13. Senior, A., Hampapur, A., Tian, Y.L., Brown, L., Pankanti, S., and Bolle, R. (2002): Tracking people with probabilistic appearance models. Proc. Interna-

tional Workshop on Performance Evaluation of Tracking and Surveillance Systems, 48–55
14. Makris, D. and Ellis, T. (2005): Learning semantic scene models from observing activity in visual surveillance. IEEE Trans. on Systems, Man, and Cybernetics – Part B: Cybernetics, **35**, 397–408
15. Su, C.-W., Liao, H.-Y.M., Tyan, H.-R., Lin, C.-W., and Fan, K.-C. (2005): A motion flow-based fast video retrieval system. Proc. 7th ACM SIGMM Workshop on Multimedia Information Retrieval, Singapore, 105–112
16. Liao, H.-Y.M., Chen, D.-Y., Su, C.-W., and Tyan, H.-R. (2006): Real-time event detection and its application to surveillance systems, to appear in Proc. IEEE International Symposium on Circuits and Systems
17. Huang, C.L. and Liao, W.C. (2004): A vision-based vehicle identification system. Proc. IEEE International Conference on Pattern Recognition, **4**, 364–367
18. Cheung, S.-C. and Kamath, C. (2004): Robust techniques for background subtraction in urban traffic video. Proc. Electronic Imaging: Visual Communications and Image Processing, **5308**, 881–892
19. Stauffer, C. and Grimson, W.E.L. (1999): Adaptive background mixture models for real-time tracking. Proc. IEEE International Conference on Computer Vision and Pattern Recognition, **19**, 23–25
20. Hammond, R. and Mohr, R. (2000): Mixture densities for video objects recognition. Proc. IEEE International Conference on Pattern Recognition, 71–75
21. Zivkovic, Z. (2004): Improved adaptive Gaussian mixture model for background substraction. Proc. IEEE International Conference on Pattern Recognition, 28–31
22. Scott, D.W. (1992): Multivariate density estimation, Wiley
23. Kailath, T. (1967): The divergence and Bhattacharyya distance measures in signal selection. IEEE Trans. on Communication Technologies, **15**, 52–60
24. Djouadi, A., Snorrason, O., and Garber, F. (1990): The quality of training-sample estimates of the Bhattacharyya coefficient IEEE Trans. on Pattern Analysis and Machine Intelligence, **12**, 92–97
25. Douglas, D.H. and Peucker, T.K. (1973): Algorithms for the reduction of the number of points required to represent a digitized line or its caricature. The Canadian Cartographer, **10**, 112–122
26. Wang, R. and Huang, T. (1999): Fast camera motion analysis in MPEG domain. Proc. ICIP, 691–694
27. Dagtas, S., Al-Khatib, W., Ghafoor, A., and Kashyap, R.L. (2000): Models for motion-based video indexing and retrieval. IEEE Trans. on Image Processing, **9**, 88–101
28. Fablet, R., Bouthemy, P., and Perez, P. (2002): Nonparametric motion characterization using causal probabilistic models for video indexing and retrieval. IEEE Trans. on Image Processing, **11**, 393–407

10

Print-to-Web Linking Technology Using a Mobile Phone Camera and its Applications in Japan

Zheng Liu[1]

C4 Technology, Inc., Meguro Tokyu Bldg., 2-13-17 Kamiosaki Shinagawa-ku, Tokyo 141-0021, Japan
zliu@c4t.jp
http://c4t.jp/

Summary. In recent years, with the rapid spread of mobile phones, the technology of print-to-web linking using mobile phone camera has attracted increasing attention. The print-to-web linking technology using a mobile phone camera is a new technique. Users can instantly link from the printed image to a related website where more information can be obtained by taking a picture with a mobile phone camera. This is an application of print-to-web linking technology using mobile phone camera. Many techniques using QR (quick response) code or bar code have been commercialized. Yet makers and advertising agencies are still trying to develop new techniques to replace them. This is because of the dull designs of QR code and bar code. The proposed methods using the watermarking techniques and image recognition techniques have been paid more attention. There are still a number of restrictions on their real applications. The general use of them remains challenging problems. A significant problem is the question of how will the future of print-to-web linking technology develop. In this chapter, I will introduce the methods of print-to-web linking technology using mobile phone camera and its applications in Japan in recent years.

10.1 Introduction

The mobile phone is one of the most significant technological advances of the 20th century. It has been reported that, in the last 10 years, the number of mobile phone subscribers has grown from 16 million in 1991 to an astounding figure of 941 million in 2001. The world mobile phone figures are estimated to grow to about 2.2 billion by 2006 [1]. An investigation done for the mobile phone market in 2005 showed that the mobile phone industry had a record first quarter with worldwide sales totaling 180.6 million units. A 17 percent increase from the first quarter of 2004, according to the report made by Screen Studio [2]. With the fast growth of mobile phone market, a mobile phone will play increasingly important roles in our daily life than a traditional phone. It

Z. Liu: *Print-to-Web Linking Technology Using a Mobile Phone Camera and its Applications in Japan*, Studies in Computational Intelligence (SCI) **58**, 261–285 (2007)
www.springerlink.com

can be used for tasks such as remote health supervision, home supervision, as an identification card and a multimedia terminal. Currently, some have already been realized in our daily life.

In addition to the mobile phone services described above, an innovation of traditional mobile phone is the appearance of the mobile phone camera. You can easily capture a picture and share it. In Japan, Sharp and J-Phone [3] introduced the first camera-phone J-SH04 [4] in September 2000. Three years later, in 2003, about 60% percent of mobile phones in Japan have cameras. It is expected that by 2005 the market penetration will about 100%. The image quality has greatly improved from the original 110k pixels of the J-SH04 in 2000 to the 4M pixels of D901iS [5] in 2005. This is as powerful as a high performance digital camera. With the rapid growth of mobile phone camera, a major topic on the Internet is the application of print-to-web linking technology using a mobile phone camera.

The print-to-web linking technology using mobile phone camera is a technique where users can instantly link from a printed image to a related website. More information can then be acquired. The QR (quick response) code and bar code have been commercialized for print-to-web linking technology using a mobile phone camera. Many makers are still trying to develop new techniques to replace the QR code and the bar code. This is because they are unsatisfied with the dull designs of the QR code and the bar code. They consider that the dull designs reduces the commercial effect of advertisements if they are printed using a QR code or bar code.

In order to develop new techniques to replace the QR code and bar code applications, in recent years, many new methods have been proposed for the applications of print-to-web linking technology using mobile phone camera. In these methods, watermarking techniques have been given much attention where the URL of a related website is acquired by extracting the watermark from the captured image by using a mobile phone camera. Their general use is still challenging problems. The major problem is the geometrical distortion of the images using a mobile phone camera.

Another new method of print-to-web technology using a mobile phone camera is that using recognition techniques. This is where the URL of a related website is acquired by using image recognition techniques. Compared with the methods using watermarking techniques, the methods using recognition techniques have high image quality and a high rate of success in print-to-web linking. This is because recognition techniques do not require embedding of information into an image. The image containing geometrical distortion can be also recognized by the use of image recognition techniques.

Although many new methods have been proposed to replace the QR code or bar code in recent years, there are still restrictions to their applications. The general uses of them are still challenging works. What is the future of print-to-web linking technology using mobile phone camera be? What market will exist in the near future? In this chapter, I introduce the development of print-to-web linking technology and their applications in Japan in recent years.

Section 10.2 presents a brief overview of techniques and applications for print-to-web linking technology using mobile phone camera. Section 10.3 introduces the inputting methods, traditional methods of print-to-web linking technology using a mobile phone. Section 10.4 introduces readable code methods, and general methods of print-to-web linking technology using mobile phone camera. Section 10.5 and Section 10.6 introduce watermarking methods and recognition methods respectively. These are the most attractive and challenging topics in the applications of print-to-web linking technology using a mobile phone camera. Section 10.7 introduces the applications of print-to-web linking technology using a mobile phone camera recently in Japan. Finally, some discussions and conclusions are given in Section 10.8.

10.2 Print-to-Web Linking Technology

Section 10.1 describes print-to-web linking technology using a mobile phone camera. This is a new technique which allows users to link from the printed image to a related website instantly where they can get more information. This is done by taking a photograph using a mobile phone camera. One can ask how does it work and what kind of applications can it serve? In this section we will give a brief answer to these questions.

10.2.1 System of Print-to-Web Linking Technology

There are basically two kinds of service system using print-to-web linking technology include a mobile phone camera. They may be categorized as those without and those with a retrieve server which is used to retrieve website URLs.

The System Without a Retrieve Server

As shown in Fig. 10.1, a system of print-to-web linking technology using a mobile phone camera without a retrieve server operates using the following steps:

Step 1: Editing the information about the URL of a website using sample pages from print media that can be done using the following methods.

(1) Embedding the information as watermark into a sample image and then printing the image on paper.

(2) Embedding the information into a bar code and then printing the bar code with the images on paper.

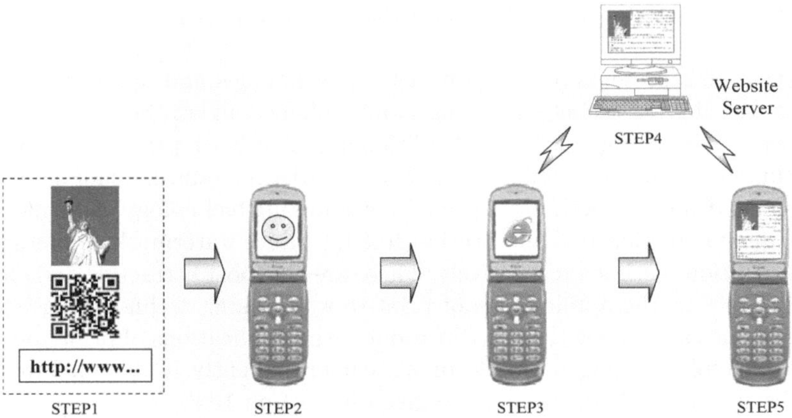

Fig. 10.1. A system of print-to-web linking technology without a retrieve server.

(3) Printing the URL with the images of the sample onto paper. The information about the URL of a website can be the n-bit stream corresponding to the URL or to the URL itself.

Step 2: Obtaining the information about the URL of a website by using a mobile phone that can be initially completed by using the following methods.

(1) Capturing printed image or bar code using the mobile phone camera and then extracting the information about the URL or using the URL from the captured image or bar code.

(2) Inputting the URL into the mobile phone directly. If the extracted information about the URL is not the URL itself, the information should be transformed to the URL by using a retrieve database that has been registered in a server or in the mobile phone previously.

Step 3: Linking the mobile phone to a related website with the URL obtained.

Step 4: Downloading the website page to the mobile phone.

Step 5: Displaying the website page on the mobile phone screen.

System With a Retrieve Server

In contrast to the system not using retrieve server, the system with a retrieve server can carry out complicated calculations. These include extracting the watermark from a captured image using complicated techniques, and retrieving the URL with a large database registered in a retrieve server. As shown in Fig. 10.2, a system with a retrieve server using these steps is given below.

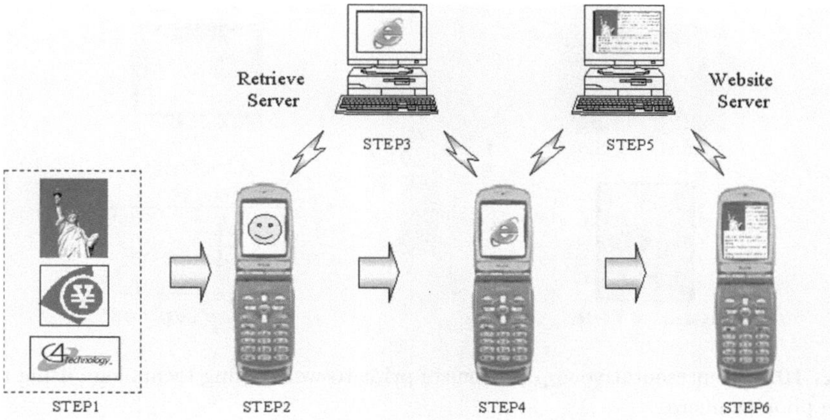

Fig. 10.2. A system of print-to-web linking technology with a retrieve server.

Step 1: Editing the information about the URL of a website on the sample pages of a printed media that can be done using the following methods.
  (1) Embedding the information as watermark into an image and then printing out the image on paper;
  (2) Representing the information using a logo mark and then printing out the logo mark with the image samples on paper. As described above, the information about URL of a website can be an n-bit stream corresponding to the URL or the URL itself.

Step 2: Obtaining the information about URL of a website by using a mobile phone can be completed by the following methods.
  (1) Capturing the printed image or logo mark using a mobile phone camera;
  (2) Sending the captured image or logo mark to a retrieve server.

Step 3: Retrieving the URL by extracting the information about the URL from the captured image or by comparing the logo mark with those registered in the database in a retrieve server, and then returning the URL to the mobile phone.

Step 4: Linking the mobile phone to a related website with the retrieved URL.

Step 5: Downloading the website page to the mobile phone.

Step 6: Showing the website page on the mobile phone screen.

10.2.2 Applications of Print-to-Web Linking Technology

With the development of the Internet, it is common in the print media, such as posters, pamphlets, magazines and corporate guidance, samples are printed with URL. Users can then access a related website where detailed information and related service can be acquired. When accessing a website with a mobile

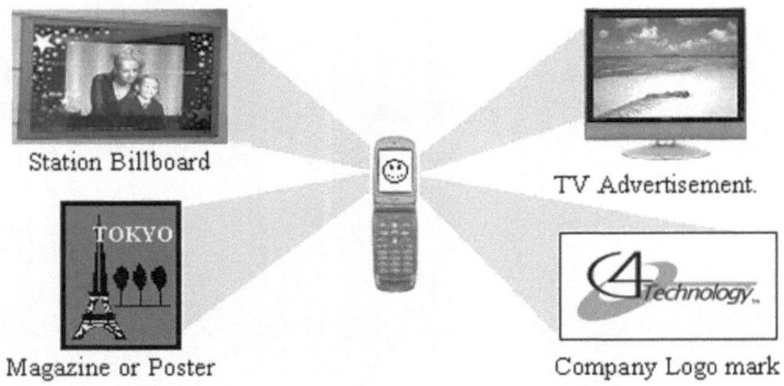

Fig. 10.3. Representative applications of print-to-web linking technology using mobile phone camera.

phone, it is usual that a long and tedious URL has often caused the operator to input the alphabets into the mobile phone until the last one, since there are few input buttons in a mobile phone. The development of print-to-web linking technology using the mobile phone, it becomes possible to link from print media to a related website. This can be done by taking a photograph with a mobile phone camera.

In our daily life, there are many possible applications of print-to-web linking technology using a mobile phone camera. Fig. 10.3 shows four representative applications of print-to-web linking technology using a mobile phone camera. They are as follows.

Magazines and Posters:

Instantly linking from a sample image printed on magazines or posters to a related website.

Television Advertisement:

Instantly linking from a still advertisement shown on a television screen to a related website instantly.

Station Signboard:

Instantly linking from a picture of a billboard to a related website instantly.

Company's Logo-mark:

Instantly linking from the company's logo mark printed on business cards or pamphlets to the company's website instantly.

In addition to the applications described above, there are many other applications that have been used or are about to be used in our daily life. These include:

(1) Buying tickets for a movie, a concert, or sport from a poster or news paper.
(2) Acquiring detail information about a movie, a concert, or sport, from the tickets.
(3) Watching a movie introduction from a DVD cover.
(4) Sampling songs from a CD cover.
(5) Watching a product demonstration from a pamphlet.
(6) Looking up product ingredients listed from a food tag.
(7) Acquiring author information from a book.
(8) Acquiring detailed information from a guide map when visiting a zoo, or visiting a famous place.
(9) Looking up the history of a handicraft, high-quality goods from the sample printed on magazine.
(10) Acquiring detailed information from the prescription of medical supplies.

10.2.3 Techniques of Print-to-Web Linking

Many techniques have been proposed for the applications of print-to-web linking technology using a mobile phone camera. They can be divided roughly into four categories as follows [6].

(1) Button inputting methods.
(2) Readable code methods.
(3) Watermarking methods.
(4) Image recognition methods.

In the following sections, we introduce these methods.

10.3 Button Inputting Methods

Button inputting methods are ways in which users can input the URL of a website into a mobile phone using the input buttons. Access to a remote service center or a website server where detailed information can be acquired. In this way, there are 3 kinds of inputting methods using a mobile phone.

(1) Inputting a telephone number.
(2) Inputting an URL.
(3) Inputting a brief code.

Inputting a Telephone Number:

The method of inputting a telephone number into a mobile phone is a traditional way of print-to-web linking technology using the telephone. Before the development of the Internet, dialing a telephone number printed with the samples on a poster or a magazine to access to a service center was a major way for users to acquire detailed information about printed samples. Currently, it is still an effective way for users to acquire detailed information about printed samples by the use of a mobile phone.

Inputting URL:

The method of inputting URL into a mobile phone is also a traditional way of print-to-web linking technology. Here users can access from print media to a related website by inputting the URL into a computer. With the development of web-enabled mobile phones, the method of inputting URL is also an effective way for users to acquire detailed information about printed samples using a mobile phone.

Inputting Brief Code:

The method of inputting a brief code is a simple way of inputting the URL. Users can have access to a related website only by inputting a brief code. i-Code [7] is an application of inputting brief code, where an URL is replaced by a brief code consisting of a sign and several digits such as `@123456`.

The system of inputting brief code method is completed with the following steps.
In preprocessing,

(1) determining a brief code to replace the URL of a website and registering the brief code to a data base in a retrieve server;
(2) printing out the brief code and the image samples on paper.

In its applications,

(1) inputting the brief code printed with an image sample on a poster or a magazine into a mobile phone with the input buttons;
(2) sending input brief code to a retrieve server where the received brief codes are compared with the brief codes in the data base a corresponded URL is retrieved;
(3) returning the retrieved URL to the mobile phone;
(4) linking the mobile phone to the website with retrieved URL.

Generally, the method of inputting brief code requires a plug-in type program to be executed on the mobile phones. These are downloaded into the mobile phones as previously done. An example is i αppli [8], BREW [9], etc.

10.4 Readable Code Methods

The readable code methods are the ways in which the URL of a website related to a printed media is encoded into a machine-readable code. It is then printed onto the paper with image samples.

Bar code is a traditional readable code that expresses numbers and characters with the combination of the "bar" and "space". It is detected optically by a read-machine. There are two kinds of bar code products, one is 1-dimensional bar code that expresses the information with a number of linear bars and a number of linear spaces. Another is a 2-dimensional bar code that arranges the information in the two directions of length and width. Fig. 10.4 shows two examples of bar code, a 1-dimensional and a 2-dimensional one.

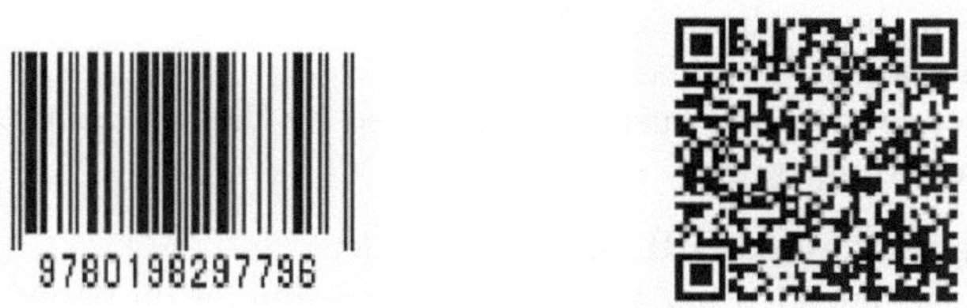

(a) JAN Code (b) QR Code

Fig. 10.4. Two examples of bar code, in which (a) is a sample of a 1-dimensional bar codes called JAN Code, and (b) is a sample of a 2-dimensional bar codes called QR Code (Quick Response Code).

Generally, the bar code is used as an input because of its efficiency, accuracy and low cost. With the appearance of mobile phone cameras, it became possible to use bar code as a method for the applications of print-to-web linking technology using mobile phone camera. At present, the function for reading a bar code has been widely supplied on mobile phones. It has become a standard function of the mobile phone.

Compared with 1-dimensional bar codes, 2-dimensional bar codes can increase the embedded amount of information 200 times or more. Since the data embedded into 2-dimensional bar codes are enciphered, the security is also improved. Therefore, 2-dimensional bar codes are more widely used in mobile phones.

In addition to the bar codes, there are some other kinds of readable codes that have been used for print-to-web linking technology. The methods of developing readable codes can be divided into 3 categories according to the dimension or design of their constructions. They are as follows.

(1) One-dimensional bar code methods;

(2) Two-dimensional bar code methods;
(3) Color code methods.

10.4.1 One-Dimensional Bar Code Methods

As shown in Fig. 10.4(a), JAN (Japan Article Number) is a 1-dimensional bar code that can be read and recognized by Barcode Reader [10]. It is a popular application for the mobile phone in Japan. JAN is standardized by JIS (JIS-X-0501) and is carried by almost all of the goods in the store.

10.4.2 Two-Dimensional Bar Code Methods

As shown in Fig. 10.4(b), QR Code (Quick Response Code) is a 2-dimensional bar code, which is also standardized by JIS (JIS-X-0501). Currently it has been widely used in the applications of print-to-web linking technology using the mobile phone camera in Japan.

The bar code method is usually completed by the following processes. In the preprocessing stage,

(1) encoding the desired URL into a bar code;
(2) printing the encoded bar code with image samples on paper.

In its application,

(1) starting a bar code reading is make by the use of a mobile phone;
(2) The bar code is printed to a mobile phone camera;
(3) the bar code is captured by the mobile phone camera and is controlled by the bar code reading solution. The URL is automatically decoded from the captured image;
(4) the mobile phone is linked to the website with decoded URL;
(5) the website page is downloaded to the screen of the mobile phone.

As an application of print-to-web linking technology using a mobile phone camera, the bar code method is a mature technique widely used in daily life. However, as shown in Fig. 10.4, the major defect of bar code may be its dull design. It was imagined that the original design of printed image would be spoiled, when the pages of a magazine have too many mosaic-like patterns. The bar code methods require additional space on paper for printing a bar code with an image sample. This will reduce the effectiveness of advertisements.

It is for the above reasons that many advertising agencies are unwilling to print bar code with the samples on their papers. The bar code is used freely on the Internet [11].

10.4.3 Color Code Methods

Considering the negative effects of the bar code methods described above, some makers are trying to use the designs with attractive patterns to replace the dull designs of bar codes. The color code method is an example. It was proposed by Colozip Media Inc. and called as ColorCode [12]. As shown in Fig. 10.5, the ColorCode consists of 5 and 5 patterns in 4 kinds of colors, red, green, blue, and black, with a black frame. Therefore, they are also known as 3-dimensional codes. As shown in Fig. 10.6, the design of ColorCode can have other kinds of patterns such as squares, hearts, characters, etc.

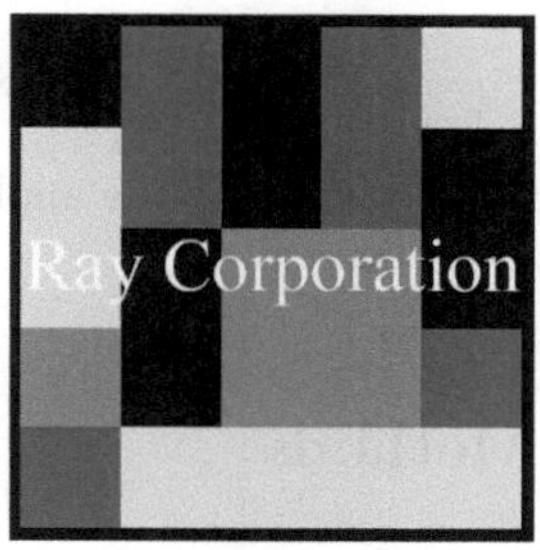

Fig. 10.5. A sample of ColorCode [12].

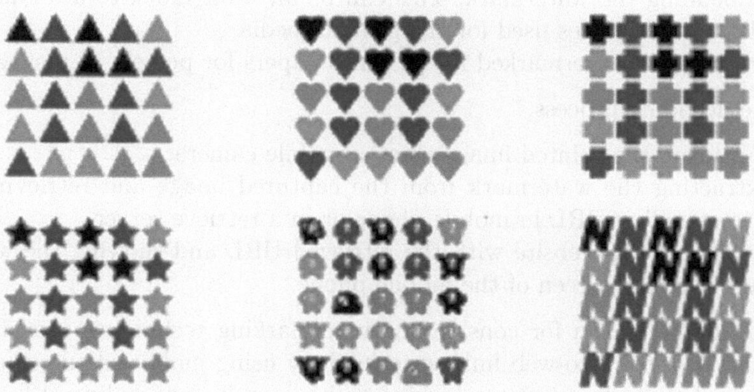

Fig. 10.6. Examples of designs of ColorCode [12].

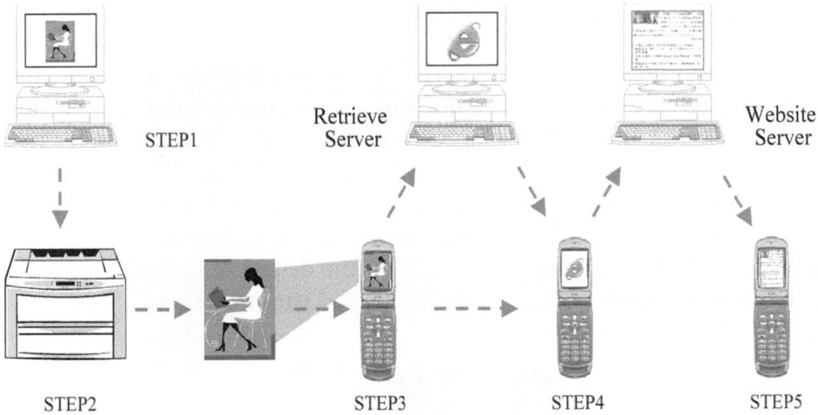

Fig. 10.7. Watermarking techniques used for the applications of print-to-web linking technology using mobile phone camera.

10.5 Watermarking Methods

The third kind of method used for the applications of print-to-web linking technology using mobile phone is the watermarking technique. As shown in Fig. 10.7, the watermarking methods are generally completed using the following processes.
The embedding process,

(1) Embedding the watermark. This can be an n-bit index to a database of URL of the images used for the printed media.
(2) Printing the watermarked images onto papers for posters or magazines.

The decoding process,

(1) Capturing the printed image using a mobile camera.
(2) Extracting the watermark from the captured image and retrieving the corresponding URL in mobile phone or in a retrieve server.
(3) Linking to the website with the retrieved URL and showing the website page onto the screen of the mobile phone.

The major reason for considering watermarking techniques used for the application of print-to-web linking technology using mobile phone camera is that one of the roles of watermarking technology is data hiding [13]. By its use we can embed the information about URL imperceptibly into an image. The URL information can then be extracted from the printed image. With the improvement of robustness in watermarking techniques, it is not a novelty to extract embedded information from a printed image by capturing the image with a PC-camera. An example of this application is Digimarc's ImageBridge [14]. This was the first application of the watermarking technique being used for printed media together with a PC-camera or a scanner.

10.5.1 Major Problems for Watermarking Methods

The major merit of using watermarking techniques is that it is unnecessary to have an additional space on paper for printing an additional mark such as with QR codes. Compared to the applications using a PC-camera or scanner, it is not easy to use watermarking techniques for the applications of print-to-web linking technology using mobile phone camera. This is because there are some strict restrictions in their applications. These are as follows.

Illumination Condition:

The embedded watermark must be extracted exactly from the image captured under the lighting conditions. When using a mobile phone camera, this include factors such as dark light indoor, or sunshine outdoor.

Photography Conditions:

Here again the embedded watermark must be extracted exactly from the image captured by those who have used the mobile phone camera. Therefore, the resolution of the captured image will be widely different depending on the photography method used.

Mobile Camera Condition:

The embedded watermark must again be extracted exactly from the image captured by the mobile phone cameras. These have different performances, and the resolutions can be very different.

Embedding Capability:

The images must have the capability to embed watermark with enough bits in order to index a wide range of websites. In general, the current mobile phone camera suffers in that the maximal image pixels and the capability of image processing are limited.

Printed Image Quality:

In order to embed more information into an image having limited image pixels is to enhance the watermark robustness. This is done at the cost of reducing image quality within the tolerable range of the human eye. The ability to reduce the image quality is very limited. This is because the precondition for using watermarking is that it should be imperceptible in the image quality.

10.5.2 Watermarking Schemes

In order to solve the problems of watermarking techniques used for the applications of print-to-web linking technology using mobile phone camera, the only way for us is to make the watermark more robust at the cost of reducing image quality within the perceptible tolerance of human eyes. As a general method for robust watermarking techniques, it is common to generate watermark into patterns that have the low perceptibility and have high correlation properties.

Many watermarking methods have been proposed for the applications of print-to-web linking technology using a mobile phone camera. These can be divided into 4 categories as follows:

(1) Watermarking in the frequency domain.
(2) Watermarking in the spatial domain.
(3) Watermarking in the color domain.
(4) Watermarking in the special design.

10.5.3 Frequency Domain Methods

A watermark generated in frequency domain is a method that inserts some special components into an image frequency domain. It then generates the watermark pattern by inverse-transforming the pattern into the spatial domain. We know that the major merit of a watermark generated in the frequency domain is the robustness to geometrical transform [15]. Fig. 10.8 shows an example of watermark generated in frequency domain. A similar method was proposed by a company in Japan. The drawback of this method is that it is time consuming during the watermark extraction process.

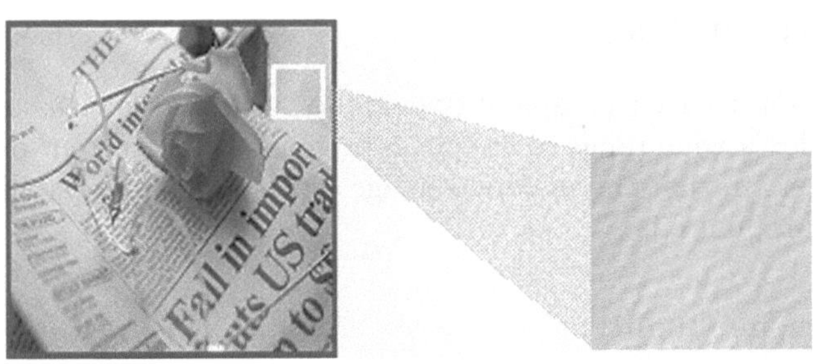

Fig. 10.8. An example of the watermark generated in frequency domain, and the right one is an expanded area in the left image.

10.5.4 Spatial Domain Methods

A watermark generated in the spatial domain is a method that generates watermark patterns using some noise patterns that possess correlation properties. For example m-sequences. The watermark patterns are then embedded into an image in spatial domain. Fig. 10.9 shows an example of a watermark pattern generated in spatial domain. A similar method was proposed by a company in Japan. The major merit of this method is fewer calculations in the process of watermark extraction. The drawback of this method is that in the process of watermark detection, the existence of the image itself will reduce the rate of detection of embedded noise patterns. Therefore, as shown in Fig. 10.9, the images are generally designed with a wide blank background where the noise patterns are embedded.

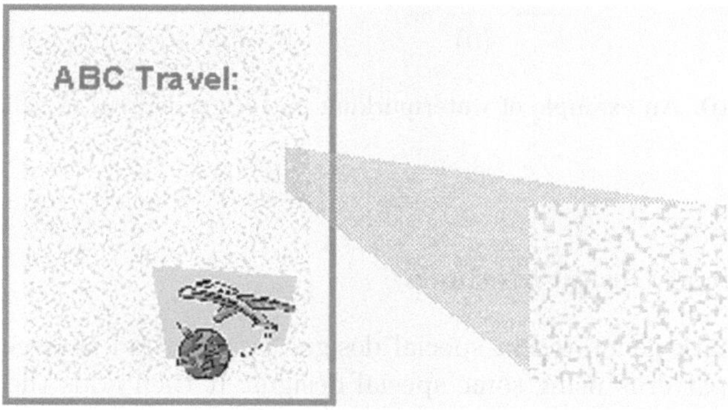

Fig. 10.9. An example of a watermark generated in spatial domain, and the right one is an expanded area in the left image.

10.5.5 Color Domain Methods

The watermark generated in the color domain is a method that generates the watermark patterns using colors that are hard to perceive by the human eye. It embeds the watermark patterns into an image in the spatial domain. Fig. 10.10 shows an example of a watermark generated using yellow colors. A similar method was proposed by a company in Japan. As shown in Fig. 10.10(b), the yellow domain of an image Fig. 10.10(a) was divided into small blocks and two adjoining blocks were indexed from left to right horizontally. These are embedded with 1 bit of information in the following way. If a bit information 1 is embedded,

- then the average yellow in left block is adjusted to be larger than that in right block.

On the other hand, if a bit information 0 is embedded,

- the average yellow in left block is adjusted to become smaller than that in right block.

The major merit of this method is that the watermarked image is barely perceptible to human eyes. When the image contains fewer yellow components, the performance of this method will be impaired.

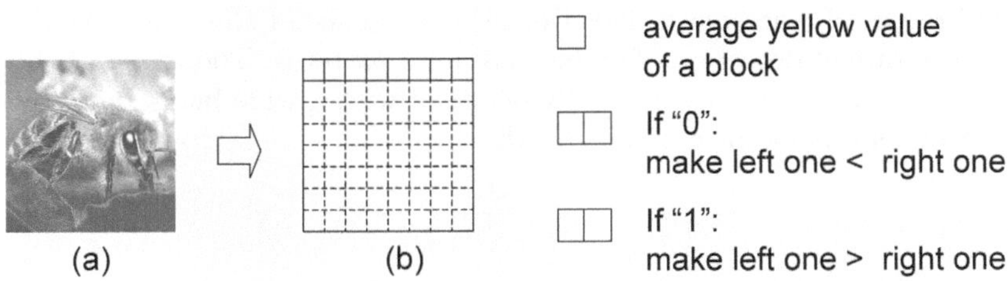

Fig. 10.10. An example of watermarking pattern generated in yellow color.

10.5.6 Special Design Methods

The watermark generated in special designs is a method that generates the watermark patterns using some special designs. It then adds the watermark patterns into an image in the spatial domain. Fig. 10.11 shows an example of watermarking patterns using a design shown in the right hand side. A similar method was proposed by a company in Japan. The major merit of this method is the robustness of pattern designs. As shown in Fig. 10.11, the drawback of this method is it can be easily seen in designed patterns. This is despite the fact that the patterns are designed to be as beautiful as possible.

10.5.7 Watermark Decoding

We know that in a watermarking technique, the watermark robustness is generally determined in watermark encoding process. The problem is how to extract the watermark from a watermarked image effectively. This is the work of watermark decoding. The embedded watermark must be detected from the image, which may be geometrically transformed with some image editing or image processing.

Currently, there are two kinds of watermark decoding methods used for the applications of print-to-web linking technology using the mobile phone camera. They are as follows:

(1) Decoding in a mobile phone;

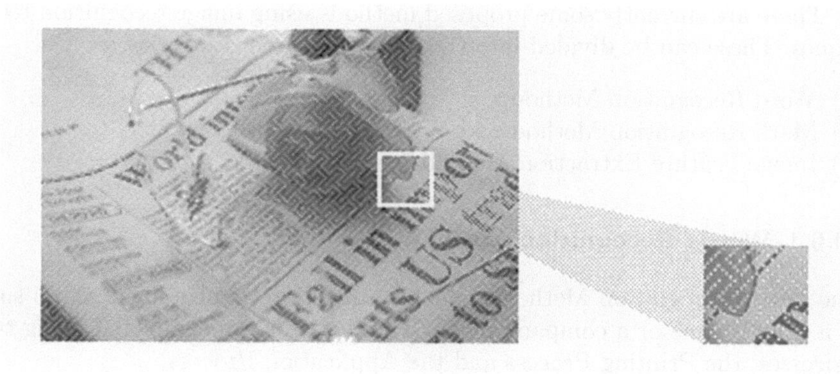

Fig. 10.11. An example of watermark generated in a special design, and the right one is an expanded area in the left image.

(2) Decoding in a server.

As shown in Fig. 10.1, the method of decoding in a mobile phone is the way in which the watermark is decoded from a captured image by a calculation in a mobile phone. The merit of this detection method is that the process of decoding will not be affected by the mobile phone communication state. The drawback of this method is that it consumes too much time for decoding calculation, because of the limited computing capability of current mobile phones.

As shown in Fig. 10.2, the method of decoding in a server is a way in which the watermark is decoded from a captured image. This is done by sending captured image to the server and by the calculation in that server. The merit of this method is that watermark can be decoded by using a highly effective scheme for the calculation. The drawback of this method is that the transmission of a picture from mobile phone to a server may be greatly changed. It may also take too much time when the communication of mobile phones is congested.

10.6 Image Recognition Methods

The fourth kind of method used for the applications of print-to-web linking technology using a mobile phone camera is the method using Image Recognition Techniques. Contrary to the watermarking methods, the major merits of image recognition techniques are their high rate of image recognition and high image quality. The reasons are that the pictures captured with mobile phone cameras are retrieved by image features without embedding and further for the image. A captured image can be easily recognized by the use of Image Recognition Techniques.

There are currently some proposed methods using image recognition techniques. These can be divided into the following three categories.

(1) Word Recognition Method;
(2) Mark Recognition Method;
(3) Image Feature Extraction Method.

10.6.1 Words Recognition Method

The Word Recognition Method is mainly used to recognize fixed words such as a brand name or a company name. The methods are completed using two processes, the Printing Process and the Application Process.
In the Printing Process, the method is as follows.

(1) Registering the special words as a pattern in a retrieve server;
(2) Printing the words with samples on the pages of publisher.

In the Application Process, the method is as follows.

(1) Captured printed words from the pages of publisher using a mobile phone camera;
(2) Cropping the word patterns pattern from the captured image and then sending it to the retrieve server;
(3) Retrieving the corresponding URL by comparing the captured words pattern with those registered in the retrieve server;
(4) Sending the retrieved URL to the mobile phone and linking mobile phone to a related website with retrieved URL.

The techniques used for recognizing words patterns can be any kind of recognition process such as the techniques of Image Matching or Pattern Recognition. The PaperClick Code [16] is an application of print-to-web linking technology using a mobile phone, which has the word reading function.

10.6.2 Mark Recognition Method

The Mark Recognition Method is mainly used to recognize special marks, such as commercial marks or company logo marks, which is a way similar to the words recognition method. The printing process and application process of mark recognition method are as same as those of the words recognition method excepting that the registered objects in the retrieved server are Mark Patterns, not Words Patterns.

10.6.3 Image Feature Extraction Method

In recognition methods, an attractive topic is the image recognition, because the original samples on printed media are images. If we can link printed image to a related website by using the image itself, it is not necessary to print the image samples with some additional patterns such as bar code, words pattern, and logo mark, etc. The realization of Image Recognition Methods will be more challenging work compared with the Words Recognition Methods. The mark recognition methods should be used and more image data should be processed. This is because in order to recognize an image, more complicated techniques are necessary in this case.

Image Feature Extraction Method:

A proposed image recognition method is called as MiLuLa [17], in which the URL is retrieved by the method of image features extraction. As principle, let us consider a pair of pictures showed in Fig. 10.12.

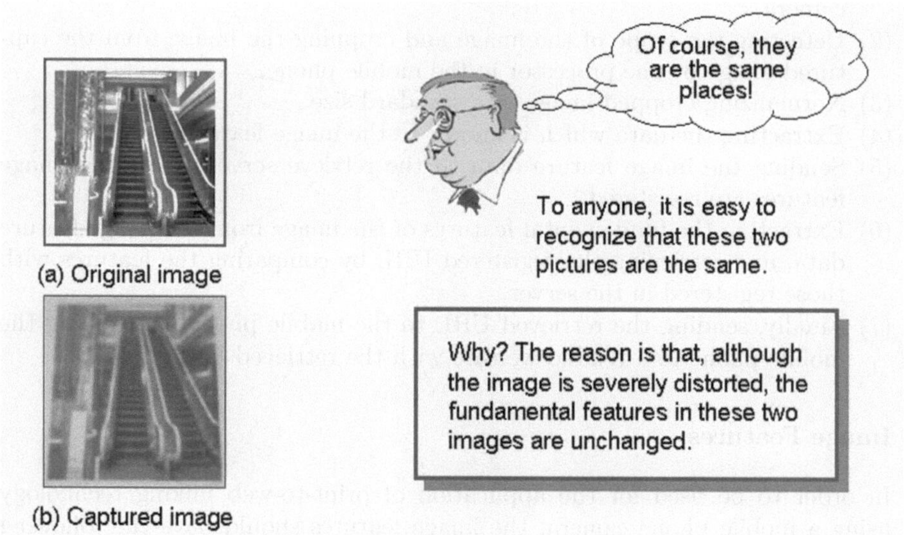

Fig. 10.12. Image (a) and (b) are an original image and an image with severe geometrical deformation which was taken by a mobile phone camera.

In Fig. 10.12, the images (a) and (b) are an original picture and a picture with severe geometrical deformation that was taken using a mobile phone camera. Generally, it is difficult for a watermarking method to extract an embedded watermark from an image with such severe deformation as in Fig. 10.12(b). With the human eye, we can easily recognize that these two images are the same pictures. Why is this? The reason is that, although the image is severely deformed, the fundamental features in the image remain unchanged. With these fundamental features we can recognize the image correctly at a short time.

According to the principle described above, the image extraction method is completed in two processes: the process of image feature registration and the process of image feature retrieval. The purpose of process of image feature registration is to extract the fundamental features from an image. This is completed as follows.

(1) Normalizing the image to a standard size.
(2) Extracting the fundamental image features from the standardized image.
(3) Registering the extracted image features in a retrieve server.

The purpose of the process of retrieving image features is to link a mobile phone to a website by extracting the fundamental features from the captured image using a mobile phone camera. It is completed as follows:

(1) Capturing an image from the printed image by using a mobile phone camera.
(2) Detecting the scope of the image and cropping the image from the captured image by the processor in the mobile phone.
(3) Normalizing cropped image to a standard size.
(4) Extracting the data which is known as the image feature data.
(5) Sending the image feature data to the retrieve server where the image features are registered.
(6) Extracting the fundamental features of the image from the image feature data, and retrieving the registered URL by comparing the features with those registered in the server.
(7) Finally, sending the retrieved URL to the mobile phone and linking the mobile phone to a related website with the retrieved URL.

Image Features:

In order to be used for the application of print-to-web linking technology using a mobile phone camera, the image features should have the following characteristics.

(1) They should represent the image characteristics as well as possible with the image data.
(2) They could be extracted from the image with less calculation.
(3) They shall be retrieved from many registered image features in the least time.
(4) They could be able to be extracted from the photographs taken under the different lighting conditions.
(5) They shall be able to be extracted from images having some geometric distortions.

Applications:

The results of actual applications proved that proposed method of image feature extraction can be effectively used for print-to-web linking technology. In March 2005, the product of MiLuLa was formally adopted as Pattobi-by-MiLuLa by NTTDATA CORPORATION [18]. This is a server service for print-to-web linking applications. The performance of MiLuLa is given in Table 10.1.

Table 10.1. The performance of MiLuLa.

Item	Data
Server CPU:	2.8 GHz (Pentium4)
Server OS:	Windows Server2003
Server RAM:	1 GB
Mobile Phone:	NTT DoCoMo
Total Registered Images:	10000 Sheets
Server Retrieval Time:	0.14 Second

10.7 Developments of Print-to-Web Linking Technology in Japan

With the rapid increase of mobile phone cameras in recent years, industrialization of the print-to-web linking technology is becoming a topic of great interest in Japan since June 2003. Each major maker has expended a great of energy on the technique and development for the applications of print-to-web linking technology using a mobile phone camera. The developed technology or products are then announced. Table 10.2 shows the techniques released by makers in Japan since June 2003.

Although each technique as shown in Table 10.2 has the required features respectively, there are still issues which must be resolved before their real utilization. With the fast development of mobile phone camera techniques, the utilization of print-to-web linking technology will become reality in the near future.

10.8 Conclusions and Discussions

In this chapter, I have introduced the techniques used in Japan for print-to-web linking applications and the development of print-to-web linking technology. As shown in Fig. 10.13, the proposed methods used for the applications

Table 10.2. The developments of print-to-web linking technology in Japan.

Release Date	Manufacturer (Product Name)	Technique/Decode Type
2003/06/16	Kyodo Printing Co., Ltd. [19]	Color Domain/Server
2003/07/07	NTT (Cyber-Squash) [20]	Spatial Domain/Server
2003/11/10	M.Ken.Co., Ltd.(i-acuaport) [21]	Frequency Domain/Local
2004/01/27	NTT (P-warp) [22]	Special Design/Server
2004/06/21	MediaGrid Inc.(ClickPix!) [23] Technique resource: Digimarc Corporation, U.S.A [14]	Spatial Domain/Server
2004/06/30	Fujitsu Laboratories Ltd. [24]	Color Domain/Local
2004/07/20	SANYO Electric Co., Ltd. [25]	Frequency Domain/Server
2004/08/12	C4 Technology, Inc.(MiLuLa) [17]	Image Feature/Server
2004/11/11	Olypus Corporation (SyncR) [26]	Image Recognize/Local
2005/03/01	Colozip Japan Inc.(ColorCode) [12] Technique resource: Colozip Media Inc. Korea [12]	Color Domain/Local

of print-to-web linking technology using mobile phone can be divided into four categories: button inputting methods, the readable code methods, the watermarking methods, and the image recognition methods.

The button inputting methods are the simplest and are used for the applications of print-to-web linking technology. The methods can be completed by only pushing buttons in a mobile phone. It is often a frequent complaint that it is too troublesome to input a long URL into a mobile phone using buttons in a mobile phone, they remain basic functions of a mobile phone used for print-to-web linking technology.

Readable code methods, especially the two-dimensional bar code methods, have been widely used in mobile phones to replace the button inputting methods. The methods can be completed with high reliability and provide website linking at a low cost. These methods require the additional space to print the sample with a bar code. Moreover, the dull design of the bar code will reduce the effectiveness of the samples when used for advertisement. It is for these reasons that many advertising agencies are still trying to find new methods to replace the bar code or to use QR code methods.

Watermarking methods are proposed to replace the bar code method. They have the merit that they do not require the additional space to print some marks with the samples on the papers. There are some restrictions on the applications of the watermarking methods, as embedding the information about URL on an image will reduce the image quality of the samples. The major problem is the geometrical distortion of the images when extracting the information of URL from a printed image captured by a mobile phone camera.

As for watermarking methods, the image recognition methods, and especially the image feature extracting methods were proposed to replace the bar

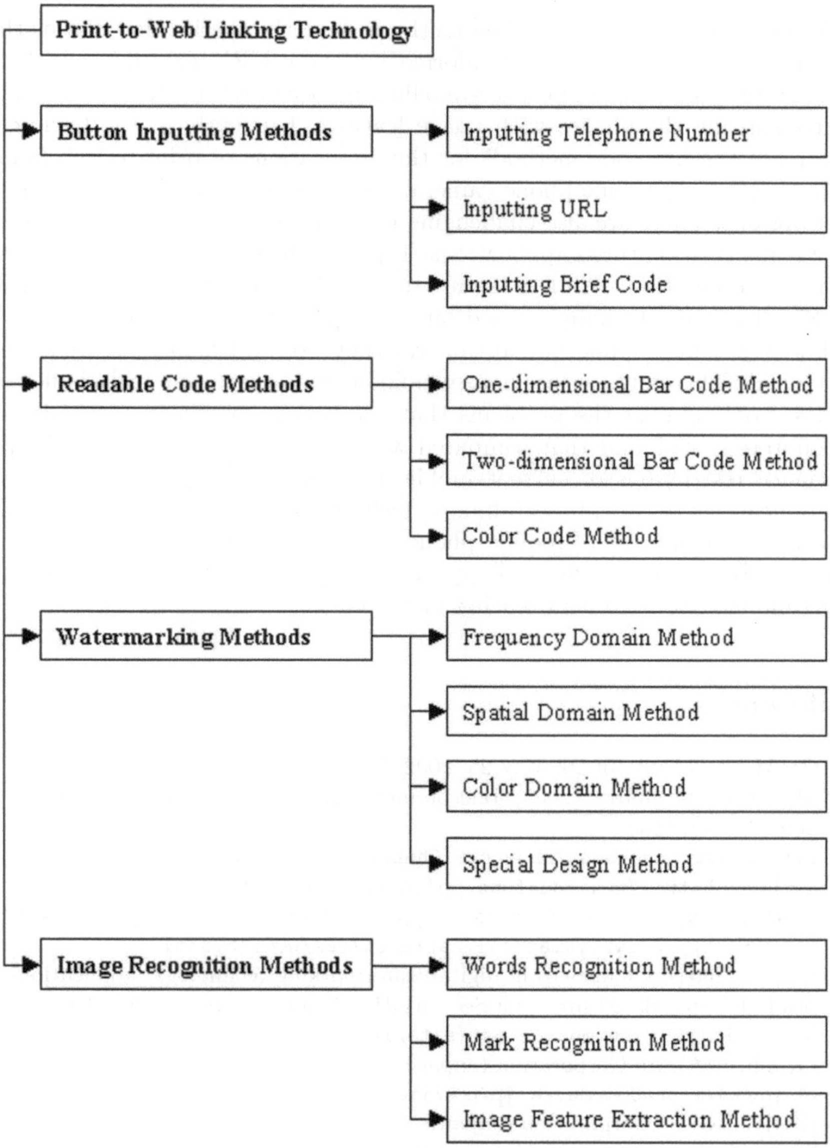

Fig. 10.13. Family tree for the applications of print-to-web linking technology using mobile phones.

code and QR code methods. The methods have the merits that the method does not require embedding any information about URL into an image. It has a high rate of a success in print-to-web linking, because the URLs are retrieved by recognizing the images with image features. Currently as the techniques to replace the bar code methods for the applications of print-to-web linking technology using mobile phone camera, the recognition methods may be the best options. There are also challenging topics for recognition methods before they reach their matured applications. Topics such as how to increase the rate of image recognition with less feature data and less computing time remain.

Finally, as the techniques used for the application of print-to-web linking technology using mobile phone camera, they are still being researched and developed. Therefore, as previously pointed out, there are still challenging topics. Looking over the problems that the various proposed methods have encountered, we found that compared with the technical problems, the performance restrictions of current mobile phones may be the major obstacle to applications of print-to-web linking technology using a mobile phone camera. The development of mobile phone techniques indicates it will not be a long time before the commercial application of print-to-web linking technology using mobile phone camera reaches maturity.

References

1. COAI News Bulletin 10: May 25, 2002, `http://www.coai.com/`
2. Mobile phone market 2005, Telecommunication Industry Report 6, February 2005, Screen Studio, `http://www.thechannelshow.com/ChannelNews/IndustryReports1386.htm`
3. J-Phone: `http://www.vodafone.jp/scripts/english/top.jsp`
4. J-SH04: `http://k-tai.impress.co.jp/cda/article/news_toppage/504.html`
5. D901iS: `http://www.yamaguchi.net/archives/000615.html`
6. Liu, Z. (2004): Challenges in digital watermarking technology: applications for printed materials. Multimedia Security Handbook, Chap. 13, CRC Press
7. i-Code: `http://www.mookde.net/site/icode.html`
8. i αppli, DoCoMo Corporation (Japan): `http://www.nttdocomo.co.jp/p_s/imode/make/java/`
9. BREW, KDDI Corporation (Japan): `http://www.au.kddi.com/ezfactory/tec/spec/brew.html`
10. Barcode Reader: `http://www.camreader.jp/eng/product/index.html`
11. QR Code used for the DoCoMo's mobile phones: `http://www.nttdocomo.co.jp/p_s/imode/barcode/`
12. ColorCode, Colorzip Japan Inc. (Japan): `http://www.colorzip.co.jp/en/company.html`
13. Liu, Z. and Inoue, A. (2004): Watermark for industrial application. Intelligent Watermarking Techniques [Pan, J.S., Huang, H.C., and Jain, L.C., Eds.], Chap. 22, World Scientific Publishing Company, Singapore
14. ImageBridge, Digimarc Corporation (U.S.A): `http://www.digimarc.com/watermark/imagebridge/`

15. Cox, I.J., Kilian, J., Leighton, F.T., and Shamoon, T. (1997): Secure spread spectrum watermarking for multimedia. IEEE Transactions on Image Processing, **6**, 1673–1687
16. PaperClick: `http://www.paperclick.com/applications.jsp`
17. C4 Technology, Inc.: `http://c4t.jp/news/press/2005/press_20050323.html`
18. Pattobi, NTT DATA Corporation (Japan): `http://pattobi.jp/`. (Pattobi-G by MiLuLa)
19. Kyodo Printing Co. Ltd. (Japan): `http://www.kyodoprinting.co.jp/release/2003/nr20030616.html`
20. Cyber-Squash, NTT Cyber Solutions Laboratory Group (Japan): `http://www.ntt.co.jp/news/news03/0307/030707.html`
21. M. Ken. Co. Ltd. (Japan) (Merged to C4 Technology, Inc. since January 16, 2004): `http://www.c4t.jp/`
22. P-warp, NTT Cyber Solutions Laboratory Group (Japan): `http://www.ntt-east.co.jp/release/0401/040127.html`
23. ClickPix!, MediaGrid Inc. (Japan): `http://www.mediagrid.co.jp/news/20040621.htm`
24. Fujitsu Research (Japan): `http://www.scinet.com/global/news/pr/archives/month/2004/20040630-01.html`
25. SANYO Electric Co., Ltd. (Japan): `http://www.sanyo.co.jp/koho/hypertext4/0407news-j/0720-3.html`
26. SyncR, Olympus Corporation (Japan): `http://www.olympus.co.jp/jp/news/2004b/nr041111syncrj.cfm`

11

Multipurpose Image Watermarking Algorithms and Applications

Zhe-Ming Lu[1,2], Hans Burkhardt[3], and Shu-Chuan Chu[4]

[1] Institute for Computer Science, University of Freiburg
Georges-Koehler-Allee 052, room 01-046
79110 Freiburg i.Br., Germany
zheminglu@informatik.uni-freiburg.de

[2] Department of Automatic Test and Control, Harbin Institute of Technology, P.O. Box 339, 150001 Harbin, China
zhemingl@yahoo.com

[3] Institute for Computer Science, University of Freiburg Georges-Koehler-Allee 052, room 01-030 79110 Freiburg i.Br., Germany
Hans.Burkhardt@informatik.uni-freiburg.de

[4] Department of Information Management Cheng-Shiu University, Kaohsiung 840, Taiwan
scchu@csu.edu.tw

Summary. The rapid growth of digital multimedia and Internet technologies has made copyright notification, copyright protection, copy protection, integrity verification and multimedia retrieval to become important issues in the digital world. To solve these problems, digital watermarking technique and content based multimedia retrieval have been presented and widely researched. In this chapter, we consider the following three applications for images: (1) to achieve the goal of content authentication and copyright protection simultaneously; (2) to notify and protect the copyright of digital images simultaneously; (3) to develop a multipurpose watermarking scheme for image retrieval. For the first application, the motivation and main idea is as follows: traditional watermarking algorithms are mostly based on discrete transform domains, such as discrete cosine transform (DCT), discrete Fourier transform (DFT) and discrete wavelet transform (DWT). Most of these algorithms are good for only one purpose. Recently, some multipurpose digital watermarking methods have been presented, which can achieve the goal of content authentication and copyright protection simultaneously. They are based on DWT or DFT. Lately, several robust watermarking schemes based on vector quantization (VQ) have been presented, but they can be used only for copyright protection. Here, we describe our multipurpose digital image watermarking method based on the multistage vector quantizer structure, which can be applied to image authentication and copyright protection. In this method, the semi-fragile watermark and the robust watermark are embedded in different VQ stages using different techniques, and both can be extracted without the original image. Simulation results demonstrate the effectiveness of this algorithm in terms of robustness and fragility. For the second application,

Z.-M. Lu et al.: *Multipurpose Image Watermarking Algorithms and Applications*, Studies in Computational Intelligence (SCI) **58**, 287–323 (2007)
www.springerlink.com

to achieve the objective of notifying and protecting the copyright of digital images simultaneously, the following is used. The DCT coefficients of each image block are divided into two parts for embedding the visible and invisible watermarks, respectively. The visible watermark is embedded in the DC DCT coefficient and most of the AC DCT coefficients of each block, and the invisible watermark in the rest. Based on the characteristics of the Human Visual System (HVS), the embedding strength of the visible watermark is varied in accordance with the underlying content of the host image. The invisible watermark is embedded in a selection of midrange frequencies. Experimental results show that the visible watermark is hard to remove and the invisible watermark is robust to common digital signal processing operations. For the third application, we deal with an image database as follows. First, several important features are computed offline for each image in the database. Then, the copyright, annotation and feature watermarks are embedded offline into all images in the database. During the online retrieval, the query image features are compared with the extracted features from each image in the database to find the similar images. Experimental results based on a database with a 1000 images in 10 classes demonstrate the effectiveness of the proposed scheme.

11.1 Introduction

Digital multimedia is today largely distributed over the Internet and via CD-ROM. The possibility of lossless and unlimited copies of digital contents is a major obstacle from the owner's viewpoint when considering entering the digital world. The amount of audiovisual information available in digital format has grown exponentially in recent years, and has resulted in information an explosion which has exceeded the limit of acceptability. Digitization, compression, and archival of multimedia information has become popular, inexpensive and straightforward. Subsequent retrieval of the stored information might require considerable, additional work in order to be effective and efficient. Copyright notification, copyright protection, copy protection, content authentication and multimedia retrieval have therefore become the five important issues in the digital world. This chapter considers following three applications for images: (1) to achieve the goal of content authentication and copyright protection simultaneously; (2) to notify and protect the copyright of digital images simultaneously; (3) provide a multipurpose watermarking scheme for image retrieval.

Conventional cryptographic systems permit only valid keyholders access to encrypted data. Once such data is decrypted there is no way to track its reproduction or retransmission. Over the last decade, digital watermarking has been presented to complement cryptographic processes. In general, there are two types of digital watermarks addressed in the existing literature, and they are visible and invisible watermarks. The invisibly watermarked digital content appears visually to be very similar to the original. Invisible watermarks can be broadly classified into two types, robust and fragile or semi-fragile watermarks. Robust watermarks [1, 2, 3, 4, 5, 6] are generally used for copyright protection and ownership verification because they are robust to nearly all kinds of image processing operations. In comparison, fragile or semi-fragile watermarks [7, 8, 9, 10] are mainly applied to content authentication and integrity attestation because they are fragile to most modifications. Most existing watermarking schemes are designed for either copyright protection or content authentication. However, we should also consider using multiple watermarks in the following cases:

1) Alice sells a digital product or artwork to Bob. Bob wants to know if the product is authentic or counterfeit. On the other hand Alice wants to know if Bob or other users have been reselling her product;
2) Alice sends Bob some important commercial information in the form of multimedia. Bob wants to know where the information is from or who makes the decision. Bob also wants to know if the information has been tampered with by others;
3) Alice sends to Bob some secret military information by securely embedding this information into an irrelevant image. Bob wants to know if the embedded information is authentic.

Thus, the watermarking algorithms that can fulfill multipurpose and are for this reason alone urgently required.

A visible watermark typically contains a visible message or a company logo indicating the ownership of the image. A visible watermark can be used to convey immediate claim of the copyright and prevent the unauthorized commercial use of images. Howsoever robust a visible watermark might be, it can always be partially or fully removed using software. To provide further protection for the image work, we give a method to embed an invisible watermark as a back-up in the host image in addition to the visible watermark.

For the third application, we should use effective retrieval methods to get the desired images. In general, the visual contents of the images in the database are extracted and are described by multi-dimensional feature vectors. The feature vectors form a feature database. To retrieve images, users provide the retrieval system with example images or sketched figures. The similarities/distances between the feature vectors of the query example or sketch and those of the images in the database are then calculated. The retrieval is also done with the aid of an indexing scheme. Recent retrieval systems have incorporated users' relevance feedback to modify the retrieval process. In general, the copyright protection and image retrieval issues are considered separately. The last part of this chapter presents a multipurpose watermarking scheme to solve these two problems simultaneously.

11.2 A Multipurpose Image Watermarking Algorithm Based on Multistage VQ for Copyright Protection and Content Authentication

Most of the existing watermarking schemes are designed for copyright protection or content authentication. In order to fulfill the multipurpose applications, several multipurpose watermarking algorithms based on wavelet transform [11] and fast Fourier transform [12] are given. Compared to traditional watermarking algorithms, there are following extra technical challenges in designing the multipurpose watermarking schemes. Firstly, the embedding order of the multiple watermarks should be analyzed in detail. Secondly, how to reduce the effect of the later embedded watermarks on the former embedded watermarks is a hard problem to solve. Thirdly, the detection or extraction of each watermark should be independent. In [11], watermarks are embedded once in the hiding process and can be blindly extracted for different applications in the detection process. This scheme has three special features:

1) The approximation information of a host image is kept in the hiding process by utilizing masking thresholds.
2) Oblivious and robust watermarking is done for copyright protection.
3) Fragile watermarking is done for detection of malicious modifications and tolerance of incidental manipulations.

In addition to images, both gray-scale and color, this method has been extended to audio watermarking [12]. It is noted that, unlike multipurpose watermarking, multiple or cocktail watermarking methods [13, 14] are mainly applied to copyright protection. This is done by embedding multiple robust watermarks, each one being robust to particular kinds of attacks.

Traditional digital watermarking schemes are mainly based on DCT and DWT transforms. Recently, some robust image watermarking techniques based on vector quantization (VQ) [15, 16, 17, 18, 19, 20, 21] have been presented. References [15, 16, 17, 18] embed the watermark information into the encoded indices under the constraint that the extra distortion is less than a given threshold. Reference [19] embeds the watermark bit in the dimension information of the variable dimension reconstruction blocks of the input image. References [20, 21] embed the watermark information by utilizing properties, such as mean and variance, of neighboring indices. In this section, we give a novel multipurpose watermarking method based on multistage vector quantization. In the proposed algorithm, the robust watermark is embedded in the first stage by using the embedding method presented in [20]. The semi-fragile watermark is embedded in the second stage by using a novel index constrained method. The remainder of this section is organized as follows. In Section 11.2.1, previous VQ-based watermarking algorithms are reviewed. In Section 11.2.2, the proposed multipurpose watermarking method is described in detail. The simulation results are given in Section 11.2.3. The conclusions are given in Section 11.2.4, respectively.

11.2.1 Previous VQ-Based Watermarking Algorithms

Vector Quantization

Vector quantization (VQ) has become an attractive block-based encoding method for image compression in the last two decades. It can achieve a high compression ratio. In environments such as image archival and one-to-many communications, the simplicity of the decoder makes VQ very efficient. In brief, VQ can be defined as a mapping from k-dimensional Euclidean space R^k into a finite subset $C = \{\mathbf{c}_i \mid i = 0, 1, \cdots, N-1\}$. That is generally called a codebook, where $\mathbf{c}_i$ is a codeword and N is the codebook size. VQ first generates a representative codebook from a number of training vectors using, for example, the iterative clustering algorithm [22]. It is often referred to as the generalized Lloyd algorithm (GLA). In VQ, the image to be encoded is first decomposed into vectors and then sequentially encoded vector by vector. In the encoding phase, each k-dimensional input vector $\mathbf{x} = (x_1, x_2, \cdots, x_k)$ is compared with the codewords in the codebook $C = \{\mathbf{c}_0, \mathbf{c}_1, \cdots, \mathbf{c}_{N-1}\}$. This is done to find the best matching codeword $\mathbf{c}_i = (c_{i1}, c_{i2}, \cdots, c_{ik})$ satisfying the following condition:

$$d(\mathbf{x}, \mathbf{c}_i) = \min_{0 \le j \le N-1} d(\mathbf{x}, \mathbf{c}_j). \tag{11.1}$$

That is, the distance between $\mathbf{x}$ and $\mathbf{c}_i$ is the smallest, where $d(\mathbf{x}, \mathbf{c}_j)$ is the distortion caused by representing the input vector $\mathbf{x}$ by the codeword $\mathbf{c}_j$. This is often measured by the squared Euclidean distance. That is,

$$d(\mathbf{x}, \mathbf{c}_j) = \sum_{l=1}^{k} (x_l - c_{jl})^2 . \tag{11.2}$$

The index i of the best matching codeword assigned to the input vector $\mathbf{x}$ is transmitted over the channel to the decoder. The decoder has the same codebook as the encoder. In the decoding phase, for each index i, the decoder performs a table look-up operation to obtain $\mathbf{c}_i$. This is then used to reconstruct the input vector $\mathbf{x}$. Compression is achieved by transmitting or storing the index of a codeword rather than the codeword itself. The compression ratio is determined by the codebook size and the dimension of the input vectors. The overall distortion is dependent on the codebook size and the selection of codewords.

Watermarking Algorithms Based on Codebook Partition

The main idea of this kind of VQ-based digital watermarking scheme [15, 16, 17, 18] is to carry secret copyright information by codeword indices. The aim of the codebook partition is to classify the neighboring codewords into the same cluster. Given a threshold $D > 0$, we denote by $S = \{S_1, S_2, \cdots, S_M\}$, which is a *standard partition* of the codebook $C = \{\mathbf{c}_0, \mathbf{c}_1, \cdots, \mathbf{c}_{N-1}\}$ for the threshold D, if S satisfies the following four conditions:

(1) $S = \bigcup_{i=1}^{M} S_i$;
(2) $\forall i, j, 1 \leq i, j \leq M$, if $i \neq j$, then $S_i \cap S_j = \emptyset$;
(3) $\forall i, 1 \leq i \leq M$, if $\mathbf{c}_l \in S_i$ and $\mathbf{c}_j \in S_i$ $(0 \leq l, j \leq N-1)$, then $d(\mathbf{c}_l, \mathbf{c}_j) \leq D$;
(4) $\|S_i\| = 2^{n(i)}$. Where $\|S_i\|$ denotes the number of codewords in S_i and $n(i)$ is a natural number.

Before the embedding process, the original image is first divided into blocks. For each block, the index of the best match codeword is found. The watermarked codeword index is then obtained by modifying the original codeword index according to the corresponding watermark bits. The modification is under the constraint that the modified index and the original are in the same partition. A further condition is that the introduced extra distortion is less than the given distortion threshold. In the decoding phase, not the original but the watermarked codeword is used to represent the input image block. Therefore, the VQ-based digital image watermarking will introduce some additional distortion. Whether the original image is required or not during the watermark extraction is dependent on the embedding method. In these algorithms, the codebook is open for users but the partition is the secret key. Experimental results show that these algorithms are robust to VQ compression with high-performance codebooks, JPEG compression and some to spatial image processing operations. These algorithms are fragile to rotation operations and to VQ compression with low-performance codebooks.

Watermarking Algorithms Based on Index Properties

To enhance the robustness to rotation operations and VQ compression operations, some image watermarking algorithms [20, 21] based on the properties of neighboring indices have been proposed. In [20], the original watermark $\mathbf{W}$ of size $A_{\mathrm{w}} \times B_{\mathrm{w}}$ is first permuted by a predetermined key, key_1, to generate the permuted watermark $\mathbf{W}_{\mathrm{P}}$ for embedding. The original image $\mathbf{X}$ with size $A \times B$ is then divided into vectors $\mathbf{x}(m,n)$ with a size $(A/A_{\mathrm{w}}) \times (B/B_{\mathrm{w}})$, where $\mathbf{x}(m,n)$ denotes the image block at the position of (m,n). After that, each vector $\mathbf{x}(m,n)$ finds its best codeword $\mathbf{c}_i$ in the codebook C and the index i is assigned to $\mathbf{x}(m,n)$. We can then obtain the indices matrix $\mathbf{Y}$ with elements $y(m,n)$, which can be represented by:

$$\mathbf{Y} = \mathrm{VQ}(\mathbf{X}) = \bigcup_{m=0}^{\frac{A}{A_{\mathrm{w}}}-1} \bigcup_{n=0}^{\frac{B}{B_{\mathrm{w}}}-1} \mathrm{VQ}(\mathbf{x}(m,n)) = \bigcup_{m=0}^{\frac{A}{A_{\mathrm{w}}}-1} \bigcup_{n=0}^{\frac{B}{B_{\mathrm{w}}}-1} y(m,n). \tag{11.3}$$

For natural images, the VQ indices among neighboring blocks tend to be very similar. We can make use of this property to generate the *polarities* $\mathbf{P}$. After calculating the variances of $y(m,n)$ and the indices of its surrounding blocks using

$$\sigma^2(m,n) = \left(\frac{1}{9} \sum_{i=m-1}^{m+1} \sum_{j=n-1}^{n+1} y^2(i,j) \right) - \left(\frac{1}{9} \sum_{i=m-1}^{m+1} \sum_{j=n-1}^{n+1} y(i,j) \right)^2 . \quad (11.4)$$

We can obtain the polarities $\mathbf{P}$ as follows

$$\mathbf{P} = \bigcup_{m=0}^{\frac{A}{A_w}-1} \bigcup_{n=0}^{\frac{B}{B_w}-1} p(m,n), \quad (11.5)$$

where

$$p(m,n) = \begin{cases} 1, & \text{if } \sigma^2(m,n) \geq T; \\ 0, & \text{otherwise.} \end{cases} \quad (11.6)$$

For convenience, we set the threshold T to be half of the codebook size, $N/2$. We are then able to generate the final embedded watermark or the secret key, key_2, with the exclusive-or operation as follows

$$key_2 = \mathbf{W}_\mathrm{P} \oplus \mathbf{P}. \quad (11.7)$$

After the inverse-VQ operation, both the reconstructed image $\mathbf{X}'$ and the secret key, key_2, work together to protect the ownership of the original image.

In the extraction process, we first calculate the estimated polarities $\mathbf{P}'$ from $\mathbf{X}'$. We then obtain an estimate of the permuted watermark by

$$\mathbf{W}'_\mathrm{P} = key_2 \oplus \mathbf{P}'. \quad (11.8)$$

Finally, we can do the inverse permutation operation with key_1 to obtain the extracted watermark $\mathbf{W}'$.

In order to embed multiple watermarks, reference [21] also uses the mean of the indices to generate another kind of polarities $\mathbf{P}_1$ for embedding. Experimental results show that these algorithms are robust to many kinds of attacks, including JPEG, VQ, filtering, blurring and rotation. These algorithms have the following two problems:

(1) We can also extract the watermark from the original image that has no embedded watermark.
(2) The codebook should be used as a key, because if the user possesses the same codebook, he can also embed his own watermark in the watermarked image without modification.

In fact, unlike traditional watermarking methods, these watermarking algorithms do not modify the VQ compressed cover work. The term "fingerprint" or "secure fingerprint" may be more appropriate. Sometimes we can call this kind of watermark "zero-watermark". In view of unification, we use the term "robust watermark" instead of "secure fingerprint" although we don't modify the VQ compressed cover work during the robust watermarking process.

11.2.2 Multistage VQ based Multipurpose Watermarking Algorithm

Multistage Vector Quantization

The basic idea of multistage VQ is to divide the encoding task into successive stages, where the first stage does a relatively crude quantization of the input vector using a small codebook. A second stage quantizer then operates on the error vector between the original and quantized first stage output. The quantized error vector then provides a second approximation to the original input vector which leads to a refined or a more accurate representation of the input. A third stage quantizer may then be used to quantize the second stage error to provide a further refinement.

In this chapter, we adopt a two-stage vector quantizer as illustrated in Fig. 11.1. It is the simplest case and can be used to generate the general multistage vector quantizer. The input vector $\mathbf{x}$ is quantized by the initial or first stage vector quantizer denoted by VQ_1 whose codebook is $C_1 = \{\mathbf{c}_{10}, \mathbf{c}_{11}, \cdots, \mathbf{c}_{1(N_1-1)}\}$ with size N_1. The quantized approximation $\hat{\mathbf{x}}_1$ is then subtracted from $\mathbf{x}$ producing the error vector $\mathbf{e}_2$. This error vector is then applied to a second vector quantizer VQ_2 whose codebook is $C_2 = \{\mathbf{c}_{20}, \mathbf{c}_{21}, \cdots, \mathbf{c}_{2(N_2-1)}\}$ with size N_2 yielding the quantized output $\hat{\mathbf{e}}_2$. The overall approximation $\hat{\mathbf{x}}$ to the input $\mathbf{x}$ is formed by summing the first and second approximations, $\hat{\mathbf{x}}_1$ and $\hat{\mathbf{e}}_2$. The encoder for this VQ simply transmits a pair of indices specifying the selected codewords for each stage. The task of the decoder is to perform two table lookups to generate and then sum the two codewords. In fact, the overall codeword or index is the concatenation of codewords or indices chosen from each of two codebooks. That is, this is a product code where the composition function g of the decoder is a summation of the reproductions from the different two VQ decoders. Thus the equivalent product codebook C can be generated from the Cartesian product $C_1 \times C_2$. Compared to the full search VQ with the product codebook C, the two-stage VQ can reduce the complexity from $N = N_1 \times N_2$ to $N_1 + N_2$.

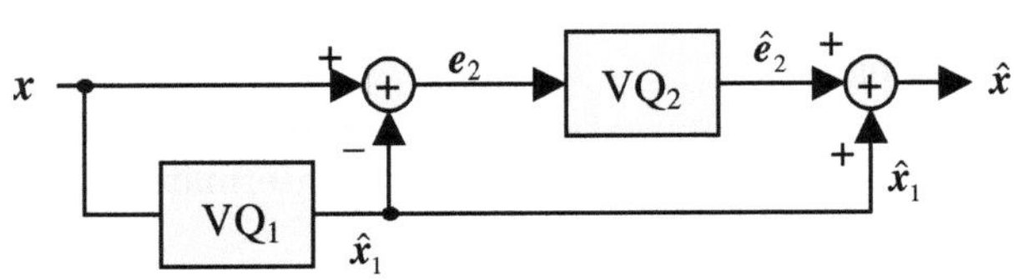

Fig. 11.1. Two-stage VQ.

The Embedding Process

Before describing the proposed algorithm, we make some assumptions. Let $\mathbf{X}$ be the original image with size $A \times B$. Let $\mathbf{W}_\mathrm{R}$ and $\mathbf{W}_\mathrm{F}$ be the binary robust and semi-fragile watermarks with the size $A_\mathrm{w} \times B_\mathrm{w}$, respectively. Here, a small visually meaningful binary image $\mathbf{V}$ with size $a \times b$ is replicated periodically to obtain the binary semi-fragile watermark $\mathbf{W}_\mathrm{F}$ with the size $A_\mathrm{w} \times B_\mathrm{w}$. That is a large enough size for embedding. In each stage of the proposed algorithm, only one bit is embedded in each input image block (or vector). The dimension of each input vector or codeword is $k = (A/A_\mathrm{w}) \times (B/B_\mathrm{w})$. Assume that the first stage codebook is $C_1 = \{\mathbf{c}_{10}, \mathbf{c}_{11}, \cdots, \mathbf{c}_{1(N_1-1)}\}$ with size $N_1 = 2^{n_1}$. The second stage codebook is $C_2 = \{\mathbf{c}_{20}, \mathbf{c}_{21}, \cdots, \mathbf{c}_{2(N_2-1)}\}$ with size $N_2 = 2^{n_2}$. Here n_1 and n_2 are natural numbers. Thus a binary number with $n_1 + n_2$ bits, in which the first n_1 bits stand for the index of Stage 1 and the last n_2 bits denote the index of Stage 2, can represent the overall index. The overall codeword can be selected from the equivalent product codebook $C = \{\mathbf{c}_0, \mathbf{c}_1, \cdots, \mathbf{c}_{(N-1)}\}$ with size $N = N_1 \times N_2$. In other words, if the index in codebook C_1 is i and the index in codebook C_2 is j, then the equivalent overall index in the product codebook C is $i + (j \times N_2)$.

In our algorithm, the robust watermark $\mathbf{W}_\mathrm{R}$ and the semi-fragile watermark $\mathbf{W}_\mathrm{F}$ are embedded in two stages respectively. We embed the robust watermark in the first stage and the semi-fragile watermark in the second stage to enhance the robustness and transparency of the proposed algorithm. In the following, we describe the two-stage embedding process.

The Robust Watermark Embedding Process:

In the proposed algorithm, we adopt the method [20] based on index properties to embed the robust watermark in the first stage as shown in Fig. 11.2. The original watermark $\mathbf{W}_\mathrm{R}$ is first permuted by a predetermined key, key_1, to generate the permuted watermark $\mathbf{W}_\mathrm{RP}$ for embedding. The polarities $\mathbf{P}$ are then calculated with Eqs. (11.3)–(11.6). Finally, we generate the final embedded watermark known as the secret key, key_2, using the exclusive-or operation in Eq. (11.7). After the first stage of embedding, we can obtain the reconstructed image $\mathbf{X}'$ and the error image $\mathbf{X}_1$ as follows:

$$\mathbf{X}' = \mathrm{VQ}_1{}^{-1}\left[\mathrm{VQ}_1\left[\mathbf{X}\right]\right]. \tag{11.9}$$

$$\mathbf{X}_1 = \mathbf{X} - \mathbf{X}'. \tag{11.10}$$

According to Section 11.2.1, we know that this method has two problems. However, in our algorithm, these two problems can be automatically solved, and this will be discussed later in the extraction process.

The Semi-Fragile Watermark Embedding Process:

To embed one bit of each index in the second stage, we can adopt the index constrained vector quantization (ICVQ) encoding scheme shown in Fig. 11.3.

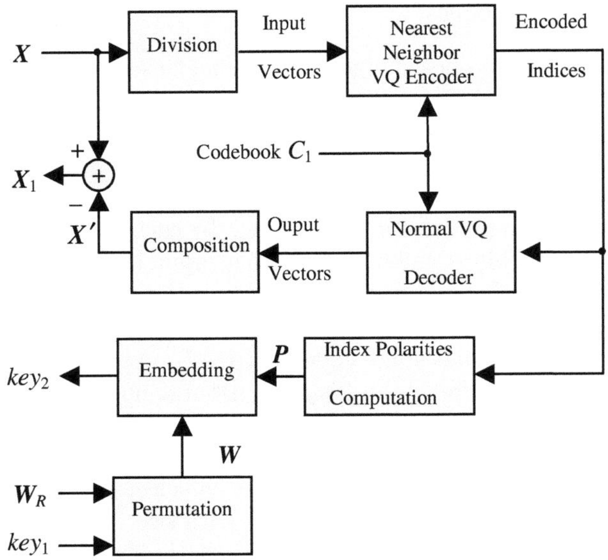

Fig. 11.2. The robust watermark embedding process of the first stage.

Because each index has n_2 bits, we can select an embedding position from n_2 candidate positions. Assume that we select Position key_3, which is considered as a key, to embed the watermark bit. Here $0 \leq key_3 \leq n_2 - 1$. Unlike the normal VQ encoder, the embedding process for each watermark bit can be done by searching for the best match codeword $\mathbf{c}_{2p}$ for each input error vector $\mathbf{x}_1$. This has the constraints that the key_3-th bit of index p is equal to the watermark bit to be embedded. After applying the normal VQ decoder, we can obtain the reconstructed error image $\mathbf{X}_1'$ as follows

$$\mathbf{X}_1' = \mathrm{VQ_2}^{-1}\left[\mathrm{ICVQ_2}\left[\mathbf{X}_1\right]\right]. \tag{11.11}$$

We can then obtain the final watermarked image $\mathbf{X}_\mathrm{W}$ as follows

$$\mathbf{X}_\mathrm{W} = \mathbf{X}' + \mathbf{X}_1'. \tag{11.12}$$

The Extraction Process

To enhance the security of the embedding process, we use the equivalent product codebook C in the extraction process as shown in Fig. 11.4. That is to say, the two-stage codebooks are used as secret keys while the product codebook is available to users. The users do not know the codebook sizes used in two-stage VQ or, how to segment the overall index into two stage indices is also a secret key, key_5. In order to make the embedding algorithm more secure, we can also permute the product codebook and then give the permuted codebook C_u for users. The extraction process can be done without the original

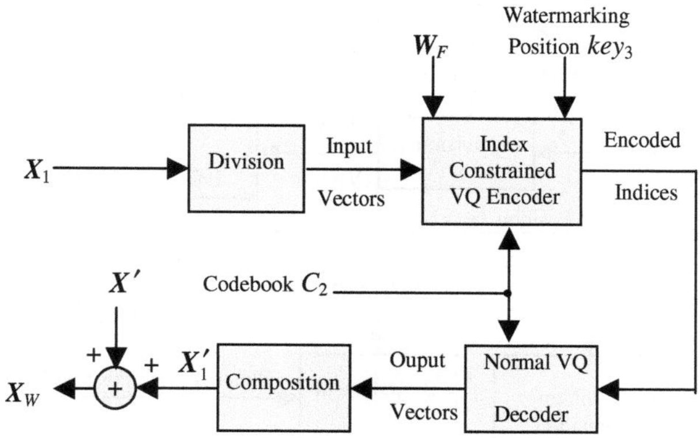

Fig. 11.3. The semi-fragile watermark embedding process in the second stage.

image and can be described as follows. First, perform the inverse permutation operation with key_4 on codebook C_{u} to obtain the product codebook C. Secondly, the watermarked image $\mathbf{X}_{\text{W}}$ is divided into blocks or vectors. Thirdly, the normal VQ encoder then does the Nearest Neighbor Codeword Search on all input vectors to obtain the encoded overall indices. Fourthly, according to the two stage codebook sizes, each overall index is segmented into two indices. One is for robust watermark extraction. The other is for semi-fragile watermark extraction. Finally, the robust and semi-fragile watermarks are extracted independently. For the robust watermark extraction, we first compute the polarities $\mathbf{P}$ from the indices of Stage 1. Then we do the XOR operation between $\mathbf{P}$ and key_2 to obtain the extracted permuted robust watermark $\mathbf{W}_{\text{EPR}}$. Finally do the inverse permutation operation with key_1 to obtain the extracted robust watermark $\mathbf{W}_{\text{ER}}$. For the semi-fragile watermark extraction, we check the key_3-th bit of each index of Stage 2 to obtain the extracted watermark bit. Here key_3 is the watermarking position. We then piece all the extracted bits together to form the extracted semi-fragile watermark $\mathbf{W}_{\text{EF}}$. From the above we can see that the advantages of using ICVQ in the semi-fragile watermarking are as follows: (1) the embedding and the extraction processes are very simple; (2) the extraction process is blind; (3) the embedded position can be controlled by a key for more security.

In Section 11.2.1, we mention two problems with the robust embedding technique [20]. In our algorithm, these two problems are automatically solved. Detecting the existence of the semi-fragile watermark in the original image provides a solution to the first problem. Two-stage codebooks are not used. The equivalent product codebook is used however to extract the watermarks and it also provides a solution to the second problem. From Fig. 11.4 we can see that the extraction time is determined by the codebook size of C. If N is very large, then the full search VQ encoding is a time-consuming process. As a consequence the fast codeword search algorithm [23] is used in this algorithm.

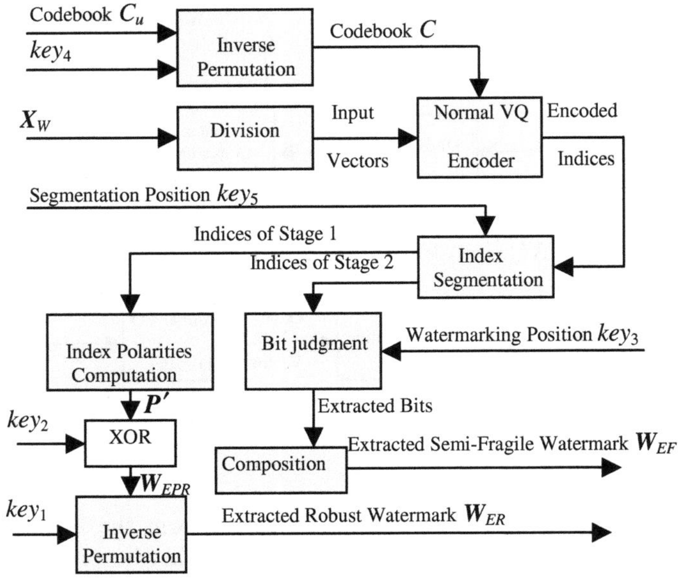

Fig. 11.4. The watermark extraction process.

11.2.3 Experimental Results

To evaluate the performance of the proposed method, the 512×512 Lena image with 8 bits/pixel resolution is used for multipurpose watermarking. The Lena image is divided into 16384 blocks of size 4×4 for VQ encoding. A binary image of size 32×32 is replicated 16 times to obtain a binary watermark $\mathbf{W}_\mathrm{F}$ with size 128×128 for semi-fragile watermarking. Another binary watermark $\mathbf{W}_\mathrm{R}$ with size 128×128 is used for robust watermarking. The original Lena image and two watermarks are shown in Figs. 11.5(a)–(c). The codebook C_1 with size 16 is used for Stage 1. The codebook C_2 of size 256 is used for Stage 2 are obtained by use of the LBG algorithm [22]. This corresponds to $4 + 8 = 12$ bits per overall index. If we embed the semi-fragile watermark in the second stage, we can randomly select the watermarking position key_3 ranging from 0 to 7 for the semi-fragile watermarking. Before extraction, the equivalent product codebook C of size $16 \times 256 = 4096$ is generated by the Cartesian product $C_1 \times C_2$.

We first make an experiment upon the order of embedding using robust and semi-fragile watermarks to show why we should embed the robust watermark in the first stage and the semi-fragile watermark in the second stage. Fig. 11.6(a) shows the watermarked image with PSNR = 30.553 dB obtained by use of the proposed method. Fig. 11.6(b) shows the watermarked image with PSNR = 26.105 dB obtained by using the algorithm in the reverse embedding order. We see that the proposed embedding order produces higher

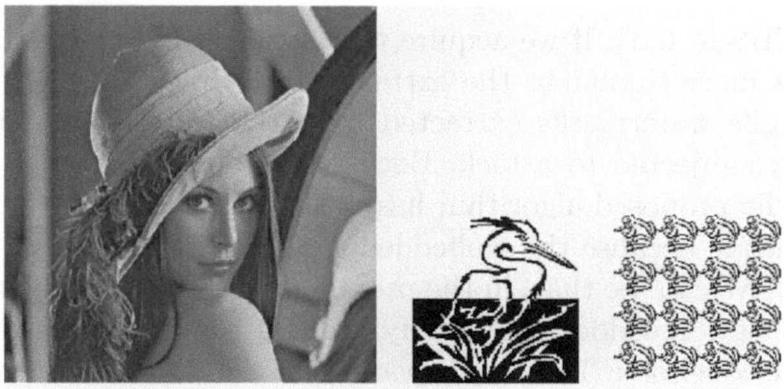

(a) (b) (c)

Fig. 11.5. Original image and watermarks. (a) Original Lena image. (b) Original robust watermark. (c) Original semi-fragile watermark.

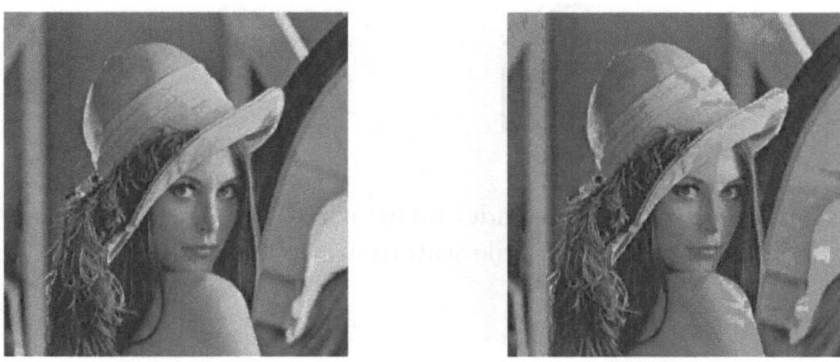

(a) (b)

Fig. 11.6. The watermarked images obtained by algorithms having different embedding orders. (a) The watermarked image with PSNR = 30.553 dB obtained by using the proposed method. (b) The watermarked image with PSNR = 26.105 dB obtained by using the algorithm in the reverse embedding order.

image quality than the alternative. The first reason for this is that the first-stage codebook is small. The second reason is that the robust embedding algorithm [20] does not modify the encoded indices at all. In contrast the semi-fragile watermarking method does. If we embed the semi-fragile watermark in the first stage, then the reconstructed error image may be very poor, which greatly affects the reconstructed image.

In this chapter, we use the *Normalized Hamming Similarity*, NHS, to evaluate the effectiveness of the proposed algorithm. The NHS between the embedded binary watermark $\mathbf{W}$ and that extracted $\mathbf{W}'$ is defined as

$$\mathrm{NHS} = 1 - \frac{\mathrm{HD}\left(\mathbf{W}, \mathbf{W}'\right)}{A_{\mathrm{w}} \times B_{\mathrm{w}}}, \tag{11.13}$$

where $\mathrm{HD}(\cdot,\cdot)$ denotes the Hamming Distance between two binary strings. That is, the number of different bits in the two binary strings. We can easily prove that NHS ∈ [0, 1]. If we acquire the higher NHS values, the embedded watermark is more similar to the extracted one. Fig. 11.7 shows the robust and semi-fragile watermarks extracted from the watermarked image which has not been subjected to attack. Both NHS values are equal to 1.0. This means that the proposed algorithm has been able to extract the watermarks perfectly. That is because the embedded watermarks and the extracted ones are identical. We can see that, in the proposed method, the robust watermark is embedded first and does not modify the VQ compressed cover work with the first stage codebook. The robust watermark doesn't affect the semi-fragile part. We do not use the two stage codebooks but we do use the product codebook in the extraction process. The semi-fragile and robust watermarks are independent as shown in Fig. 11.7.

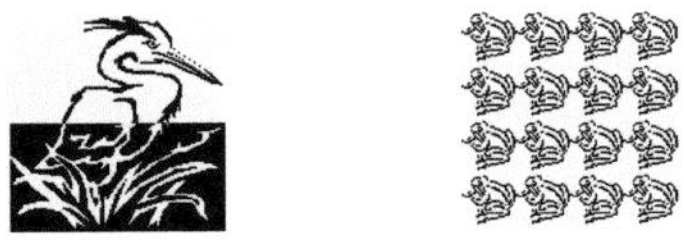

(a) (b)

Fig. 11.7. Extracted watermarks under no attack. (a) Extracted robust watermark, NHS = 1.0. (b) Extracted semi-fragile watermark, NHS = 1.0.

To check the robustness and fragility of our algorithm, we have made several attacks on the watermarked image. These include JPEG compression, VQ compression, spatial image processing and rotation. We also do the experiment of watermark extraction from the original image in which no watermark is embedded. We now give the experimental results in five subsections.

Watermark Extraction from the Original Image

The experimental results of watermark extraction from the original image are shown in Fig. 11.8. In this experiment, we use not the product codebook in the extraction process but the two-stage VQ codebooks. From the results, it is clear that, although we can extract the robust watermark using NHS = 1.0 from the original image, we cannot extract the semi-fragile watermark from the original image. For the first stage, each original image block can be encoded using the same codeword as the watermarked compressed image block with the first stage VQ codebook. Note that the robust watermarking does not modify the compressed image and the watermarked image is the same as the VQ compressed image in the first stage. The index properties of the original image are the same as that of the compressed image using the first stage VQ codebook. We can extract the exact robust watermark from the original image. For the fragile part, the un-watermarked index obtained is different from that of the watermarked compressed image of the second

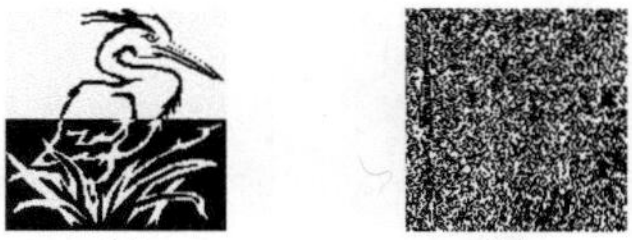

(a) (b)

Fig. 11.8. The watermarks extracted from the original image using the two-stage codebooks. (a) Extracted robust watermark, NHS = 1.0. (b) Extracted semi-fragile watermark, NHS = 0.047.

stage VQ codebook. The fragile watermark cannot be extracted from the original image. We can decide that there are no watermarks embedded in the original image. The first problem of algorithm [20] described in Section 11.2.1 is therefore solved.

JPEG Compression Attacks

In this experiment, we perform JPEG compression using different quality factors (QF) on the watermarked image as shown in Fig. 11.9. Here QF = 100%, 80%, 50% and 30%, respectively. The extracted watermarks and NHS values are depicted in Fig. 11.10. From these results, we see that the proposed algorithm is robust to JPEG compression. Where QF is larger than 80%, the extracted watermarks, both robust and semi-fragile, are similar to the embedded ones. For all cases, the extracted robust watermarks have relatively high NHS values. From these results, we see that the VQ indices can, to some extent, tolerate the incidental distortions produced by high-quality JPEG compression.

VQ Compression Attacks

We now use four different codebooks to compress the watermarked image. Codebook 1 is the product codebook used in our method. Codebook 2 with a size of 8192 and Codebook 3 with a size of 256 are both trained from the Lena image. The corresponding PSNRs of the encoded Lena images are 37.08 dB and 30.39 dB respectively. Codebook 4 with a size of 4096 is trained from the Pepper image. The corresponding PSNR of the encoded Pepper image is 33.74 dB. Fig. 11.11 shows the four VQ-attacked watermarked images, and Fig. 11.12 shows the watermarks extracted from these images. We can see that from these results the proposed algorithm can extract the same watermarks as the embedded ones from the VQ compressed watermarked image with the product codebook. The reason for this is that the watermarked image is not modified under the VQ compression with the product codebook. For the other cases, the robust watermark can tolerate the VQ compression, while the semi-fragile watermark cannot. The higher the codebook performance is, the larger the NHS value of the semi-fragile watermark.

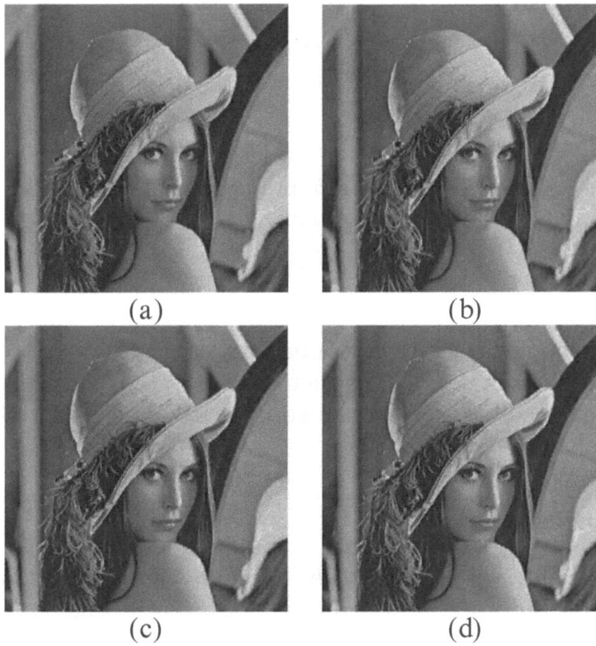

Fig. 11.9. The JPEG compressed watermarked images. (a) QF = 100%. (b) QF = 80%. (c) QF = 50%. (d) QF = 30%.

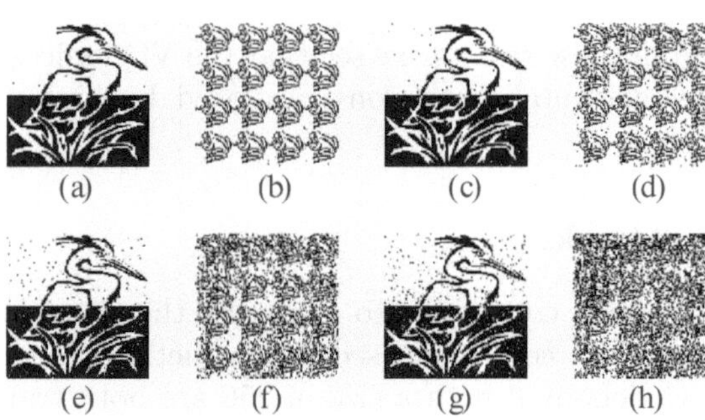

Fig. 11.10. The watermarks extracted from JPEG compressed watermarked images. (a) The robust one from Fig. 11.9(a), NHS = 0.999. (b) The semi-fragile one from Fig. 11.9(a), NHS = 0.990. (c) The robust one from Fig. 11.9(b), NHS = 0.988. (d) The semi-fragile one from Fig. 11.9(b), NHS = 0.874. (e) The robust one from Fig. 11.9(c), NHS = 0.968. (f) The semi-fragile one from Fig. 11.9(c), NHS = 0.663. (g) The robust one from Fig. 11.9(d), NHS = 0.937. (h) The semi-fragile one from Fig. 11.9(d), NHS = 0.400.

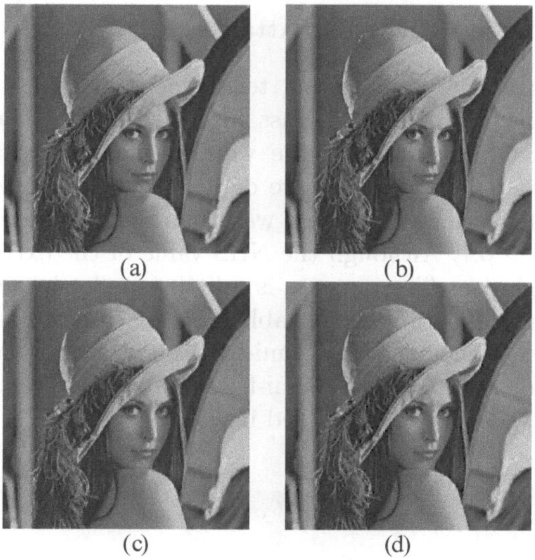

Fig. 11.11. The VQ compressed watermarked images. (a) By Codebook 1. (b) By Codebook 2. (c) By Codebook 3. (d) By Codebook 4.

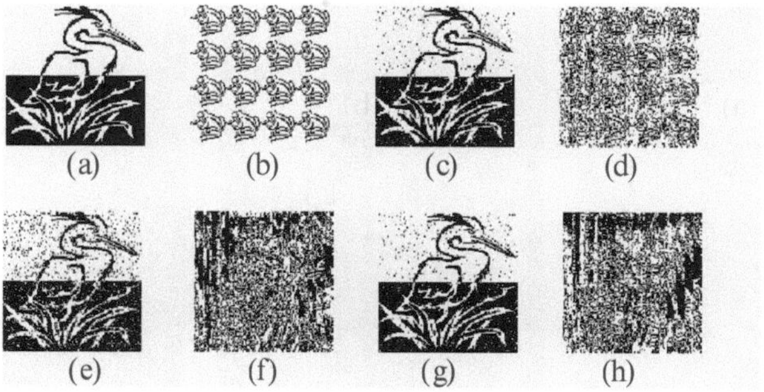

Fig. 11.12. The watermarks extracted from VQ compressed watermarked images. (a) The robust one extracted from Fig. 11.11(a), NHS = 1.0. (b) The semi-fragile one extracted from Fig. 11.11(a), NHS = 1.0. (c) The robust one extracted from Fig. 11.11(b), NHS = 0.945. (d) The semi-fragile one extracted from Fig. 11.11(b), NHS = 0.604. (e) The robust one extracted from Fig. 11.11(c), NHS = 0.851. (f) The semi-fragile one extracted from Fig. 11.11(c), NHS = 0.069. (g) The robust one extracted from Fig. 11.11(d), NHS = 0.943. (h) The semi-fragile one extracted from Fig. 11.11(d), NHS = 0.189.

Spatial-Domain Image Processing Attacks

Several spatial-domain image processing techniques, including image cropping, median filtering, blurring, high-pass filtering, contrast enhancement, brightness enhancement are done on the watermarked image as shown in Fig. 11.13. The extracted watermarks are depicted in Fig. 11.14. Except in the case of high-pass filtering, the robust watermark can successfully survive with a value of NHS > 0.7. Although the NHS value of the extracted robust watermark in the high-pass filtering case is a little smaller in our algorithm, the information conveyed is still recognizable. For the case of image cropping in the upper-left corner, the extracted semi-fragile watermark can locate the cropping position. For each case, the semi-fragile watermark can be used to verify the authenticity of the watermarked image.

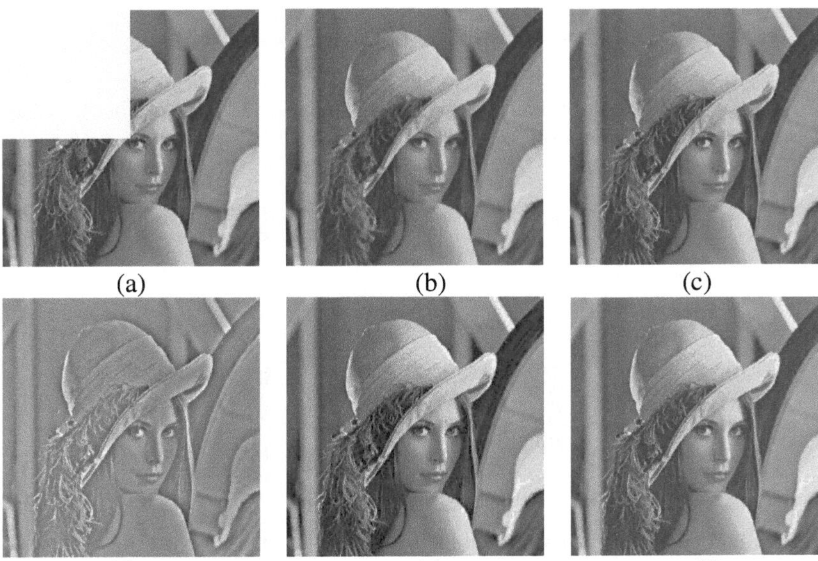

(a) (b) (c) (d) (e) (f)

Fig. 11.13. The spatial-domain-attacked watermarked images. (a) Image cropping in the upper-left corner. (b) Median filtering with the radius of 2 pixels. (c) Blurring with radius = 1.0 and a threshold = 10.0. (d) High-Pass filtering with radius = 10.0. (e) Contrast Enhancement by 10%. (f) Brightness Enhancement by 10%.

Rotation Attacks

With StirMark, we can perform the geometric attack by rotating the watermarked image with using different angles. We rotate the watermarked image by 0.5° and 1° in clockwise and counter-clockwise directions as shown in

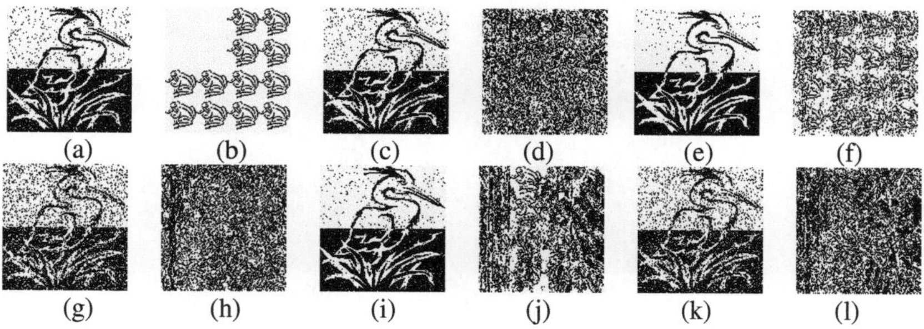

Fig. 11.14. Watermarks extracted from spatial-domain-attacked watermarked images. (a) The robust one from Fig. 11.13(a), NHS = 0.887. (b) The semi-fragile one from Fig. 11.13(a), NHS = 0.901. (c) The robust one from Fig. 11.13(b), NHS = 0.868. (d) The semi-fragile one from Fig. 11.13(b), NHS = 0.164. (e) The robust one from Fig. 11.13(c), NHS = 0.954. (f) The semi-fragile one from Fig. 11.13(c), NHS = 0.645. (g) The robust one from Fig. 11.13(d), NHS = 0.647. (h) The semi-fragile one from Fig. 11.13(d), NHS = 0.103. (i) The robust one from Fig. 11.13(e), NHS = 0.926. (j) The semi-fragile one from Fig. 11.13(e), NHS = 0.245. (k) The robust one from Fig. 11.13(f), NHS = 0.710. (l) The semi-fragile one from Fig. 11.13(f), NHS = 0.035.

Fig. 11.15. The extracted watermarks are shown in Fig. 11.16. From these results, we demonstrate the robustness of the robust watermark and the fragility of the semi-fragile watermark to rotation.

In order to show the effectiveness of the proposed algorithm for other images using the watermarks above, we do the similar experiments based on the other two test images. That is the Pepper and F16 images. The experimental results are shown in Table 11.1, where the rotation angles are $0.5°$ and $3°$. This is done in order to show the robustness of the proposed algorithm to rotation operations. For the cover images, the product Codebook C_1 has a size of 16 for Stage 1, and the Codebook C_2 has a size of 256 for Stage 2. The codebook used in the watermarking algorithm is the same as Codebook 1 used in VQ compression attacks. This is trained from the cover image. The Codebook 2 has a size of 8192 and the Codebook 3 has a size of 256. The Codebooks 2 and 3 used in VQ compression attacks are trained from the cover image itself. The Codebook 4 has a size of 4096 used in VQ compression attacks is trained from the Lena image. The parameters of the spatial-domain attacks are the same as that in Lena image watermarking.

11.2.4 Conclusions

An efficient multipurpose watermarking algorithm based on multistage VQ has been presented. In the proposed algorithm, the robust watermark is embedded in the first stage using the robust watermarking method based on index properties [20]. The semi-fragile watermark is embedded in the sec-

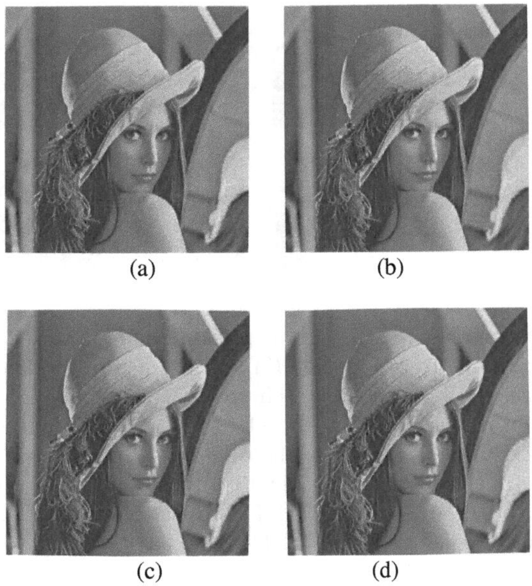

Fig. 11.15. The rotated watermarked images. (a) Rotation by 0.5° in the clockwise direction. (b) Rotation by 0.5° in the counter-clockwise direction. (c) Rotation by 1° in the clockwise direction. (d) Rotation by 1° in the counter-clockwise direction.

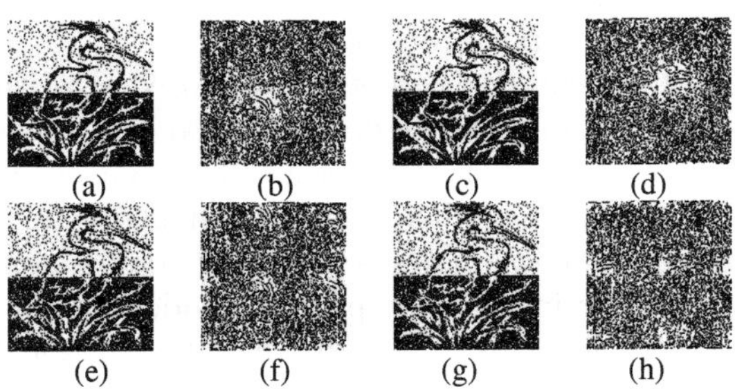

Fig. 11.16. The watermarks extracted from rotated watermarked images. (a) The robust watermark extracted from Fig. 11.15(a), NHS = 0.805. (b) The semi-fragile watermark extracted from Fig. 11.15(a), NHS = 0.063. (c) The robust watermark extracted from Fig. 11.15(b), NHS = 0.783. (d) The semi-fragile watermark extracted from Fig. 11.15(b), NHS = 0.067. (e) The robust watermark extracted from Fig. 11.15(c), NHS = 0.724. (f) The semi-fragile watermark extracted from Fig. 11.15(c), NHS = 0.047. (g) The robust water-mark extracted from Fig. 11.15(d), NHS = 0.713. (h) The semi-fragile watermark extracted from Fig. 11.15(d), NHS = 0.047.

Table 11.1. Experimental Results for the Pepper and F16 Images.

Operations	Image			
	Pepper		F16	
Embedding (PSNR in dB)	29.879		29.901	
	Robust (NHS)	Semi -Fragile (NHS)	Robust (NHS)	Semi -Fragile (NHS)
Extraction (no attack)	1.000	1.000	1.000	1.000
JPEG (QF = 100%)	0.998	0.955	0.990	0.940
JPEG (QF = 80%)	0.969	0.861	0.964	0.824
JPEG (QF = 50%)	0.951	0.705	0.949	0.683
JPEG (QF = 30%)	0.939	0.388	0.937	0.387
VQ (Codebook 1)	1.000	1.000	1.000	1.000
VQ (Codebook 2)	0.901	0.518	0.889	0.500
VQ (Codebook 3)	0.830	0.049	0.791	0.089
VQ (Codebook 4)	0.912	0.177	0.890	0.189
Image cropping	0.789	0.948	0.857	0.921
Median filtering	0.871	0.132	0.888	0.124
Blurring	0.925	0.634	0.932	0.615
High-Pass filtering	0.614	0.049	0.627	0.093
Contrast Enhancement	0.918	0.254	0.920	0.215
Brightness Enhancement	0.701	0.045	0.713	0.035
Rotation by 0.5° clockwise	0.801	0.069	0.732	0.143
Rotation by 0.5° counterclockwise	0.782	0.058	0.693	0.120
Rotation by 3° clockwise	0.621	0.091	0.604	0.098
Rotation by 3° counterclockwise	0.601	0.089	0.598	0.084

ond stage using a simple index constrained method. Although the encoded indices of the attacked watermarked image may be very different from the original ones, the variance of neighboring indices does not vary a great deal. The first-stage watermarking method is therefore robust. The second-stage watermarking method is based on an index constrained codeword search procedure, in which the index is modified according to the bit to be embedded. Any change in the encoded indices may introduce the change in the extracted watermark bit. In other words, the second-stage watermarking method can tolerate few modifications, which means is fragile to most intentional attacks. Experimental results demonstrate that the proposed method can be used for copyright protection by extracting the first-stage watermark. It can also be used for image authentication by extracting the second-stage watermark.

Compared with existing multipurpose watermarking algorithms, the advantages of the proposed algorithm are as follows:

1) The proposed algorithm can tolerate rotation attacks with having larger angles.

2) The semi-fragile and robust watermarks are extracted independently and blindly.
3) Different codebooks are used for the embedding and the extraction processes. The first uses the two stage codebook and the second the product codebook. The final product codebook can be made public for users, so that the extraction process sometimes can be performed publicly for special applications.
4) Because the embedded position in the VQ index for the semi-fragile watermark is secret, the two stage codebooks used in the embedding process are secret. The product codebook used for extraction is encrypted and not the same as that for users, it is hard for the attacker to forge a valid semi-fragile watermark in the tampered watermarked image.
5) The proposed algorithm can be extended to meet three purposes. These are (a) A digital fingerprint, (b) copyright protection, and (c) image authentication, by embedding three watermarks in a three-stage VQ.
6) The VQ-based watermarking algorithm can also reduce the amount of the data needed or transmitted.

There are some disadvantages or problems remaining which need to be solved in the future. These are as follows:

1) The quality of the watermarked image obtained by use of the existing VQ-based watermarking algorithms is not high enough for copyright protection. We may use other kinds of vector quantizers or combine it with DWT or DCT to improve the image quality.
2) The semi-fragile watermark used in the proposed algorithm does not know the kind of attack the watermarked image is under.
3) Human visual characteristics are not adopted in the VQ-based watermarking systems.
4) The extraction process is based on the product codebook. It is therefore time-consuming if we use the full-search encoding algorithm.
5) From the experimental results, we see that in the proposed algorithm, the robust watermark should be embedded in the first stage to obtain a high quality. The method of analyzing the embedding order in general sense is a problem yet to be solved.

11.3 DCT Based Multipurpose Watermarking Technique for Image Copyright Notification and Protection

A visible watermark can act as an advertisement while the invisible watermark can be used for copyright protection or content authentication. Relatively, only a few researches [24, 25, 26, 27, 28] have focused on visible watermarking. This may be due to the fact that the visible watermark will reduce the commercial value of the watermarked content. It can also reduce the intention of the intruder to illicitly possess the visibly watermarked content. The visibly watermarked content can be used as in sales promotion or to publicize a reduced-price product. Now, consider that the provider may advertise on the Internet in order to sell an image that is visibly watermarked. Someone wants to buy this image through Internet by using a credit card. Under the circumstances, three serious problems may be encountered. The first is, if the customer wants to buy the image without the visible watermark, the provider or the authorized buyer can automatically remove this from the watermarked image. However, the customer may illicitly resell the one without visible watermark to others. Secondly, someone may directly download the visibly watermarked image and sell it to others in a low price. Thirdly, someone may illicitly embed the provider's visible watermark in his own products for sales promotion.

In fact however despite the robust properties of a visible watermark, it can always be partially or fully removed or tampered with using software. To provide further protection for the image work, this section gives a method to embed an invisible watermark as a back-up in the host image. This is in addition to the visible watermark. The two watermarks are embedded in the image simultaneously and independently. The visible watermark is embedded in the DC DCT coefficient and most of the AC DCT coefficients of each block. The invisible watermark in the rest. Based on the characteristics of Human Visual System (HVS), the embedding strength of the visible watermark is varied in accordance with the underlying content of the host image. We embed the invisible watermark in a number of midrange frequencies. Since the invisible watermarks inserted in the high frequency components are vulnerable to attack but the low frequency components are perceptually significant. Alterations to the low frequency components may become visible.

11.3.1 Watermarking Algorithm

In [26], a visible watermarking technique that modifies all the DCT coefficients of each host image block using the following equation is proposed:

$$c'_{ij}(n) = \alpha_n \cdot c_{ij}(n) + \beta_n \cdot w_{ij}(n), \tag{11.14}$$

where α_n and β_n are respectively the scaling factor and the embedding factor for block n. The $c_{ij}(n)$ are the DCT coefficients of the block n in the host image and $w_{ij}(n)$ are the DCT coefficients of block n in the watermark image. The α_n and β_n values are found by using a mathematical model developed by exploiting the texture sensitivity of the HVS. We can embed more information in the block where energy tends to be evenly distributed. That is, the AC DCT coefficients have small variances. For convenience, the scaling factor α_n is assumed to be proportional to the variance σ_n^2 and the embedding factor β_n to be inversely proportional to σ_n. The blocks with mid-intensity gray scales are more sensitive to noise than those of low intensity blocks as well as high intensity blocks. If the mean gray scale of each image block is denoted as μ_n

and that of the image as μ, then the relationship between α_n and μ_n can be taken to be truncated Gaussian. The variation of β_n with respect to μ_n is the reverse of that of α_n. So α_n and β_n can be computed as:

$$\alpha_n = \sigma'_n \exp\left(-\left(\mu'_n - \mu'\right)^2\right), \tag{11.15}$$

$$\beta_n = \frac{1 - \exp\left(-\left(\mu'_n - \mu'\right)^2\right)}{\sigma'_n}, \tag{11.16}$$

where μ'_n, μ' are the normalized values of μ_n and μ, respectively, and σ'_n is normalized logarithm of σ_n. This is the variance of the AC DCT coefficients. Lastly, α_n and β_n are scaled to the ranges $(\alpha_{\min}, \alpha_{\max})$ and $(\beta_{\min}, \beta_{\max})$ respectively. Here $\alpha_{\min}$ and $\alpha_{\max}$ are the minimum and maximum values of the scaling factor, and $\beta_{\min}$ and $\beta_{\max}$ are the minimum and maximum values of the embedding factor. In this chapter, four mid-frequency AC DCT coefficients are chosen to embed the invisible watermark. Thus in Equation (11.14), the resultant α_n and β_n affect the DCT coefficients except for the four chosen coefficients.

When embedding the visible watermark, the invisible watermark should be embedded in the blocks where α_n have smaller values. This is in order to improve the robustness of the invisible watermark. The embedding process is based on quantization index modulation (QIM) techniques [15, 29, 30]. Each selected AC DCT coefficient is used to embed one watermark bit, so if a 512×512 host image is decomposed into nonoverlapping 8×8 blocks. Only a quarter of the blocks are required to embed a 64×64 binary watermark. We distinguish those blocks having a smaller α_n and randomly select a quarter of all of the blocks from them.

To determine the selected coefficient $c_{ij}(n)$, first compute the integer quotient $q_{ij}(n)$ and the remainder $r_{ij}(n)$ as follows:

$$q_{ij}(n) = \text{Int}\left[c_{ij}(n)/L\right], \tag{11.17}$$

$$r_{ij}(n) = c_{ij}(n) - q_{ij}(n) \times L, \tag{11.18}$$

where L is the quantization step, which in this chapter is equal to 24. Then modify the coefficient $c_{ij}(n)$ according to the value of invisible watermark bit W by using the following equations.
If $c_{ij} \geq 0$, then

$$c'_{ij}(n) = \begin{cases} q_{ij}(n) \times L + \frac{L}{2}, & \text{if } (q_{ij}(n)\%2) = \overline{W}; \\ q_{ij}(n) \times L + \frac{3L}{2}, & \text{if } (q_{ij}(n)\%2) = W \text{ AND } |r_{ij}(n)| > \frac{L}{2}; \\ q_{ij}(n) \times L - \frac{L}{2}, & \text{if } (q_{ij}(n)\%2) = W \text{ AND } |r_{ij}(n)| < \frac{L}{2}; \end{cases} \tag{11.19}$$

else if $c_{ij} < 0$, then

$$c'_{ij}(n) = \begin{cases} q_{ij}(n) \times L - \frac{L}{2}, & \text{if } (q_{ij}(n)\%2) = W; \\ q_{ij}(n) \times L - \frac{3L}{2}, & \text{if } (q_{ij}(n)\%2) = \overline{W} \text{ AND } |r_{ij}(n)| > \frac{L}{2}; \\ q_{ij}(n) \times L + \frac{L}{2}, & \text{if } (q_{ij}(n)\%2) = \overline{W} \text{ AND } |r_{ij}(n)| < \frac{L}{2}; \end{cases} \tag{11.20}$$

where $c'_{ij}(n)$ denotes the modified coefficient, % denotes the modulo operation and $|r|$ the absolute value of r.

Finally, use the inverse DCT operation to obtain the dual watermarked image.

In the invisible watermark extraction process, the invisible watermark bit W' is extracted from the modified coefficient $c'_{ij}(n)$ by using

$$W' = \begin{cases} \left(\mathrm{Int}\left[c'_{ij}(n)/L\right]\right)\%2, & \text{if } c'_{ij}(n) < 0; \\ 1 - \left(\mathrm{Int}\left[c'_{ij}(n)/L\right]\right)\%2, & \text{if } c'_{ij}(n) \geq 0. \end{cases} \tag{11.21}$$

11.3.2 Experimental Results

In our experiments, the 512×512 256-grayscale Lena image, a 512×512 256-grayscale visible watermark, a 64×64 binary invisible watermark are used. The visible and invisible watermarks are shown in Fig. 11.17 We decompose the Lena image and the visible watermark into nonoverlapping 8×8 blocks. The invisible watermark is embedded in the selected AC DCT coefficients of midrange frequencies, and the visible watermark is embedded in others. The dual watermarked image and the corresponding extracted invisible watermark are shown in Fig. 11.18. To test the robustness of the proposed algorithm, we made several attacks on the watermarked image. These include JPEG compression, median filtering and Gaussian filtering in Stirmark [31] benchmark software, together with contrast enhancement and cropping in Adobe Photoshop 5.0 software. Visible watermark removal was done by exploiting the original visible watermark. The extracted invisible watermarks are shown in Figs. 11.19(a)–(h) and evaluated by normalized Hamming similarity (NHS). The results show that the proposed algorithm is robust to normal attacks. The invisible and visible watermarks are independent of each other and the quality of the watermarked image is well preserved. The invisible watermark extraction is blind as the original image is not required during the extraction process.

11.3.3 Conclusion

A novel multipurpose image watermarking technique based on DCT is presented. The basic idea is to embed the invisible watermark in some frequency bands, and embed the visible watermark in others. Future work will be focused on improving the robustness of the invisible watermark to geometric attacks.

11.4 Image Retrieval Based on a Multipurpose Watermarking Scheme

Due to the development of computer, multimedia, and network technologies, two important issues have arisen nowadays. The first problem is that the

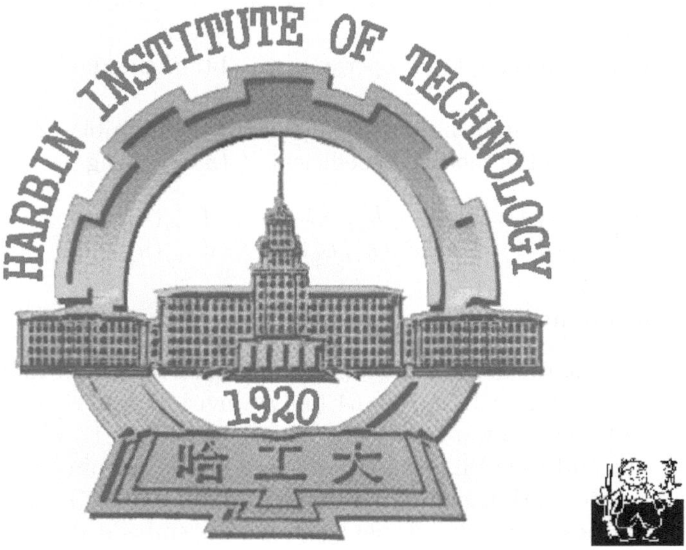

Fig. 11.17. Visible and invisible watermarks.

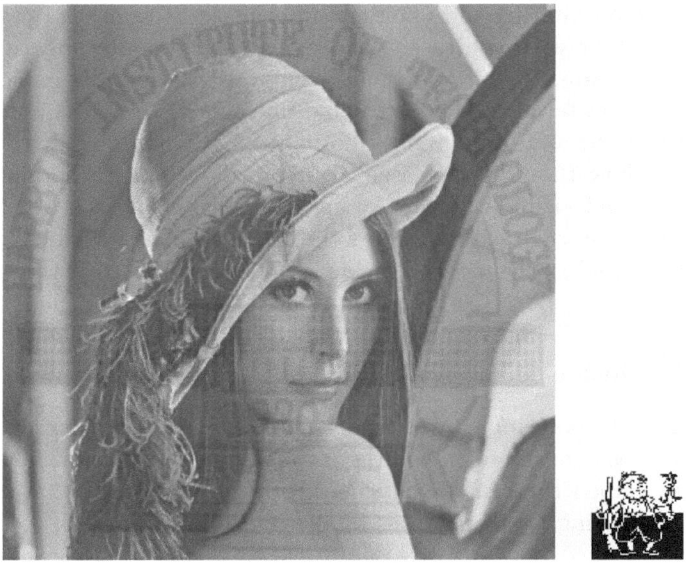

Fig. 11.18. Dual watermarked image and extracted invisible watermark, NHS = 1.0000

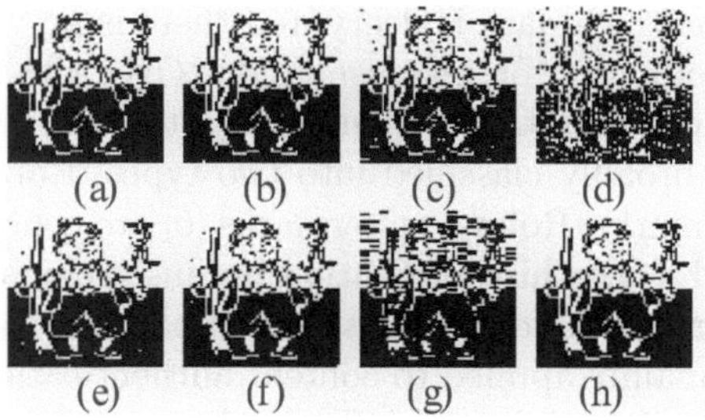

Fig. 11.19. Invisible watermarks extracted from the attacked watermarked images. (a) JPEG compression QF = 70%, NHS = 1.0000; (b) JPEG compression QF = 60%, NHS = 0.9976; (c) 3 × 3 median filtering, NHS = 0.9744; (d) 2 × 2 median filtering, NHS = 0.8723; (e) Gaussian filtering 3 × 3, NHS = 0.9954; (f) Contrast enhancement by 30%, NHS = 0.9966; (g) A quarter of the image in the upper-left corner cropped, NHS = 0.8549; (h) Visible watermark removing, NHS = 1.0000.

amount of audiovisual information available in digital format has grown exponentially in recent years. This has resulted in an information explosion that has exceeded the limit of human capability. Digitization, compression, and archival of multimedia information has become popular, inexpensive and straightforward. Subsequent retrieval of the stored information may require considerable additional work in order for it to be effective and efficient. The second problem is that there is almost no limit for anyone to make unlimited copies of digital contents on the Internet and by means of CD-ROM. This is a major disadvantage from the owner's viewpoint when entering the digital world. Copyright protection has therefore been one of the most important issues in the digital world. This chapter is concerned with the problems in image retrieval and copyright protection. The first question is whether we should use some effective retrieval methods to get the desired images. In typical Content-Based Image Retrieval (CBIR) systems [32], the visual contents of the images in the database are extracted and are described by multi-dimensional feature vectors. The feature vectors form a feature database. To retrieve images, users provide the retrieval system with example images or sketched figures. The similarities and distances between the feature vectors of the query example or sketch and those of the images in the database are then calculated. Retrieval is accomplished with the aid of an indexing scheme. Recent retrieval systems have incorporated users' relevance feedback to modify and improve the retrieval process. The existing image retrieval algorithms can be classified into two classes. That is, Low-Level Based and High-Level (semantic) Based. The low-level features include color [33], texture [34], shape [35] and spatial relationships [36]. Some retrieval methods based on semantic-level [37] have been recently proposed.

On the latter issue, encryption may provide one of solutions. However, conventional cryptographic systems permit only valid keyholders access to encrypted data. Once such data is decrypted there is no way to keep track of its subsequent reproduction or retransmission. Over the last decade, digital watermarking has been used to complement cryptographic processes. Invisible watermarks can be broadly classified into two types, Robust and Fragile (or Semi-Fragile) watermarks. Robust watermarks [6] are generally used for copyright protection and ownership verification because they are robust to nearly all kinds of image processing operations. In comparison, fragile or semi-fragile watermarks [9] are mainly applied to content authentication because they are fragile to most types of modifications. To fulfill copyright protection and content authentication simultaneously, the multipurpose watermarking algorithm based on wavelet transform [11] has been suggested.

In general, the above two issues are separately taken into account. This chapter presents a simple multipurpose watermarking scheme which is able to solve these two problems simultaneously. The main idea is to embed offline three watermarks. These are the Copyright, the Denotation, and Features into each of the images in the database. During the online retrieval, we can make queries based on the Copyright, the Denotation and the Features, or the combination of them. In the following sections, we describe the features which we use. Then we give the proposed Offline Multipurpose Watermarking Scheme. We then discuss how to make the query and how to retrieve online. We next provide the experimental results and conclusions.

11.4.1 Feature Extraction

In general, we should extract as many as possible of the available features. In our system, because the embedding of watermarks will affect the image quality, we should select as few as possible of the best representative features. We use three kinds of features, that is, the Global Invariant Feature based on the Haar Integral [38], Statistical Moments of the Color Histogram and the Hu Moments, which are now described in detail.

Global Invariant Feature

Invariant features remain unchanged even when the image is transformed according to a group of transformations. In [38], an example of global feature invariant to rotations and translations is considered. Given a gray-scale image

$$\mathbf{M} = \{\mathbf{M}(\mathbf{x}), \mathbf{x} = (x_0, x_1), 0 \le x_0 < N_0, 0 \le x_1 < N_1\}, \tag{11.22}$$

and an element $g \in G$ of the group of image translations and rotations. The transformation can be expressed as follows.

$$\begin{aligned} &(g\mathbf{M})(\mathbf{x}) = \mathbf{M}(\mathbf{x}'), \\ &\text{with} \quad \mathbf{x}' = \left\{ \begin{pmatrix} \cos\phi & \sin\phi \\ -\sin\phi & \cos\phi \end{pmatrix} \mathbf{x} + \begin{pmatrix} t_0 \\ t_1 \end{pmatrix} \right\} \bmod \begin{pmatrix} N_0 \\ N_1 \end{pmatrix}. \end{aligned} \tag{11.23}$$

Based on above definition, an invariant transformation T must satisfy

$$T(g\mathbf{M}) = T(\mathbf{M}), \quad \forall g \in G. \tag{11.24}$$

For a given gray-scale image $\mathbf{M}$ and an arbitrary complex-valued function $f(\mathbf{M})$, it is possible to construct an invariant transformation T by using the Haar integral:

$$\begin{aligned} T[f](\mathbf{M}) &:= \frac{1}{|G|}\int_G f(g\mathbf{M})\,\mathrm{d}g \\ &= \frac{1}{2\pi N_0 N_1}\int_{t_0=0}^{N_0}\int_{t_1=0}^{N_1}\int_{\phi=0}^{2\pi} f(g(t_0,t_1,\phi)\mathbf{M})\,\mathrm{d}\phi \mathrm{d}t_1 \mathrm{d}t_0. \end{aligned} \tag{11.25}$$

Because this integral is of linear complexity in the number of pixels and in the maximum radius of the kernel function's support, we need to reduce the calculation complexity. For discrete images, because we can choose integers for (t_0, t_1) and use K steps for ϕ, the following formula can be obtained.

$$T[f](\mathbf{M}) \approx \frac{1}{KN_0N_1}\sum_{t_0=0}^{N_0-1}\sum_{t_1=0}^{N_1-1}\sum_{k=0}^{K-1} f\left(g\left(t_0,t_1,\phi=\frac{2\pi k}{K}\right)\mathbf{M}\right). \tag{11.26}$$

The calculation strategy can be illustrated by Fig. 11.20. If we select a simple function

$$f(\mathbf{M}) = \sqrt{\mathbf{M}(0,1)\times\mathbf{M}(2,0)}, \tag{11.27}$$

then

$$\begin{aligned} T[f](\mathbf{M}) = &\frac{1}{2\pi N_0 N_1}\int_{t_0=0}^{N_0}\int_{t_1=0}^{N_1}\int_{\phi=0}^{2\pi}\sqrt{\mathbf{M}(\sin\phi+t_0,\cos\phi+t_1)} \\ &\times\sqrt{\mathbf{M}(2\sin(\phi+\pi/2)+t_0, 2\cos(\phi+\pi/2)+t_1})\mathrm{d}\phi\mathrm{d}t_1\mathrm{d}t_0. \end{aligned} \tag{11.28}$$

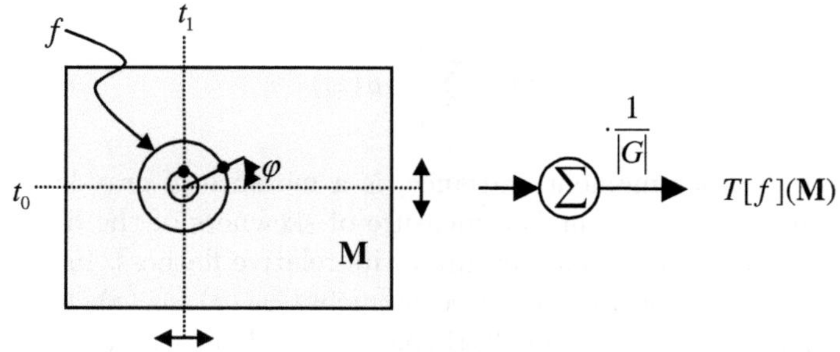

Fig. 11.20. Calculation strategy for invariant integration in the case of Euclidean motion.

We can apply the Monte-Carlo method for the calculation of multi-dimensional integrals as follows:

Step 1: Generate a set of n random vectors $\mathbf{P} = \{\mathbf{p}_0, \mathbf{p}_1, \cdots, \mathbf{p}_{n-1}\}$ that are equally distributed in $\{(t_0, t_1, \phi) \,|\, 0 \le t_0 < N_0,\ 0 \le t_1 < N_1,\ 0 \le \phi \le 2\pi\}$.

Step 2: Evaluate

$$\mathbf{Q} = \{f(g(t_0, t_1, \phi)\mathbf{M}) \mid (t_0, t_1, \phi) \in \mathbf{P}\} = \{q_0, q_1, \cdots, q_{n-1}\}$$

Here $q_i, i = 0, 1, \cdots, n-1$ are scalars. Here inter-grid positions are handled applying bilinear interpolation.

Step 3: Approximate $T[f](\mathbf{M})$ by $\overline{q} = \frac{1}{n}\sum_{i=0}^{n-1} q_i$.

In this chapter, we only use the global feature, that is one floating-typed value, calculated from luminance component of the color image.

Statistical Moments of the Color Histogram

Generally speaking, texture feature extraction methods can be classified in three major categories. These are as follows, Statistical, Structural and Spectral. In statistical approaches, texture statistics such as the moments of the gray-level histogram, or statistics based on the gray-level co-occurrence matrix are computed to discriminate different textures. In this chapter, statistical moments of the gray-level histogram are used to describe texture. Let z be a discreet random variable representing gray-levels in the range $[0, L-1]$, where L is the maximum gray value. Let $p(z_i), i = 0, 1, \cdots, L-1$ be a normalized histogram. Then the n-th moment with respect to the mean is given by:

$$\mu_n(z) = \sum_{i=0}^{L-1} (z_i - m)^n p(z_i) \tag{11.29}$$

where m is the mean value of z, that is, the average gray level

$$m = \sum_{i=0}^{L-1} z_i p(z_i) \tag{11.30}$$

The second-order moment, variance, is a measure of gray-level contrast. And the third-order moment is a measure of skewness of the histogram and the fourth-order moment is a measure of its relative flatness. In this chapter, we use the mean value m and three moments $\mu_2(z), \mu_3(z), \mu_4(z)$ of each color component's histogram in RGB color space. That is, four floating-typed values per color-component, as the features which are to be embedded.

Hu Moments

Hu moments are a set of algebraic invariants that combine regular moments [39]. They are invariant under a change of size, translation, and rotation. Hu moments have been widely used in pattern recognition and have proved to be successful in various applications. These moments can be used to describe the shape of the information of the image. For the digital image $\mathbf{M}$, considered in this chapter, we only use the first 4 moments for the luminance component. That is the four following floating-typed values.

$$\begin{cases} \phi_1 = \eta_{20} + \eta_{02}, \\ \phi_2 = (\eta_{20} - \eta_{02})^2 + 4\eta_{11}^2, \\ \phi_3 = (\eta_{30} - 3\eta_{12})^2 + (\eta_{03} - 3\eta_{21})^2, \\ \phi_4 = (\eta_{30} + \eta_{12})^2 + (\eta_{03} + \eta_{21})^2, \end{cases} \tag{11.31}$$

where

$$\begin{cases} \eta_{pq} = \mu_{pq}/\mu_{00}^{\gamma}; \\ \mu_{pq} = \sum_{x_0} \sum_{x_1} (x_0 - \bar{x}_0)^p (x_1 - \bar{x}_1)^q \mathbf{M}(x_0, x_1); \\ \bar{x}_0 = m_{10}/m_{00}; \\ \bar{x}_1 = m_{01}/m_{00}; \\ m_{pq} = \sum_{x_0} \sum_{x_1} x_0^p x_1^q \mathbf{M}(x_0, x_1). \end{cases}$$

11.4.2 Offline Multipurpose Watermarking

In our system, before we do the online retrieval, we first embed three watermarks into each image in the database. Because these three watermarks possess different purposes, we call our watermarking a Multipurpose Watermark Scheme. The first watermark is a Copyright Watermark, which is used for copyright protection. The second is the Annotation Watermark, which is the name of the image or the semantic meaning of the image. The last is the Feature Watermark, which is composed of the extracted features. These are all robust watermarks.

In our watermarking system, the famous Dither Modulation Method [30] is used to embed the three watermarks into the DCT block of each image's luminance component. We transform from RGB space to YUV space, only the Y component is used, and the U, V components remaining are unchanged. The watermark's bits are distributed image orientated, so that cropping the image will crop the watermark in the same way as the host-image. The dither modulation algorithm encodes each watermark bit in a Middle-Frequency DCT coefficient. Assume a DCT coefficient DCT_i in an even interval representing the bit '0' and in an odd interval representing the bit '1.' An interval is even, if, by using a given Δ, $\lfloor \mathrm{DCT}_i/\Delta \rfloor = \text{even}$, or else it is odd. If a DCT coefficient is already in an interval which represents its bit, we move it in the middle of the interval. Alternatively, we move it to the middle of the nearest interval adjacent to its current interval. Using our system, we embed twelve bits into each 8×8 DCT block.

The key problem is how to embed a floating-typed value into the image. For simplicity, we embed the 4 bytes (i.e., 32 bits) which represents the floating value directly into the image. A problem arising is the error in bits. Even one bit may make the extracted value very different from the embedded one. To overcome this problem, we embed each floating value multiple times into the image. During the extraction, we determine the extracted bits in the majority cases. This process can be shown in Fig. 11.21. A further problem is how to guarantee the security of the watermarks. This is especially important for the copyright watermark. In our system, we use the Interleaving Embedding Technique. We randomly select the columns of DCT blocks to embed one of the watermarks, so perhaps the first column is used to embed the feature watermark. The second column may be used to embed the annotation watermark, and so on. The selection scheme can be viewed as an embedding key.

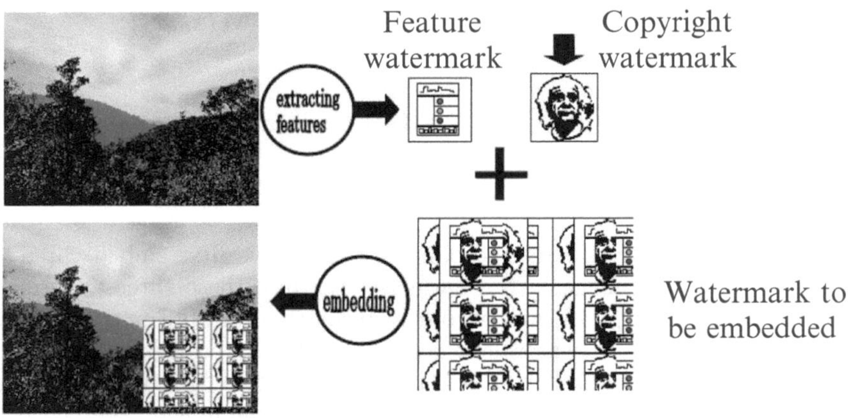

Fig. 11.21. The embedding strategy.

11.4.3 Online Image Retrieval with Various Query Strategies

After embedding the watermarks into all the images in the database, we can now do the online retrieval. Here we can use several kinds of queries. The most normal is feature-based. We can also use copyright-based and annotation-based, or alternatively we can use the combination query schemes.

For the feature-based query scheme, we first extract the features from the query image. Note that if the query image is without a feature watermark, we should compute the feature online for it. Then we compare the query feature vector with the feature watermark in each database image to find the most desired similar images. For the feature-and-annotation-based query scheme, we can only search the desired images with the same annotation. In general, it is the semantic of the image. For the feature-and-copyright-based query scheme, we can only search the desired images having the same copyright. For the feature-annotation-copyright-based query scheme, we can only search the desired images having the same copyright and the same annotation.

11.4.4 Experimental Results

We did the experiments on a test database of 1000 images in 10 classes, each class including 100 images. They are with size of 384×256 or 256×384. During the offline process, we extract and embed three kinds of features. These are, one Global Invariant Feature, four Hu Moments and 12 Histogram-Based Moments (this is for the three R, G, and B Color Components) for each database image. For the Global Invariant Feature, we use $n = 10000$ and $f(\mathbf{M}) = \mathbf{M}(0,1) \times \mathbf{M}(2,0)$. We embed a 48×48 sized binary copyright watermark, 17 floating-typed (68 bytes) feature values and 16-bytes annotation text. In our system, we can embed up to 288 bytes. In the experiment, we view the annotation text as part of the Feature Watermark. We combine the feature watermark and the Copyright Watermark to construct the watermark to be embedded for each database image. We then embed the watermark in the corresponding image. After we obtain a watermarked image database, we can perform the online retrieval to obtain answers to various queries.

For a query based on features, we show an example of retrieval results in Fig. 11.22. The average precision and recall for each class is shown in Table 11.2. The average precision and recall for each class can be obtained as follows. We first randomly select ten images from the class. We then use each image as the query image. For each query image, we obtain the "recall" by finding the ratio of returned images in this class in the first 100 returned images. We then find the position of the first returned image which is not in this class and divide it by 100 to obtain the "precision." After finding ten recalls and ten precision values, we average them to get the average recall and precision.

For the image retrieval system, the most important operation to which our system should be able to resist is the high-quality compression. Other attacks are not so important. To show the performance of the system in resisting the JPEG compression, we give some results in Figs. 11.23 and 11.24. Under the condition that we can extract the watermark which is more than 80% similar to the original embedded information, Fig. 11.23 gives the minimum compression quality factors to which the system can resist with. It uses a number of different modulation steps. Fig.11.24 shows the average watermarked image qualities obtained under different modulation steps. In previous sections, we have mentioned that the extracted feature watermark should not be responsible for bit loss. With regard to this, in the case of 100% recovery, the experimental results show that the average lowest JPEG compression quality factor to which the feature watermark can resist is 90.

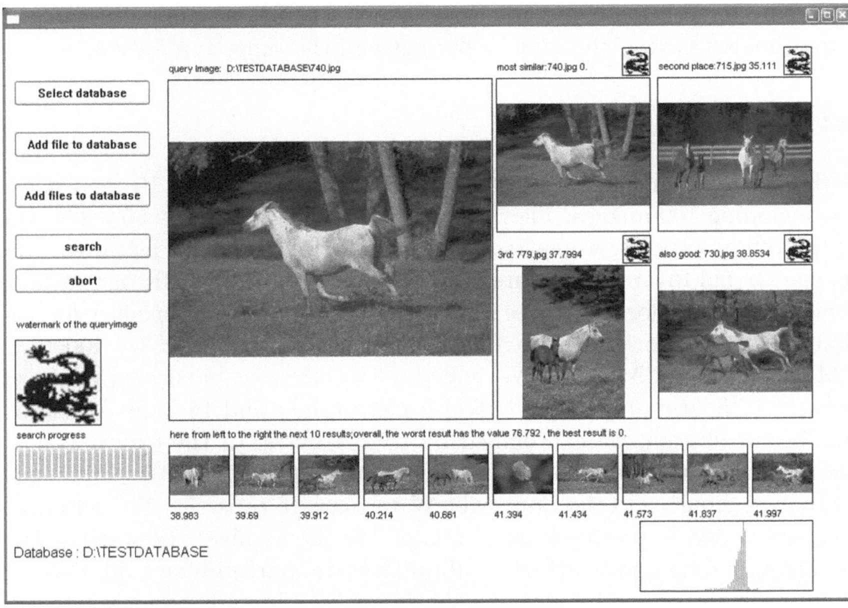

Fig. 11.22. The retrieval interface of our system.

Table 11.2. The average recall and precision for each class.

Class number	Semantic	Recall	Precision
1	People	0.27	0.02
2	Beach	0.14	0.01
3	Building	0.20	0.01
4	Bus	0.24	0.02
5	Dinosaur	0.67	0.29
6	Elephant	0.35	0.02
7	Flower	0.24	0.04
8	Horse	0.48	0.12
9	Mountain	0.18	0.02
10	Food	0.20	0.01

11.4.5 Conclusions

This chapter outlines an image retrieval system based on a multipurpose watermarking scheme. The advantages of this scheme are in three areas. The first is that the system embeds the features in the images, and no extra space is required to save the feature data. The second is that the image file can be copied to other database without recomputing the corresponding features. The thirdly is that the image is copyrighted and annotated, and the retrieval system can confirm that the image and the semantic are original.

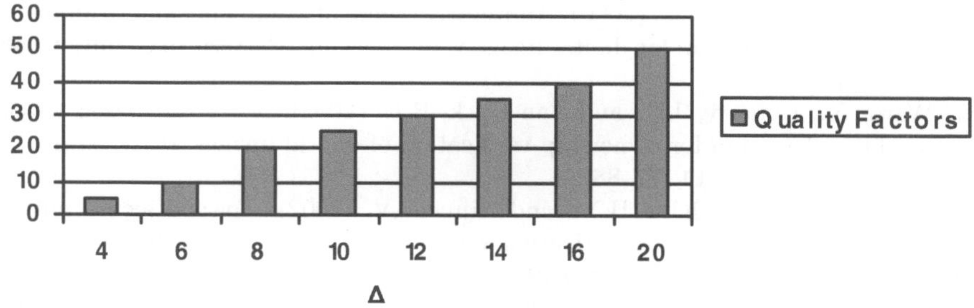

Fig. 11.23. JPEG Quality factors vs. the modulation steps in the case of more than 80% recovery.

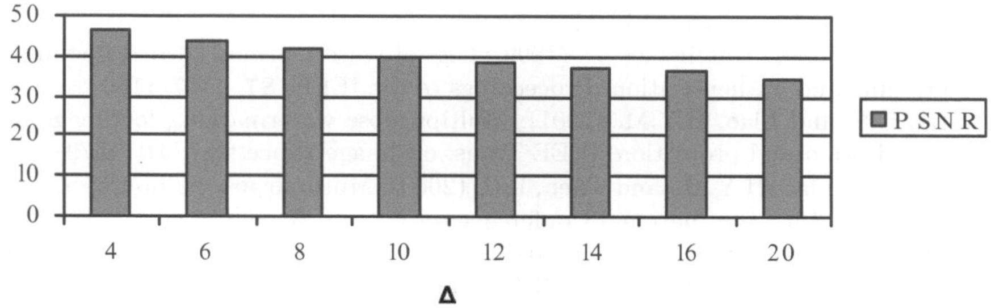

Fig. 11.24. PSNRs vs. the modulation steps.

Acknowledgement

The research work related to this chapter was supported by Alexander von Humboldt Foundation Fellowship(Germany), ID: CHN 1115969 STP and the National Natural Science Foundation of China under grant 60272074 and the Spaceflight Innovation Foundation of China under grant [2002]210-6.

References

1. O'Ruanaidh, J.J.K., Dowling, W.J., and Boland, F.M. (1996): Watermarking digital images for copyright protection. IEE Proceedings – Vision, Image and Signal Processing, **143**, 250–256
2. Cox, I.J., Kilian, J., Leighton, F.T., and Shamoon, T. (1997): Secure spread spectrum watermarking for multimedia. IEEE Trans. on Image Processing, **6**, 1673–1687
3. Swanson, M.D., Zhu, B., and Tewfik, A.H. (1998): Multiresolution scene-based video watermarking using perceptual models. IEEE Journal on Selected Areas in Communications, **16**, 540–550
4. Voyatzis, G., and Pitas, I. (1999): The use of watermarks in the protection of digital multimedia products. Proceedings of the IEEE, **87**, 1197–1207

5. Pereira, S., and Pun, T. (2000): An iterative template matching algorithm using the chirp-Z transform for digital image watermarking. Pattern Recognition, **33**, 173–175
6. Wang, Y., Doherty, J.F., and Van Dyck, R.E. (2002): A wavelet-based watermarking algorithm for ownership verification of digital images. IEEE Trans. on Image Processing, **11**, 77–88
7. Barreto, P.S.L.M., Kim, H.Y., and Rijmen, V. (2002): Toward secure public-key blockwise fragile authentication watermarking. IEE Proceedings – Vision, Image and Signal Processing, **149**, 57–62
8. Celik, M.U., Sharma, G., Saber, E., and Tekalp, A.M. (2002): Hierarchical watermarking for secure image authentication with localization. IEEE Trans. on Image Processing, **11**, 585–595
9. Lee, J. and Won, C.S. (2000): A watermarking sequence using parities of error control coding for image authentication and correction. IEEE Trans. on Consumer Electronics, **46**, 313–317
10. Kundur, D. and Hatzinakos, D. (1999): Digital Watermarking for telltale tamper proofing and authentication. Proceedings of the IEEE, **87**, 1167–1180
11. Lu, C.S. and Liao, H.Y.M. (2001): Multipurpose watermarking for image authentication and protection. IEEE Trans. on Image Processing, **10**, 1579–1592
12. Lu, C.S., Liao, H.Y.M., and Chen, L.H. (2000): Multipurpose audio watermarking. Proc. 15th International Conference on Pattern Recognition, **3**, 282–285
13. Lu, C.S., Huang, S.K., Sze, C.J., and Liao, H.Y.M. (2000): Cocktail watermarking for digital image protection. IEEE Trans. on Multimedia, **2**, 209–224
14. Busch, C., and Wolthusen, S.D. (2001): Tracing data diffusion in industrial research with robust watermarking. Proc. 2001 IEEE Fourth Workshop on Multimedia Signal Processing, 207–212
15. Lu, Z.M. and Sun, S.H. (2000): Digital image watermarking technique based on vector quantisation. Electronics Letters, **36**, 303–305
16. Lu, Z.M., Pan, J.S., and Sun, S.H. (2000): VQ-based digital image watermarking method. Electronics Letters, **36**, 1201–1202
17. Lu, Z.M., Liu, C.H., and Sun, S.H. (2002): Digital image watermarking technique based on block truncation coding with vector quantization. Chinese Journal of Electronics, **11**, 152–157
18. Jo, M. and Kim, H. (2002): A digital image watermarking scheme based on vector quantization. IEICE Transactions on Information and Systems, **E85-D**, 1054–1056
19. Makur, A. and Selvi, S.S. (2001): Variable dimension vector quantization based image watermarking. Signal Processing, **81**, 889–893
20. Huang, H.C., Wang, F.H., and Pan, J.S. (2002): A VQ-based robust multi-watermarking algorithm. IEICE Transactions on Fundamentals, **E85-A**, 1719–1726
21. Huang, H.C., Wang, F.H., and Pan, J.S. (2001): Efficient and robust watermarking algorithm with vector quantisation. Electronics Letters, **37**, 826–828
22. Linde, Y., Buzo, A., and Gray, R.M. (1980): An algorithm for vector quantizer design. IEEE Trans. on Communications, **28**, 84–95
23. Lu, Z.M., Pan, J.S., and Sun, S.H. (2000): Efficient codeword search algorithm based on hadamard transform. Electronics Letters, **36**, 1364–1365
24. Hu, Y.J. and Kwong, S. (2001): Wavelet domain adaptive visible watermarking. Electronics Letters, **37**, 1219–1220

25. Chen, P.M. (2000): A visible watermarking mechanism using a statistic approach. Proceedings of IEEE 5th International Conference on Signal Processing (WCCC-ICSP2000), **2**, 910–913
26. Mohanty, S.P., Ramakrishnan, K.R., and Kankanhalli, M.S. (2000): A DCT domain visible watermarking technique for images. Proceedings of IEEE International Conference on Multimedia and Expo (ICME2000), **2**, 1029–1032
27. Kankanhalli, M.S., Rajmohan, and Ramakrishnan, K.R. (1999): Adaptive visible watermarking of images. Proceedings of IEEE International Conference on Multimedia Computing and Systems, **1**, 568–573
28. Meng, J.H. and Chang, S.F. (1998): Embedding Visible Video Watermarks in the Compressed Domain. In Proceedings of IEEE International Conference on Image Processing (ICIP'98), **1**, 474–477
29. Chen, B. and Wornell, G.W. (2001): Quantization index modulation: a class of provably good methods for digital watermarking and information embedding. IEEE Trans. on Information Theory, **47**, 1423–1443
30. Chen, B. and Wornell, G.W. (1998): Digital watermarking and information embedding using dither modulation. IEEE Second Workshop on Multimedia Signal Processing, 273–278
31. Petitcolas, F.A.P., Anderson, R.J., and Kuhn, M.G. (1998): Attack on copyright marking systems. Proceedings of 2nd International Workshop on Information Hiding, 218–238
32. Long, F.H., Zhang, H.J., and Feng, D.D. (2003): Fundamentals of content-based image retrieval. Multimedia Information Retrieval and Management — Technological Fundamentals and Applications [Feng, D.D., Siu, W.C., and Zhang, H.J. Eds.], Springer-Verlag, Berlin Heidelberg
33. Smith, J.R. (2002): Color for image retrieval. Image Databases-Search and Retrieval of Digital Imagery [Castelli, V., and Beagman L.D., eds.] John Wiley & Sons, Inc. 285–311
34. Sebe, N., Lew, M.S. (2001): Texture features for content based retrieval. Principles of Visual Information Retrieval [Lew, M.S. ed.], Springer, 51–85
35. Lee, K.M., Street, W.N. (2002): Incremental feature weight learning and its application to a shape based query system. Pattern Recognition Letters, **23**, 265–274
36. Sciascio, E.D., Donini, F.M., and Mongiello, M. (2002): Spatial layout representation for query by sketch content-based image retrieval. Pattern Recognition Letters, **23**, 1599–1612
37. Lew, M.S. (2001): Features selection and visual learning. Principles of Visual Information Retrieval [Lew, M.S., ed.], Springer, 297–318
38. Siggelkow, S. and Burkhardt, H. (2001): Fast invariant feature extraction for image retrieval. State-of-the-Art in Content-Based Image and Video Retrieval [Veltkamp R. C., Burkhardt H., Kriegel, H. P. ed.], Kluwer Acadenic Publishers
39. Belkasim, S.O., Shridhar M., and Ahmadi, M. (1991): Pattern recognition with moment invariants: a comparative study. Pattern Recognition, **24**, 1117–1138

12

Tabu Search Based Multi-Watermarking over Lossy Networks

Hsiang-Cheh Huang[1], Jeng-Shyang Pan[2], Chun-Yen Huang[2], Yu-Hsiu Huang[3], and Kuang-Chih Huang[3]

[1] Department of Electrical Engineering, National University of Kaohsiung, 700 University Rd., Kaohsiung 811, Taiwan, R.O.C.
huang.hc@gmail.com
http://hchuang.ee.nuk.edu.tw/

[2] Department of Electronic Engineering, National Kaohsiung University of Applied Sciences,
415 Chien-Kung Rd., Kaohsiung 807, Taiwan, R.O.C.
jspan@cc.kuas.edu.tw
http://bit.kuas.edu.tw/~jspan/
piscehuang@gmail.com

[3] Department of Electronic Engineering, Cheng-Shiu University,
840 Cheng-Ching Rd., Kaohsiung 833, Taiwan, R.O.C.
yhhuang@csu.edu.tw
kchuang@csu.edu.tw

Summary. Digital watermarking is one of the useful solutions for digital copy rights management systems, and it has been a popular research topic in the last decade. Most watermarking related literature focus on how to resist deliberate attacks by applying benchmarks to watermarked media to assess the effectiveness of the watermarking algorithm. Only a few have concentrated on the error-resilient transmission of watermarked media. In this chapter, we propose an innovative algorithm on vector quantization (VQ) based image watermarking, which is suitable for error-resilient transmission over lossy networks and noisy channels. By incorporating watermarking with Multiple Description Coding (MDC), our proposed schemes for embedding multiple watermarks can efficiently overcome channel impairments while retaining the capability for copyright and ownership protection. In addition, we employ an optimization technique, called tabu search, to optimize both the watermarked image quality, and the robustness of the extracted watermarks. We have obtained promising results. Simulations demonstrate the utility and practicability of our proposed algorithm.

12.1 Introduction

Digital watermarking is one useful solution for digital rights management (DRM) systems [1, 2, 3, 4]. It embeds secret information into the digital

H.-C. Huang et al.: *Tabu Search Based Multi-Watermarking over Lossy Networks*, Studies in Computational Intelligence (SCI) **58**, 325–355 (2007)
www.springerlink.com

contents in order to protect intellectual properties or the ownership of the original multimedia sources [5]. Typical watermarking schemes were based on transform-domain techniques using discrete cosine transform (DCT) [6], discrete wavelet transform (DWT) [7] and discrete Fourier transform (DFT) [8], spatial-domain methods [9], VQ domain schemes [10, 11], for example, to embed the watermark into certain coefficients in their respective domains. These schemes have been popular research topics in the last decade.

As we stated in Chapter 1, the three most critical requirements for designing watermarking algorithms are: *watermark imperceptibility*, *watermark robustness*, and *watermark capacity*. After considering the three fundamental requirements for watermarking, we determine in this chapter, how to fix the watermark capacity, and how to employ tabu search [12, 13] to find a tradeoff between watermark imperceptibility and watermark robustness. Tabu search is an evolutionary algorithm, a meta-heuristic approach, and is characterized by the use of a flexible memory. It is able to eliminate local minima and to search areas beyond a local minimum. There are few research papers concentrating on designing watermarking algorithms with optimization techniques [14, 15] in literature. One of the contributions in this chapter is how to employ tabu search, an optimization technique, to obtain an optimal, watermarked image.

Different from conventional schemes used to perform watermarking in the spatial or transform domains, we propose in this chapter an innovative algorithm concentrating on vector quantization (VQ) [16]. This is the VQ-based image watermarking, suitable for error-resilient transmission over lossy networks and noisy channels. Searching research literature relating to digital watermarking, only a few research papers concentrate on the error resilient transmission of watermarked media [17, 18, 19, 20]. In addition, most of the watermarking related literature focus on how to resist intentional attacks by applying benchmarks to watermarked media in order to assess the effectiveness of the watermarking algorithm. Therefore, we provide another viewpoint to protect the ownership of the original, and simultaneously retain the reconstructed image quality with error-resilient coding.

At the beginning of watermarking research in mid-1990's, researchers examined the robustness of watermarking algorithms by imposing some attacking schemes, including the low-pass filtering, compression, geometric distortion, flipping, for example, into the watermarked media. These attacking schemes were integrated into several benchmarks like Stirmark [21]. These benchmarks seldom consider the scenario of transmitting the watermarked media over the communication channels [22]. This is the motivation of the research in this chapter. With the inspiration that there is little research relating to transmission of watermarked media over the transmission channels, we combine the two topics. That is, watermarking and error resilient coding, and this has led to promising results. By using tabu search, we obtain an optimized solution suitable for the transmission of watermarked images over lossy channels.

The aim is to transmit watermarked images over noisy channels. Our proposed schemes for embedding single or multiple watermarks using tabu search can effectively overcome channel impairments and reproduce a good reconstructed image, while still retaining the capability for ownership and copyright protection.

12.2 Backgrounds of Multiple Description Coding and Its Generic Model

During transmissions of data, losses are inevitable due to channel errors or lost packets under different types of transmission channels. In contrast to the conventional schemes such as progressive transmission, Multiple Description Coding (MDC) offers an alternative method for the effective transmission of compressed multimedia information.

MDC is an error resilient coding technique, which can be used as a source coding method for a channel whose end-to-end performance includes uncorrected erasures. This channel is encountered in a packet communication system that has effective error detection but does not have the features which permit the retransmission of incorrect or lost packets. MDC uses diversity to overcome channel impairments so that a decoder, which receives an arbitrary subset of the channels, may reproduce a useful reconstruction [23]. Information-theoretic issues of MDC have been studied extensively since the early eighties [24, 25]. In Multiple Description (MD) coders, the same source material is coded into several chunks of data, called *descriptions*, such that each description can be decoded independently in order to obtain minimum fidelity. It also combines with other descriptions to achieve a better quality. The goals for MDC and channel coding are to make effective transmission of data, the MDC offers a totally different perspective from that of channel coding [26].

MDC is suitable for transmission with noisy channels with long bursts of errors. To gain robustness of the loss of descriptions in spite, MDC must sacrifice some compression efficiency while still retaining the capability of error resilience. Fig. 12.1 depicts the generic model for MD source coding with two channels and three decoders. The Encoder is denoted by α_0. Decoder 0, denoted by β_0, is called the *central decoder*, and Decoders 1 and 2, are denoted by β_1 and β_2 respectively, are the *side decoders*. The Euclidean distance between $\boldsymbol{X}$ and $\hat{\boldsymbol{X}}^{(0)}$ is the *central distortion*, while the errors between $\boldsymbol{X}$ and $\hat{\boldsymbol{X}}^{(i)}, i = 1, 2$, are the *side distortions*. It suggests a situation in which there are three separate users or three classes of users, which could arise when broadcasting on two channels. The same abstraction holds if there is a single user that can be in one of three states depending on which descriptions are received. Generally speaking, if we extend the number of transmission channels in Fig. 12.1 to K, there will be $2^K - 1$ receivers that decode with different number of descriptions received, and obtain different qualities of the reconstructed image.

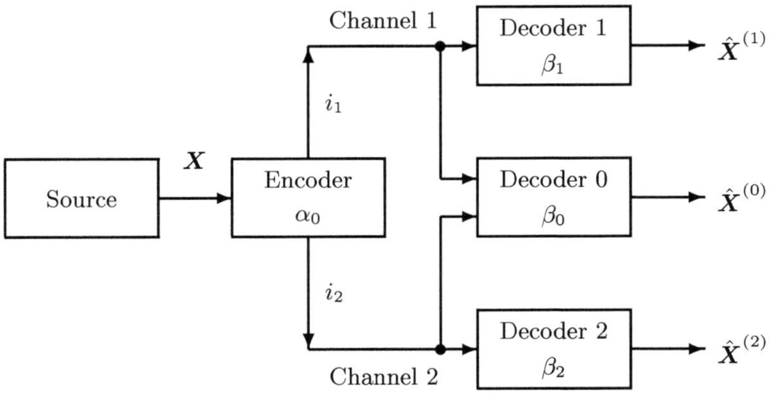

Fig. 12.1. The generic model for MD source coding with two channels and three receivers. The general case has K channels and $2^K - 1$ receivers.

In addition to making theoretic researches, it is also important to devise practical designs to make MDC applicable with the situation depicted in Fig. 12.1. Practical applications and implementations of MDC emerged in the nineties. Two major categories for MDC applications are:

(i) *quantization based* schemes, such as Multiple Description Scalar Quantization (MDSQ) [27] and Multiple Description Vector Quantization (MDVQ) [28], and
(ii) *transform-domain based* schemes, called Multiple Description Transform Coding (MDTC) [29, 30].

In this chapter, we focus on quantization based MD schemes for watermarking. Operations and realizations of quantization-based MDC will be described in Sec. 12.3. The idea for watermarking with MDTC is basically the same as that with MDVQ. However, even though watermarking with MDTC has the same design as MDVQ conceptually, the design and implementation of algorithm needs to be done by other means. These will not be addressed here. We will concentrate in watermarking with quantization-based MDC.

12.3 Quantization Based Multiple Description Coding

Applications of MDC focus on error concealment and error resilience. In this chapter, we introduce an idea of how to apply MDC with watermarking schemes to cover both the reconstructed image quality after reception, and the ownership of the original image.

Fig. 12.1 is the generic structure of MDC, which can also be applied to quantization based multiple-description (MD). Taking scalar quantization for example because MDSQ is the first practical design of MDC, employing different quantization levels into the MD structure is a straightforward solution. Also, MDSQ is flexible in that it allows a designer to choose the relative importance of the central distortion and each side distortion. The basic structure for MDSQ with two descriptions is illustrated in Fig. 12.2. The input $\boldsymbol{X}$ is first quantized into a scalar i, using the scalar quantization function α. Then, the encoder produces from each scalar sample i a pair of quantization indices (i_1, i_2). This step is called "index assignment." In [27], the author described in detail how to perform quantization using an invertible function, and introduced a convenient way to visualize the encoding operation. The way in which to turn the scalar sample into the indices by carrying out the index assignment process was also developed. The encoding is first decomposed into two steps:

$$\alpha_0 = l \circ \alpha. \tag{12.1}$$

The initial encoder α is a regular scalar quantizer. That is, it partitions the real line into cells that are each intervals. The index assignment l uses the index produced by the ordinary quantizer α, and the resulting encoder α_0 to produce the pair of indices (i_1, i_2). After transmission of the indices over different channels with mutually independent breakdown probabilities p_1 and p_2, the three decoders produce estimates from received indices. That is, $(\hat{i}_1, \hat{i}_2)$ for Decoder 0, $\hat{i}_1$ for Decoder 1, and $\hat{i}_2$ for Decoder 2, respectively. The index assignment must be invertible. That is necessary in order for the central decoder to recover the output of α. The visualization technique is to write l^{-1}, forming the index assignment matrix. Therefore, the β_1 and β_2 decoder mappings are indicated by the row and column positions in the MDSQ index assignment in Fig. 12.3. The action of β_0 is implicit. By performing the inverse quantization process, the output of the central decoder which is the reconstructed sample $\hat{\boldsymbol{X}}^{(0)}$ has a low central distortion. The side decoders output the reconstructions $\hat{\boldsymbol{X}}^{(1)}$ and $\hat{\boldsymbol{X}}^{(2)}$ with somewhat higher side distortions.

Fig. 12.3 gives a simple example of MDSQ to help visualize the encoding operation in the *index assignment* portion of Fig. 12.2. This has a codebook size $L = 8$. In designing an MD scalar quantizer, one can optimize α_0, β_0, β_1, and β_2 quite easily as in Fig. 12.2. The optimization of the index assignment l is very difficult. Instead of addressing the exact optimal index assignment problem, in [27], the author gave several heuristic techniques, for example, the nested index assignment, that had an output close to the best possible performance. The dimension of the matrix is denoted by K. It equals the number of descriptions, or the number of channels available for transmission in Fig. 12.1. We will set $K = 2$ in this chapter. Thus, for $K = 2$, the descriptions of the MDSQ can be interpreted as the row and column indices of a matrix, where the codewords, or respectively, their indices, are placed. The basic ideas

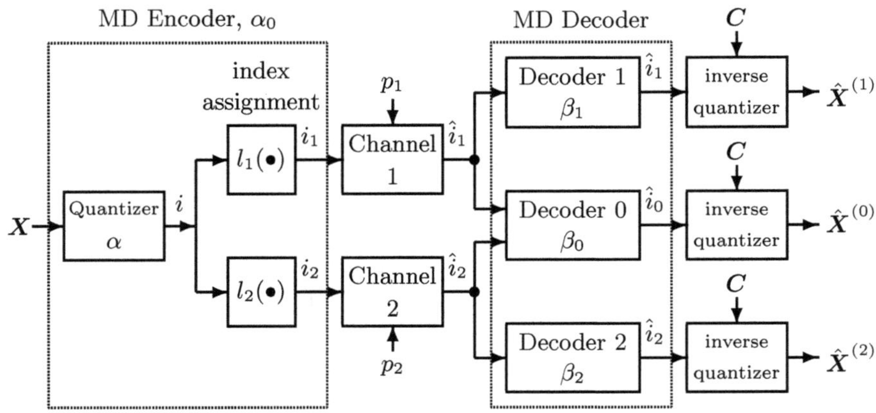

Fig. 12.2. The structure for MDSQ for two descriptions over two independent channels with mutually independent breakdown probabilities.

are to number the index assignment matrix from upper-left corner to lower-right corner and to fill in from the main diagonal outward. In [27], the author considered a set of index pairs constructed from those that lie on the main diagonal and on the $2k$ diagonals closest to the main diagonal. The parameter k is called *spread.* The index assignment shown in Fig. 12.3 is called the "Nested Index Assignment," where the row and column indices, i_1, and i_2, are transmitted over two independent channels.

The cells of the encoder α, are used in increasing values of i, and are numbered from j_0 to j_7 in Fig. 12.3(a), and j_0 to j_{21} in Fig. 12.3(b), respectively. Fig. 12.3(a) is an index assignment scheme with a spread of $k = 0$. Only eight samples, or $j_0, j_1, \cdots, j_7$, are the valid scalar samples for transmission. Generally speaking, the eight samples can be represented by 3-bit strings. Thus, if j_3 is the scalar sample to be transmitted, then after the index assignment step l, we obtain $i_1 = 011$ and $i_2 = 011$ represented in their binary forms. The central distortion is the quantization error between the input and the quantized samples. This configuration with a spread of $k = 0$ can be regarded as repetition of samples. It means that a total of 6 bits will be received if no channel breakdown occurs. Consequently, 6 bits need to be transmitted over two different channels to describe 3 bits information. It produces a redundancy of $\left(\frac{6-3}{3}\right) \times 100\% = 100\%$. In decoding the received descriptions, if both channels are alive, then by calculating the conditional expectation, and as depicted in [27], the reconstructed image decoded from both descriptions can be obtained. The conditional probabilities for receiving both descriptions in Fig. 12.3(a) are:

$$p\left(j_t \mid i_1 = 011,\ i_2 = 011\right) = \begin{cases} 1, & \text{if } t = 3; \\ 0, & \text{otherwise.} \end{cases} \tag{12.2}$$

i_1 \ i_2	000	001	010	011	100	101	110	111
000	j_0							
001		j_1						
010			j_2					
011				j_3				
100					j_4			
101						j_5		
110							j_6	
111								j_7

(a)

i_1 \ i_2	000	001	010	011	100	101	110	111
000	j_0	j_1						
001	j_2	j_3	j_4					
010		j_5	j_6	j_7				
011			j_8	j_9	j_{10}			
100				j_{11}	j_{12}	j_{13}		
101					j_{14}	j_{15}	j_{16}	
110						j_{17}	j_{18}	j_{19}
111							j_{20}	j_{21}

(b)

Fig. 12.3. The illustrations of the nested index assignment in MDSQ for two channels with the codebook size $L = 8$. (a) With spread $k = 0$. (b) With spread $k = 1$.

Because the conditional probability for transmitting j_3 is 1 given the received conditions, we determine that the transmitted index is j_3. If one of the channels breaks down, say, Channel 1, only $i_2 = 011$ is received. Using Fig. 12.3(a) and calculating the conditional probability at the decoder as indicated in Eq. (12.2), we visualize the column containing '011.' We can then determine that the transmitted scalar is j_3 with probability 1. This is the same as when both descriptions are received. In this circumstance, the central distortion is the same as the side distortion at a cost of 100% redundancy when the spread $k = 0$ in MDSQ.

Fig. 12.3(b) is an index assignment scheme with a spread of $k = 1$. There are only 22 samples, or $j_0, j_1, \cdots, j_{21}$, which are the valid scalar samples for transmission. It shows that the quality of side reconstructions needs to be represented by the small ranges of values in any row or any column depending on the received description from any one channel. An index assignment matrix with a higher fraction of occupied cells leads to a quantizer pair with lower redundancy. From theoretical point of view, the 22 samples can be represented by $\log_2(22)$-bit strings. If j_7 is the scalar sample to be transmitted in Fig. 12.3(b), then after the index assignment step l, we obtain $i_1 = 010$ and $i_2 = 011$. By doing this and when both descriptions are received, the transmitted sample j_7 is determined with probability 1 with Fig. 12.3(b). That is,

$$p\left(j_t \mid i_1 = 010,\ i_2 = 011\right) = \begin{cases} 1, & \text{if } t = 7; \\ 0, & \text{otherwise.} \end{cases} \tag{12.3}$$

and the redundancy is reduced to $\left(\frac{6-\log_2(22)}{\log_2(22)}\right) \times 100\% = 34.55\%$. If one of the channels breaks down, say, Channel 1, then only $i_2 = 011$ is received. With the aid of Fig. 12.3(b), we visualize the column containing '011,' and estimate that there are three possible candidates. These are j_7, j_9, and j_{11}, that may be transmitted with the conditional probabilities:

$$p\left(j_t \mid i_2 = 011\right) = \begin{cases} \frac{1}{3}, & \text{if } t = 7 \text{ or } 9 \text{ or } 11; \\ 0, & \text{otherwise.} \end{cases} \tag{12.4}$$

The side distortion would be larger than the central distortion, because the side distortion is the error between the transmitted j_7 and the conditional expectation in Eq. (12.4), $\frac{1}{3}\left(j_7 + j_9 + j_{11}\right)$. Comparing this to the case when $k = 0$, the redundancy is greatly reduced, while the side distortion gets somewhat increased.

It is a straightforward task to extend MDSQ to MDVQ. The index assignment of MDVQ becomes more difficult than MDSQ. Fig. 12.4 demonstrates that the MDVQ structure with two descriptions. Here, the input $\boldsymbol{X}_k$ denotes the small block or code vector. For example, the 4×4 block for VQ operation. The reconstruction $\hat{\boldsymbol{X}}_k^{(0)}$ from the central decoder has less distortion than that from each of the side decoder, $\hat{\boldsymbol{X}}_k^{(1)}$ or $\hat{\boldsymbol{X}}_k^{(2)}$. In this chapter, we follow the MDSQ in [27] and MDVQ algorithm in [28], and devise a robust multi-watermarking algorithm suitable for both error resilient transmission and copyright protection.

12.4 The MDC-Based Single Watermarking Algorithm

The algorithm for single-watermark embedding and extraction with MDC is described as follows.

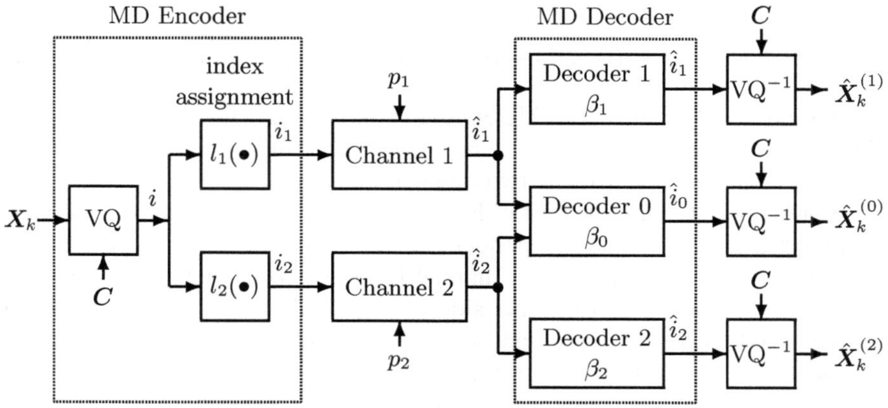

Fig. 12.4. The structure for MDVQ for two descriptions over two independent channels with mutually independent breakdown probabilities.

12.4.1 The Single Watermark Embedding Algorithm

We demonstrate the structure of our single watermarking system with MDVQ in Fig. 12.5, by introducing the watermark embedding and extraction components into Fig. 12.4 [18]. We modify the MDVQ algorithm and the index assignment process in [27] and [28] for watermark embedding. Our watermarking structure can be divided into three parts:

(i) MD encoder with watermark embedding,
(ii) multiple channels or lossy networks for transmission,
(iii) MD decoder with watermark extraction.

Our goal is to focus on using MDVQ and to incorporate with robust watermarking techniques. Our scheme provides both the error-resilient transmission of a watermarked image over different channels having independent breakdown probabilities, and the capability for copyright protection.

Let the input image be $\boldsymbol{X}$ with size $M \times N$. In the left part of Fig. 12.5, we perform the VQ operation first [16] to train the codebook for $\boldsymbol{X}$. We obtain the codebook with length L, $\boldsymbol{C} = \{c_0, c_1, \cdots, c_{L-1}\}$. Each index in $\boldsymbol{C}$ is represented by a $\lceil \log_2 L \rceil$-bit binary string, where $\lceil \bullet \rceil$ denotes a ceiling function. $\boldsymbol{X}$ is divided into non-overlapping blocks $\boldsymbol{X}_k$ with a size $\frac{M}{M_W} \times \frac{N}{N_W}$, $0 \le k \le M_W \cdot N_W - 1$. Each $\boldsymbol{X}_k$ finds its nearest codeword c_i in the codebook $\boldsymbol{C}$, and the index i is assigned to $\boldsymbol{X}_k$.

Let the watermark for embedding be $\boldsymbol{W} = \{W_0, W_1, \cdots W_{M_W \cdot N_W - 1}\}$, with a size $M_W \times N_W$. Each element in $\boldsymbol{W}$, $W_k \in \{0,\ 1\}$, $k \in [0, M_W \cdot N_W - 1]$, represents one watermark bit to be embedded into the corresponding index of $\boldsymbol{X}_k$. For watermarking purposes, the new index representing $\boldsymbol{X}_k$ is generated from two parts: This is done to shift the original index i to the left by one bit, and to tag watermark bit to the end of the shifted index. That is,

$$i_W = (i \ll 1) + W_k, \quad k \in [0, M_W \cdot N_W - 1] . \tag{12.5}$$

We next make use of the MDSQ algorithms in [27] for index assignment. The index assignments in Fig. 12.5, $i_1 = l_1(i_W)$ and $i_2 = l_2(i_W)$, map the quantizer output index to the two descriptions i_1 and i_2.

Referring to the middle part of Fig. 12.5, i_1 and i_2 are transmitted over two memoryless and mutually independent channels, or the lossy packet networks, with erasure probabilities p_1 for Channel 1, and for p_2 Channel 2, respectively.

Finally, referring to the right side of Fig. 12.5, both of the transmitted indices need to be reconstructed, and the embedded watermark needs to be extracted. At the MD decoder, it first shifts received binary indices i'_1 and i'_2 to the right by one bit to smooth away the effects from watermark embedding. It determines the outcome i' from the received indices with the MDSQ decoder. Next, it does a table look-up process on the determined i' using the codebook $\boldsymbol{C}$ to obtain c'_i and then to obtain the reconstructed block $\boldsymbol{X}'_k$. After gathering all the blocks, the reconstruction image $\boldsymbol{X}'$ is obtain.

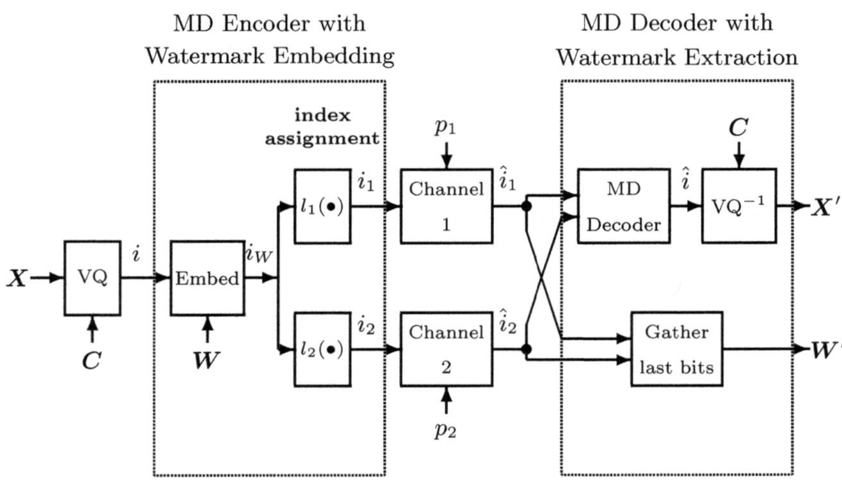

Fig. 12.5. The structure for embedding one watermark with two descriptions for transmission in MDC. The two independent channels have mutually independent breakdown probabilities.

12.4.2 The Single Watermark Extraction Algorithm

In watermark extraction, we do the estimation criterion from received indices for determining the value of the watermark bits. With MDC, if both descriptions for one block $\boldsymbol{X}_k$ are received, then the resulting index decoded by MDSQ can be uniquely determined, and the watermark bit is extracted by taking out the last bit. Because of the error concealment capability for index assignment, when only one description is received, the block can be partly reconstructed, and the watermark bit needs to be determined from several possible indices assigned in the MDSQ row or column matrix [27]. We first use a majority vote to determine the watermark bit '0' or '1'. If there are equal numbers of 0's and 1's obtained in MDSQ decoding process, we assign the watermark bit randomly. If none of the description is received, the watermark bit is randomly assigned. By gathering all the extracted watermark bits W'_k, we obtain the extracted watermark $\boldsymbol{W}'$.

12.5 The MDC-Based Multiple Watermarking Algorithm

The multiple watermarking algorithm is derived and implemented based on the single watermarking algorithm described in Sec. 12.4.

12.5.1 The Multiple Watermarks Embedding Algorithm

We propose our watermarking algorithm for embedding two watermarks with VQ and MDC in this section. The structure for our proposed watermarking system is demonstrated in Fig. 12.6. It is an extension to Fig. 12.5. That is, the multiple watermarks embedding algorithm is based on the single watermark embedding algorithm. Our goal is to focus on using MDVQ to incorporate with robust watermarking techniques to provide both an error-resilient transmission of watermarked image over different channels with independent breakdown probabilities, and to provide ownership protection.

Similar to the notations used in Sec. 12.4.1, let the input image be $\boldsymbol{X}$ with a size $M \times N$. VQ operation is performed [16] and the codebook has a length L, $\boldsymbol{C} = \{c_0, c_1, \cdots, c_{L-1}\}$ is obtained. $\boldsymbol{X}$ is divided into non-overlapping blocks $\boldsymbol{X}_k$ with a size $\frac{M}{M_W} \times \frac{N}{N_W}$, $0 \leq k \leq M_W \cdot N_W - 1$. Each $\boldsymbol{X}_k$ finds its nearest codeword c_i in the codebook $\boldsymbol{C}$, and the index i is assigned to $\boldsymbol{X}_k$. Let the watermarks for embedding be $\boldsymbol{W}_1 = \{W_{1,0}, W_{1,1}, \cdots W_{1,M_W \cdot N_W - 1}\}$ and $\boldsymbol{W}_2 = \{W_{2,0}, W_{2,1}, \cdots W_{2,M_W \cdot N_W - 1}\}$, both having sizes $M_W \times N_W$. Each element in $\boldsymbol{W}_1$ and $\boldsymbol{W}_2$ represents one watermark bit to be embedded into $\boldsymbol{X}_k$. Embedding of the two watermarks will now be described.

Embedding the First Watermark

When embedding the first watermark $\boldsymbol{W}_1$, we split $\boldsymbol{C}$ into two sub-codebooks $\boldsymbol{C}' = \left\{c'_0, c'_1, \cdots c'_{\frac{L}{2}-1}\right\}$ and $\boldsymbol{C}'' = \left\{c''_0, c''_1, \cdots c''_{\frac{L}{2}-1}\right\}$. This is known as the "codeword selection" portion in Fig. 12.6. We can see that $\boldsymbol{C}' \bigcup \boldsymbol{C}'' = \boldsymbol{C}$ and

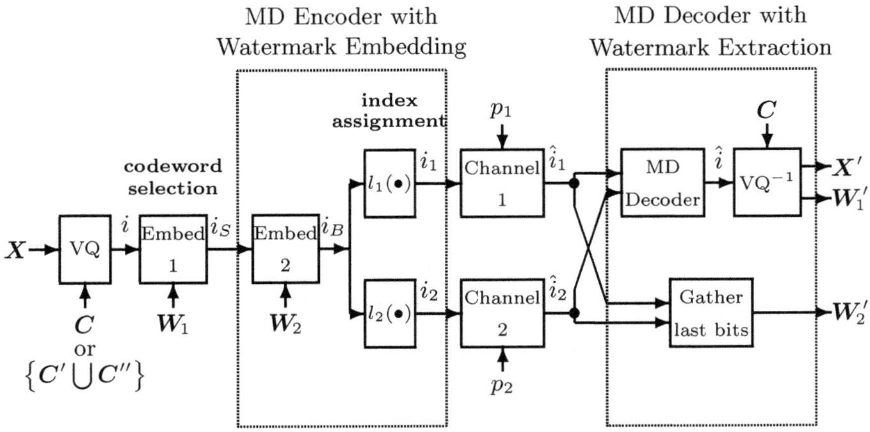

Fig. 12.6. The structure for embedding two watermarks with two descriptions for transmission in MDC. The two independent channels have mutually independent breakdown probabilities.

$\boldsymbol{C}' \bigcap \boldsymbol{C}'' = \emptyset$. We employ tabu search to split $\boldsymbol{C}$ into $\boldsymbol{C}'$ and $\boldsymbol{C}''$, and will search for the tradeoff between watermark imperceptibility and watermark robustness, in Sec. 12.7. For one index in $\boldsymbol{C}'$, there is a one-to-one corresponding counterpart, with the same subscript, in $\boldsymbol{C}''$. For example, let c_t' denote the index for the current block $\boldsymbol{X}_k$, $t \in \left[0, \frac{L}{2} - 1\right]$. When embedding the first watermark, the output index i_S, which denotes the index containing ***Single*** watermark for representing $\boldsymbol{X}_k$, is generated according to the value of the watermark bit $W_{1,k}$:

$$i_S = \begin{cases} c_t', \text{ if } W_{1,k} = 0; \\ c_t'', \text{ if } W_{1,k} = 1; \end{cases} \quad t \in \left[0, \frac{L}{2} - 1\right], \ k \in [0, M_W \cdot N_W - 1]. \quad (12.6)$$

Then, i_S is fed into the MD encoder in Fig. 12.6 to embed the second watermark.

Embedding the Second Watermark

We employ the watermarking algorithm in Sec. 12.4 for embedding the second watermark. It contains two parts. The first is to shift the watermarked index i_S to the left by one bit, and the second is to tag watermark bit $W_{2,k}$ to the end of the shifted index. That is,

$$i_B = (i_S \ll 1) + W_{2,k}, \quad k \in [0, M_W \cdot N_W - 1], \quad (12.7)$$

where i_B denotes the index containing ***Both*** watermarks. This step is the same as that in Eq. (12.5). Next, we make use of the MDSQ algorithms in Fig. 12.3(b) for index assignment. The index assignments in Fig. 12.6, are

$i_1 = l_1(i_B)$ and $i_2 = l_2(i_B)$. They map the quantizer output index i_B to the two descriptions i_1 and i_2.

After completing the embedding of $W_{1,k}$ and $W_{2,k}$ in $\boldsymbol{X}_k$, i_1 and i_2 are transmitted over two memoryless and mutually independent channels with erasure probabilities p_1 for Channel 1, and p_2 for Channel 2, respectively. This procedure finishes when all the blocks $\boldsymbol{X}_k$, $k \in [0, M_W \cdot N_W - 1]$, are processed and the relating indices are transmitted.

12.5.2 The Multiple Watermarks Extraction Algorithm

Corresponding to the watermark embedding algorithm, we describe the schemes used for extracting the two embedded watermarks. It is an inverse procedure to the multiple-watermark embedding process. We first extract the second embedded watermark, then the first embedded one.

Extracting the Second Watermark and Obtaining the Watermarked Reconstruction Containing $\boldsymbol{W}_1$

At the decoder side in Fig. 12.6, the first step is to determine the outcome i'_B from the received indices i'_1 and i'_2 with the MDSQ decoder by doing the inverse of the index assignment process, l^{-1}. Then, i'_B is shifted to the right by one bit to smooth away the effects of watermark embedding,

$$i'_S = (i'_B \gg 1)\,. \tag{12.8}$$

It next does a table look-up process on i'_S to obtain the codeword $\tilde{c}_i$, $0 \le i \le L-1$. Then we find the block $\boldsymbol{X}'_k$ that contains the watermark bit $W_{1,k}$. By gathering all the blocks $\boldsymbol{X}'_k$, $0 \le k \le M_W \cdot N_W - 1$, we obtain the watermarked reconstruction $\boldsymbol{X}'$, which contains the watermark $\boldsymbol{W}_1$.

When extracting $\boldsymbol{W}_2$, we do the estimation using the received indices to determine the value of the watermark bits by using

$$W'_{2,k} = i'_B \bmod 2, \quad k \in [0, M_W \cdot N_W - 1]\,, \tag{12.9}$$

where "mod" denotes the modulus operation. Fig. 12.7 is a demonstration of how $W'_{2,k}$ is extracted. From Fig. 12.7, and by calculating the conditional probabilities with two descriptions in MDC, one of the following conditions will be satisfied.

(1) If both descriptions for one block $\boldsymbol{X}_k$ are received, then the resulting index decoded by using MDSQ can be then determined uniquely as shown in Fig. 12.7. By visualizing the intersection between the row of the received i_1, and the column of the received i_2. The estimated watermark bit $W'_{2,k}$ is extracted by taking out the last bit from i'_B using Eq. (12.9).

(2) Because of the error concealment capability for index assignment in MDSQ, when only one description is received, the block can be partly reconstructed. The watermark bit needs to be determined from several possible indices assigned in MDSQ row or column matrix [27].
   a) If Channel 1 breaks down, then i_2 will be received. By visualizing Fig. 12.7, we choose the column containing i_2 and infer that the transmitted description should be one of the several possible indices on the column. We use a majority vote to estimate the watermark bit $W'_{2,k}$ by checking whether the subscripts of the possible indices are odd or even. If there are more odd indices, we set $W'_{2,k} = 1$. Otherwise, we set $W'_{2,k} = 0$ with the modulus operation in Eq. (12.9). After checking, if there are equal numbers of 0's and 1's in the MDSQ matrix in Fig. 12.7, we randomly assign the watermark bit. On the other hand, we calculate the conditional expectation from the possible indices, and produce the reconstructed block $\boldsymbol{X}'_k$.
   b) If Channel 2 breaks down, then i_1 will be received. By visualizing Fig. 12.7, we choose the row containing i_2 and infer that the transmitted description should be one of the several possible indices on the row. With the same procedures in the previous case, we can obtain the extracted watermark bit $W'_{2,k}$ and the reconstructed block $\boldsymbol{X}'_k$.

(3) If no description is received, the value of watermark bit $W'_{2,k}$ is randomly assigned. With no received information, the block $\boldsymbol{X}'_k$ cannot be reconstructed, and the luminance of that block is set to 128 for the 8-bit per pixel grey level images.

By gathering all the extracted watermark bits $W'_{2,k}$, we obtain the extracted watermark $\boldsymbol{W}'_2$. By gathering all the reconstructed blocks $\boldsymbol{X}'_k$, we obtain the reconstructed image $\boldsymbol{X}'$ which contains the first watermark. We proceed with watermark extraction as shown in Sec. 12.5.2 in order to extract the first watermark embedded from the received descriptions.

Extracting the First Watermark

After obtaining the codeword i'_S in Sec. 12.5.2, we are prepared to extract $\boldsymbol{W}_1$. Assuming that $i'_S = \tilde{c}_i$. We examine whether the codeword $\tilde{c}_i$ belongs to the sub-codebook $\boldsymbol{C}'$ or $\boldsymbol{C}''$, and the extract watermark bit $W'_{1,k}$. This can be estimated with Eq. (12.10), which is an inverse operation of Eq. (12.6):

$$W'_{1,k} = \begin{cases} 0, \text{ if } \tilde{c}_i \in \boldsymbol{C}'; \\ 1, \text{ if } \tilde{c}_i \in \boldsymbol{C}''; \end{cases} \quad i \in [0, L-1]\,, \; k \in [0, M_W \cdot N_W - 1]\,. \tag{12.10}$$

By gathering all the extracted watermark bits $W'_{1,k}$, we obtain an estimate of the first embedded watermark $\boldsymbol{W}'_1$.

i_1 \ i_2	0000	0001	0010	0011	0100	0101	0110	0111	1000	1001	1010	1011	1100	1101	1110	1111
0000	j_0	j_1														
0001	j_2	j_3	j_4													
0010		j_5	j_6	j_7												
0011			j_8	j_9	j_{10}											
0100				j_{11}	j_{12}	j_{13}										
0101					j_{14}	j_{15}	j_{16}									
0110						j_{17}	j_{18}	j_{19}								
0111							j_{20}	j_{21}	j_{22}							
1000								j_{23}	j_{24}	j_{25}						
1001									j_{26}	j_{27}	j_{28}					
1010										j_{29}	j_{30}	j_{31}				
1011											j_{32}	j_{33}	j_{34}			
1100												j_{35}	j_{36}	j_{37}		
1101													j_{38}	j_{39}	j_{40}	
1110														j_{41}	j_{42}	j_{43}
1111															j_{44}	j_{45}

Fig. 12.7. An example of the combination of MDC and watermarking, an extension to Fig. 12.3(b).

12.6 An Example for Watermarking with MDC

Fig. 12.7 is the example that follows Fig. 12.3(b). Here the codebook size is $L = 8$, and each codeword is 3-bit in length. Consequently, when using the watermarking scheme in Eq. (12.7), Fig. 12.7 is a direct extension of Fig. 12.3(b). This is because each watermarked codeword is 4-bit in length. The codebook with length $2^4 = 2L = 16$ is trained in advance to deal with watermark embedding. From another perspective, for watermarking purposes, the effective length of the codebook for reconstructing the compressed image is halved. The watermarked image quality with MDC is somewhat degraded.

The original image $\boldsymbol{X}$ employed has size 512×512. The two watermarks, $\boldsymbol{W}_1$ and $\boldsymbol{W}_2$, both have sizes 128×128. In VQ encoding, the original image is divided into 4×4 blocks $\boldsymbol{X}_k$, and each block is represented by one codeword

c_i, where $i \in [0, L-1]$. For watermarking, two bits can be embedded into one block, one from $\boldsymbol{W}_1$ and the other from $\boldsymbol{W}_2$.

Assuming that $W_{1,k} = 0$ and $W_{2,k} = 1$ are the two watermark bits to be embedded into $\boldsymbol{X}_k$. With the algorithm given in Sec. 12.5.1 and Eq. (12.6), and after searching for the nearest codeword in $\boldsymbol{C}'$, we conclude that the resulting codeword containing the first watermark is $i_S = 101$. According to Eq. (12.7), we embed the second watermark and obtain $i_B = 1011$. Because the binary form of 1011 has a decimal form of 19, we conclude that j_{19} is the codeword to be transmitted in Fig 12.6. Referring to Fig. 12.7, the two descriptions for transmission are $i_1 = 0110$ and $i_2 = 0111$.

In extracting the watermark, for both descriptions, or $K = 2$ in Fig. 12.1, there will be four possible cases that can occur.

(1) If both descriptions are received, then both $i_1 = 0110$ and $i_2 = 0111$ can be used for extracting the watermark bit $W_{2,k}$ and reconstructing the image. By performing the inverse operation of index assignment l^{-1} in Eq. (12.1) and computing the conditional probability, we can exactly determine that the codeword j_{19} is transmitted with probability 1, thus, the watermark bit is $W_{2,k} = 1$. In reconstructing the block from the received descriptions, we use the look-up table, and determine $\hat{\boldsymbol{X}}^{(0)} = j_{19}$. We employ the spatial domain representations of j_{19} to represent the reconstructed block $\boldsymbol{X}'_k$.

(2) If Channel 1 breaks down, then only $i_2 = 0111$ is received. By performing the inverse operation of index assignment l^{-1}, we find that j_{19}, j_{21}, and j_{23} are the three possible candidates transmitted. Because 19, 21, and 23 are odd numbers, and by using a majority vote, the embedded bit can be estimated to be $W_{2,k} = 1$. In reconstructing the received image, we need to calculate the conditional probability using the given conditions:

$$p\left(j_t \mid i_2 = 0111\right) = \begin{cases} \frac{1}{3}, & \text{if } t = 19 \text{ or } 21 \text{ or } 23; \\ 0, & \text{otherwise.} \end{cases} \tag{12.11}$$

Thus, with Eq. (12.11), the reconstructed vector is the conditional expectation $\hat{\boldsymbol{X}}^{(2)} = \frac{1}{3}\left(j_{19} + j_{21} + j_{23}\right)$. We use the spatial domain representations of j_{19}, j_{21}, and j_{23} to calculate their average to complete the reconstruction of $\hat{\boldsymbol{X}}^{(2)}$.

(3) If Channel 2 breaks down, then only $i_1 = 0110$ is received. By doing the inverse operation of index assignment, we find that j_{17}, j_{18}, and j_{19} are the three possible candidates transmitted. Using a majority vote, the embedded bit can be estimated to be $W_{2,k} = 1$. In some situations where there are two candidates, we use random selection to determine the watermark bit. In reconstructing the received image, we need to calculate the conditional probability at the given conditions:

$$p\left(j_t \mid i_1 = 0110\right) = \begin{cases} \frac{1}{3}, & \text{if } t = 17 \text{ or } 18 \text{ or } 19; \\ 0, & \text{otherwise.} \end{cases} \tag{12.12}$$

Thus, with Eq. (12.11), the reconstructed vector is the conditional expectation $\hat{\boldsymbol{X}}^{(1)} = \frac{1}{3}(j_{17} + j_{18} + j_{19})$.

(4) If both channels break down, no description is received. We randomly choose '0' or '1' to represent the embedded watermark bit $W_{2,k}$. Also, because no description is received, nothing can be reconstructed, hence we set the luminance of that block to 128 for the 8-bit per pixel grey level images.

12.7 Optimization with Tabu Search

12.7.1 Tabu Search Fundamentals

Tabu search is the meta-heuristic approach, or a kind of iterative search, and is characterized by the use of a flexible memory. It is able to eliminate local minima and to search areas beyond a local minimum [12, 13].

The process with which tabu search overcomes the local optima problem is based on an evaluation function that chooses the highest evaluation solution at each iteration. The building blocks of tabu search are stated as follows.

Forbidding strategy: This strategy is employed to avoid cycling problems by forbidding certain moves or classifying them as forbidden, or *tabu*. To prevent the cycling problem, it is sufficient to check whether a previously visited solution is revisited or not. An alternative way might be by not visiting the solutions already visited during the last T_S iterations. T_S is normally named the *tabu list length* or *tabu list size*. With the help of an appropriate value of T_S, the likelihood of cycling effectively vanishes.

Aspiration criteria and tabu restrictions: An aspiration criterion is applied to make a tabu solution which is not a forbidden state. That is if this solution is of sufficient quality and is is able to prevent cycling. A solution is acceptable if the tabu restrictions are satisfied. However, a tabu solution is also assumed acceptable if an aspiration criterion applies regardless of the tabu status. We also make use of tabu restrictions to avoid repetitions but not reversals. A tabu restriction is typically activated only when its attributes occur within a limited number of iterations prior to the present iteration. Or they have occurred with a certain frequency over a larger number of iterations. Finally, the appropriate use of aspiration criteria can be very significant for enabling a tabu search to achieve its best performance.

Freeing strategy: The freeing strategy is taken into account in order to decide what can exit the tabu list. This strategy removes tabu restrictions of the solutions so that they can be reconsidered in further steps of the search. The attributes of a tabu solution remain on the tabu list for a duration of T_S iterations.

Intermediate and long-term learning strategies: These strategies are implemented with intermediate and long-term memory functions. Their operations are to record good features of a selected number of moves generated during the execution of the algorithm.

Short-term strategy or overall strategy: This strategy manages the interplay between the different strategies listed above. A candidate list is a sub-list of the possible moves which are generally problem dependent.

The best-solution strategy: This strategy selects an admissible solution from the current solutions if it yields the greatest improvement or the least distortion in the cost function. This is provided that the tabu restrictions and aspiration criterion are satisfied.

Termination: A stopping criterion terminates the tabu search procedure either after a specified number of iterations has been performed, or the currently best solution has shown no improvement for a given number of iterations.

Using the background information presented in this section, we are able to apply the tabu search algorithm to digital watermarking.

12.7.2 Multiple Watermarking with Tabu Search

When embedding multiple watermarks with MDC in Sec. 12.5.1, the main problem for embedding the first watermark is how to split the codebook $\boldsymbol{C}$ into two sub-codebooks $\boldsymbol{C}'$ and $\boldsymbol{C}''$. The result for splitting $\boldsymbol{C}$ will not only influence the watermark imperceptibility and the robustness of the first watermark, but it will also effect the robustness of the second watermark. All the problems can be optimized using tabu search [12] by offering the reasonable fitness function. Using the fundamentals of tabu search described in Sec. 12.7.1, and the watermarking requirements depicted in Sec. 12.1, we can consider both the imperceptibility of the watermarked image, represented by Peak Signal-to-Noise Ratio (PSNR), and the robustness of the extracted watermarks, represented by Bit Correct Rates (BCR), for optimization. The fitness function with this system is:

$$f_i = \mathrm{PSNR}_i + \lambda_1 \cdot \mathrm{BCR}_{1,i} + \lambda_2 \cdot \mathrm{BCR}_{2,i} \tag{12.13}$$

where f_i denotes the fitness score in the i-th iteration, PSNR_i, $\mathrm{BCR}_{1,i}$ and $\mathrm{BCR}_{2,i}$ denote Peak Signal-to-Noise Ratio (PSNR) and Bit Correct Rates (BCR), respectively. Because the PSNR values are generally many times larger than the BCR values, we include λ_1 and λ_2 to represent the weighting factors to balance the effects of PSNR and BCR. The objective is to maximize

f_i in our system. The PSNR in the i-th iteration between the original and watermarked images can be represented by

$$\text{PSNR}_i = 10 \cdot \log_{10} \left(\frac{255^2}{\frac{1}{M \cdot N} \sum_{m=0}^{M-1} \sum_{n=0}^{N-1} \left(X(m,n) - X_i'(m,n) \right)^2} \right) \quad (12.14)$$

where $X(m,n)$ and $X_i'(m,n)$ denote the pixel values at position (m,n) of the original image $\boldsymbol{X}$ and watermarked image $\boldsymbol{X}_i'$ in the i-th iteration, where $M \cdot N$ denotes the image size. The BCR between the embedded and extracted watermarks can be defined by

$$\text{BCR}_i = \left(\frac{1}{M_W \cdot N_W} \sum_{b=0}^{M_W \cdot N_W - 1} \overline{\left(w_{b,i} \oplus w_{b,i}' \right)} \right) \cdot 100\% \quad (12.15)$$

where $w_{b,i}$ and $w_{b,i}'$ represent the embedded watermark bit and the extracted one in the i-th iteration, $M_W \cdot N_W$ denotes the watermark size, $\oplus$ indicates the "exclusive-or operation," and the line above the exclusive-or operation means the "not" operation in logic design.

Given the preliminaries in Sec. 12.1, by fixing the watermark capacity, both the watermark imperceptibility and watermark robustness can be improved after tabu search optimization. Parameters employed in the tabu search are:

- there are 20 candidate solutions trained for each iteration;
- the tabu list length T_S is set to 10;
- the weighting factors are set to $\lambda_1 = \lambda_2 = 10$;
- the aspiration value is set to 40, with $\text{PSNR}_i \geq 26$, $\text{BCR}_{1,i} \geq 0.7$, and $\text{BCR}_{2,i} \geq 0.7$ in Eq. (12.13);
- watermark embedding and extraction are performed in every training iteration to obtain the updated PSNR_{i+1}, $\text{BCR}_{1,i+1}$, and $\text{BCR}_{2,i+1}$ in the next iteration;
- the number of total training iterations is set to 100.

The above parameters were chosen carefully. In this chapter, we choose 20 candidates for training with tabu search. After considering the computation time, the memory consumption, and the convergence rate in tabu search, we choose 20 candidates for each training iteration based on the fitness function. If we choose too many candidates, the computation time per iteration will be increased, and memory allocation might become a problem. In contrast, if we choose too few candidates, the output result might be a locally optimal one, which is generally encountered in the optimization problems. Therefore, in this chapter, we have 20 candidates to be a reasonable number for training with tabu search.

Moreover, we set the tabu list length $T_S = 10$ by considering the tradeoff between the computation time and the convergence rate in the optimization process. We can also find that PSNR values are many times larger than the BCR values, hence, the weighting factors, λ_1 and λ_2, need to be included in

Eq. (12.13), the fitness function, in order to balance the effects from the PSNR, representing the image quality, and the BCR, representing the watermark robustness.

12.8 Other Related Watermarking Algorithms

To demonstrate the effectiveness of the proposed algorithm, we compare two VQ-based watermarking algorithms given in the literature. The two watermarking algorithms are described as follows.

(1) **Review of Watermarking Algorithm in [10].**
The algorithm in [10] is one of the pioneering VQ-based watermarking methods proposed in literature. The authors trained the codebook $\boldsymbol{C}$ with length L in advance. Then, $\boldsymbol{C}$ is partitioned into N groups, $\{\boldsymbol{G}_0, \boldsymbol{G}_1, \cdots, \boldsymbol{G}_{N-1}\}$, where
a) $\boldsymbol{C} = \bigcup_{i=0}^{N-1} \boldsymbol{G}_i$;
b) $\bigcap_{i=0}^{N-1} \boldsymbol{G}_i = \emptyset$;
c) $\boldsymbol{G}_i = \{\boldsymbol{c}_0^i, \boldsymbol{c}_1^i\}, \ i \in [0, N-1]$.
For a given input vector $\boldsymbol{X}_k$, we assume that the codeword $\boldsymbol{c}_t^p \in \boldsymbol{G}_p$, $p \in [0, N-1]$, $t \in \{0, 1\}$, is the nearest codeword. To embed the corresponding watermark bit $w \in \{0, 1\}$ in $\boldsymbol{X}_k$, the j-th codeword of $\boldsymbol{G}_p$ is the output as the watermarked vector $\boldsymbol{X}'_k$:

$$j = (t + w) \bmod \|\boldsymbol{G}_p\|, \tag{12.16}$$

$$\boldsymbol{X}'_k = \boldsymbol{c}_j^p, \tag{12.17}$$

where $j \in [0, \|\boldsymbol{G}_p\|]$, and $\|\boldsymbol{G}_p\|$ denotes the number of codewords contained in group $\boldsymbol{G}_p$, and "mod" means the modulus operation. For embedding only one bit into each vector, $\|\boldsymbol{G}_p\| = 2$.
After all of the watermark bits have been embedded into the corresponding vectors, the output vectors are pieced together to form the watermarked image, $\boldsymbol{X}'$. In addition, due to the embedding strategy employed, this method requires the original cover image to be presented during extraction, or otherwise the hidden information cannot be obtained. This is a fatal disadvantage for the practical application of this algorithm.

(2) **Review of Watermarking Algorithm in [11].**
The algorithm described in this sub-section is an improvement on some existing schemes for VQ-based watermarking given in literature [31]. The trained codebook has a length L which is an even number, then $\boldsymbol{C} = \{c_0, c_1, \cdots, c_{L-1}\}$ is employed for vector quantization. In [11], the authors propose a method to partition the codebook according to the watermarking bits '0' or '1' to be embedded. They divide $\boldsymbol{C}$ into the odd-indexed and even-indexed sub-codebooks $\boldsymbol{C}_o$ and $\boldsymbol{C}_e$, with $\boldsymbol{C}_o = \{c_1, c_3, c_5, \cdots, c_{L-1}\}$ and $\boldsymbol{C}_e = \{c_0, c_2, c_4, \cdots, c_{L-2}\}$. Thus, $\boldsymbol{C}_o \cup \boldsymbol{C}_e = \boldsymbol{C}$ and $\boldsymbol{C}_o \cap \boldsymbol{C}_e = \emptyset$.

In embedding the watermark, if the codeword for the current block is $c_k, k \in [0, L-1]$, and if the watermark bit is '0', $\boldsymbol{C}_e$ is adopted for watermark embedding because 0 is an even number, and the nearest codeword in $\boldsymbol{C}_e$ is found to replace the original codeword. If the watermark bit is '1', $\boldsymbol{C}_o$ is used, and the same scheme is applied for embedding watermark bit '1'. Finally, with the codewords in $\boldsymbol{C}_o$ and $\boldsymbol{C}_e$, the watermarked image $\boldsymbol{X}'$ is reconstructed.

In extracting the watermark, the codebook plays an essential role. Suppose that the watermarked image $\boldsymbol{X}'$ is transmitted over the packet loss channel, and the received image is denoted by $\boldsymbol{X}''$. In the receiver side, the same sub-codebooks $\boldsymbol{C}_o$ and $\boldsymbol{C}_e$ are employed to extract the watermark. The authors used table look-up to find the VQ indices of the received image $\boldsymbol{X}''$. For every block in vector quantization, if the index belongs to $\boldsymbol{C}_o$, then the extracted watermark bit is determined to be '0'; if not, the bit is '1'. By gathering all the extracted watermark bits, the extracted watermark $\boldsymbol{W}'$ can be obtained.

12.9 Simulation Results

In our simulations, we take the test image, Lena, with size 512 × 512, as the original source. We have the embedded watermarks with size 128 × 128, shown in Fig. 12.8. For embedding a single watermark, we employ 'watermark 1' only; for embedding multiple watermarks, we employ both the watermarks. The original source is divided into 4 × 4 blocks for VQ compression, which also meets the number of bits required for watermark embedding. The codebook sizes are $L = 512$ and $L = 1024$, and indices therein are represented by 9-bit or 10-bit strings, respectively.

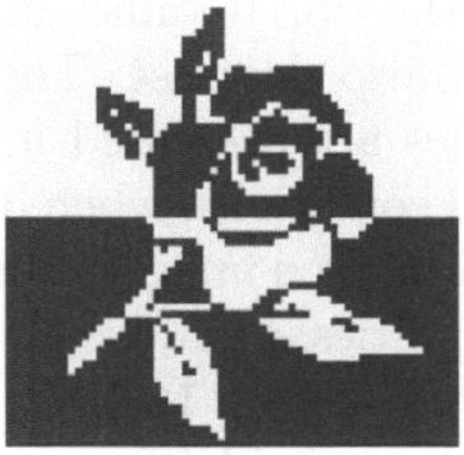

watermark 1

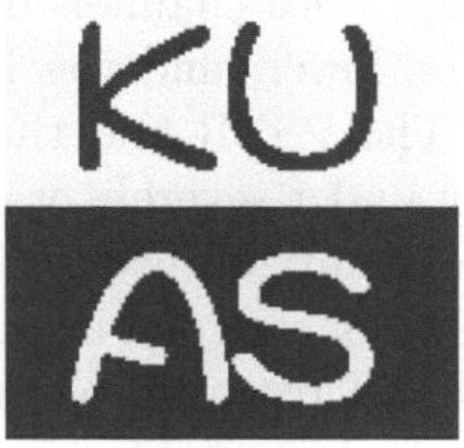

watermark 2

Fig. 12.8. The two watermarks used for embedding in this chapter, both have sizes 128 × 128. Watermark 1 shows a flower, while watermark 2 denotes the characters KUAS, representing the author's affiliation.

Two quantities are considered for evaluating the proposed algorithms. We employ the watermarked image quality as the first metric for evaluation. The watermarked image quality, measured by Peak Signal-to-Noise Ratio (PSNR) between the watermarked image $\boldsymbol{X}'$ and the original $\boldsymbol{X}$ can be calculated using Eq. (12.14). $\boldsymbol{X}'$ is reconstructed from the received descriptions which are transmitted over two mutually independent, erasure channels. The second metric, the Bit Correct Rates (BCR), of the one extracted watermark in Sec. 12.4.2, or the two extracted watermarks in Sec. 12.5.2, are employed to evaluate the robustness of the algorithm. They can be calculated using Eq. (12.15). Generally speaking, the desirable results are to obtain both the higher PSNR value in the watermarked image quality, and the higher BCR values in the extracted watermarks. We also make comparisons with other existing VQ-based watermarking schemes [10, 11] described in Sec. 12.8. Simulations show the practicality and usefulness of our method.

As shown in Figs. 12.5 and 12.6, only the watermarked VQ codewords are transmitted over the noisy channels. Therefore, attacking schemes such as low-pass filtering, or those employed in the Stirmark benchmark [21], are not suitable when applied into our scheme. Therefore, we only use the situations where the descriptions can be transmitted over mutually independent channels.

12.9.1 Results with Single Watermarking

For the single watermarking algorithm in Sec. 12.4.1, simulations with different channel erasure probabilities are now presented. The two memoryless and mutually independent channels for transmitting bitstreams in Fig. 12.5 have different erasure probabilities, p_1 for Channel 1, and p_2 for Channel 2. In Table 12.1, we perform a series of simulations by varying p_1 and p_2 for each transmitted index. Under the no loss condition, $p_1 = p_2 = 0$, and we obtain the watermarked image with PSNR = 32.53 dB, and have an extracted watermark with BCR = 100%. This is identical with that embedded. When p_1 and p_2 increase, both channels deteriorate, the PSNR values of watermarked images become lower, and the BCR values also decrease. This is as shown in Fig. 12.9. The PSNR and the BCR values are presented in detail in Table 12.1. Even under severely erased channel conditions, where $p_1 = p_2 = 0.5$, the subjective quality of reconstructed, watermarked image is acceptable. This is because MDC offers good error resilient abilities. In addition, the extracted watermark is still recognizable. As illustrated in Fig. 12.9(d), it shows that the capability for copyright protection is still retained using our scheme.

In addition, MDC is suitable for coping with severe channel conditions. We simulate the instances where one of the channels is totally broken down. The results are in Fig. 12.10 and Table 12.1. In Fig. 12.10(a), where Channel 1 is broken down, only the bitstreams transmitted over Channel 2 can be received. The extracted watermark is recognizable with a BCR value of 80.55%. The resulting watermarked reconstruction is 26.09 dB with the ability of MDC. In Fig. 12.10(b), Channel 2 is broken down, and the extracted watermark is

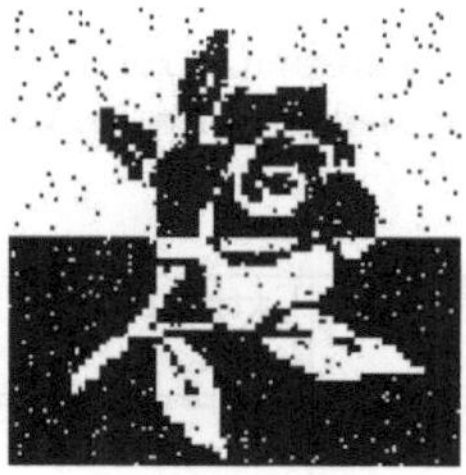

(a)
$p_1 = 0.05$, $p_2 = 0.05$,
BCR = 97.56%

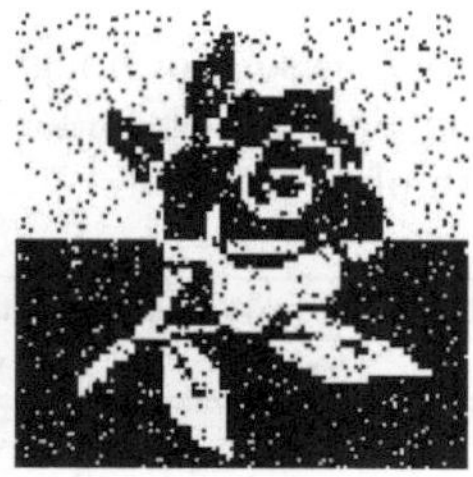

(b)
$p_1 = 0.1$, $p_2 = 0.1$,
BCR = 95.14%

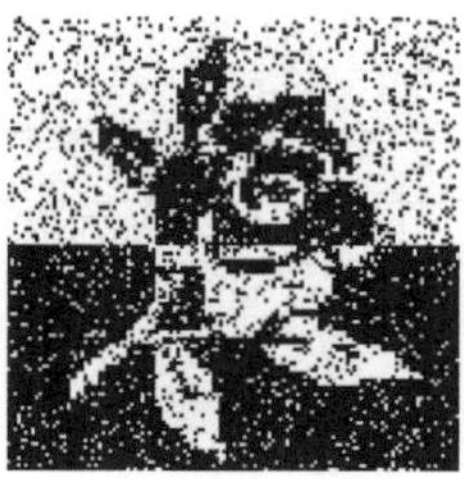

(c)
$p_1 = 0.25$, $p_2 = 0.25$,
BCR = 88.18%

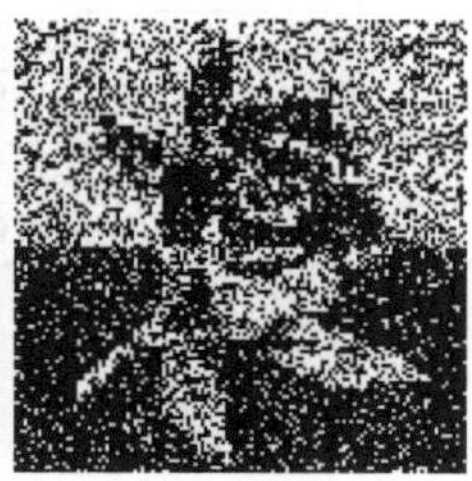

(d)
$p_1 = 0.5$, $p_2 = 0.5$,
BCR = 76.25%

Fig. 12.9. The extracted watermark under different channel erasure probabilities in Sec. 12.4.2, with acodebook size of $L = 512$. The watermark is still recognizable even under these severely erased channels in (d).

recognizable with a BCR value of 73.34%. The resulting watermarked reconstruction is 26.18 dB with MDC.

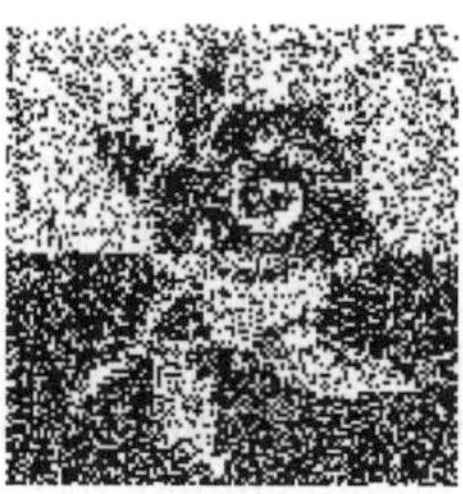

(a)
$p_1 = 0.0$, $p_2 = 1.0$,
BCR = 73.34%

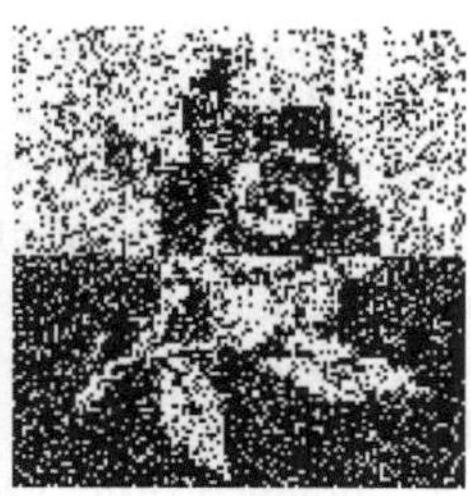

(b)
$p_1 = 1.0$, $p_2 = 0.0$,
BCR = 80.55%

Fig. 12.10. The extracted watermark under the case when one channel is total breakdown in Sec. 12.4.2, with a codebook size of $L = 512$. Both the extracted watermarks are recognizable.

Table 12.1. Comparisons of image quality and watermark robustness with single watermarking in Sec. 12.4.1 under different channel erasure probabilities with a codebook length of $L = 512$.

Channel erasure probability		Watermarked image quality (in dB)	Extracted BCR (in %)
p_1	p_2		
0	0	32.53	100
0.05	0.05	30.69	97.56
0.1	0.1	28.90	95.14
0.25	0.25	24.59	88.18
0.3	0.3	23.14	86.04
0.4	0.4	21.52	81.46
0.5	0.5	19.98	76.25
0	1	26.18	73.34
1	0	26.09	80.55

12.9.2 Results with Multiple Watermarking

For the multiple watermarking algorithm in Sec. 12.4.1, simulations with different channel erasure probabilities are presented in Fig. 12.11 and Fig. 12.12 with a codebook of length $L = 512$, and in Fig. 12.13 and Fig. 12.14 for the codebook of length $L = 1024$. We also use tables to make comparisons with the results obtained from other existing algorithms. In Table 12.2 and Table 12.3, we present the watermarked PSNR values and the BCR values of the extracted watermarks with a codebook with length of $L = 512$. Table 12.4 and Table 12.5 are their counterparts with the codebook with length of $L = 1024$.

In Fig. 12.11, p_1 and p_2 denote the erasure probabilities with Channel 1 and Channel 2. Fig. 12.11(a) shows that the extracted watermarks under error-free transmission. These are identical to those embedded in Fig. 12.8. In Fig. 12.11(b)–(d), they represent the results when transmitting over lightly to heavily erased channels. The BCR values are high and the extracted watermarks are recognizable even when $p_1 = p_2 = 0.5$. In Fig. 12.12, we demonstrate the case when one of the channels experiences a total breakdown. When Channel 2 breaks down, as shown in Fig. 12.12(a), the first watermark is recognizable, while the second cannot be distinguished. When Channel 1 breaks down, as shown in Fig. 12.12(b), we obtain similar results to those in Fig. 12.12(a).

In Table 12.2 and Table 12.3, the PSNR and the BCR values under different erasure probabilities are indicated. Comparisons with the results in [10] and [11] are also made. The PSNR values in Table 12.2 show error-resilient capabilities with MDVQ under severely erased channels. The PSNR values with our algorithm outperform others in most cases. Under the error free condition, the watermarked PSNR using our algorithm has the best performance.

(a) $p_1 = 0$, $p_2 = 0$, $\mathrm{BCR}_1 = 100\%$, $\mathrm{BCR}_2 = 100\%$

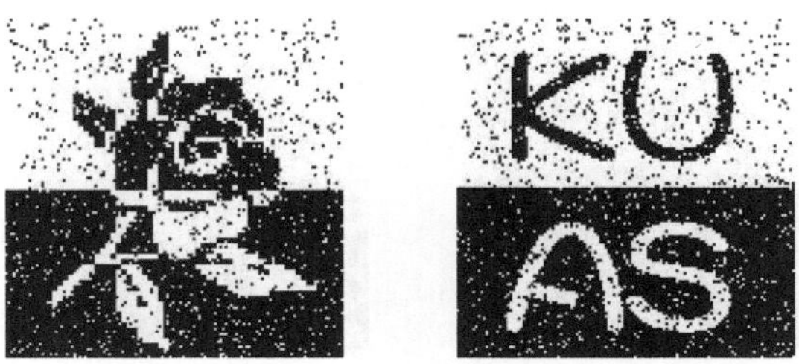

(b) $p_1 = 0.1$, $p_2 = 0.1$, $\mathrm{BCR}_1 = 94.12\%$, $\mathrm{BCR}_2 = 93.60\%$

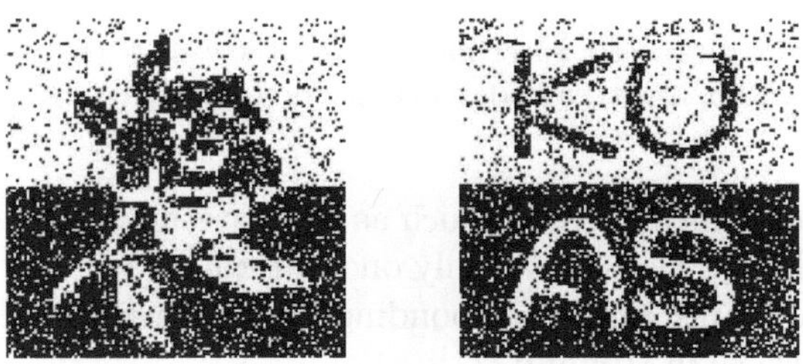

(c) $p_1 = 0.25$, $p_2 = 0.25$, $\mathrm{BCR}_1 = 87.50\%$, $\mathrm{BCR}_2 = 85.64\%$

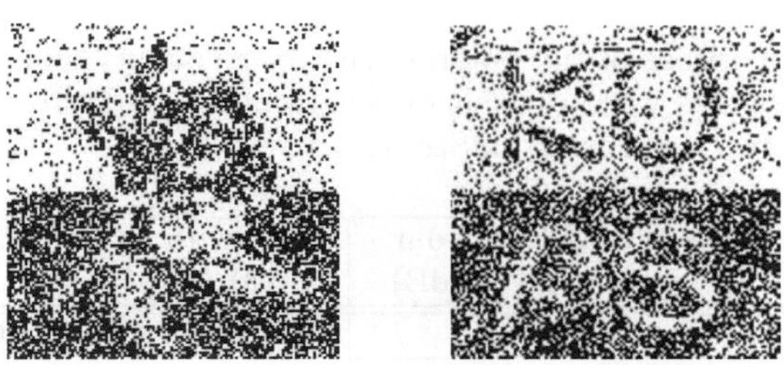

(d) $p_1 = 0.5$, $p_2 = 0.5$, $\mathrm{BCR}_1 = 74.30\%$, $\mathrm{BCR}_2 = 72.08\%$

Fig. 12.11. The two extracted watermarks under different channel erasure probabilities in Sec. 12.5.2, with a codebook size of $L = 512$.

Also, the BCR values in Table 12.3 are acceptable even with heavily erased channels, and the corresponding watermarks can all be subjectively recognized. The only situation when only one of the channels breaks down, it is not possible to recognize the second watermark. More importantly, using our

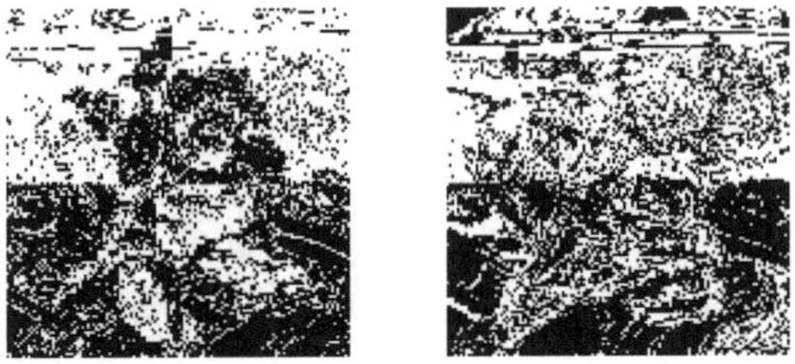

(a) $p_1 = 0.0$, $p_2 = 1.0$, $\mathrm{BCR}_1 = 81.03\%$, $\mathrm{BCR}_2 = 68.23\%$

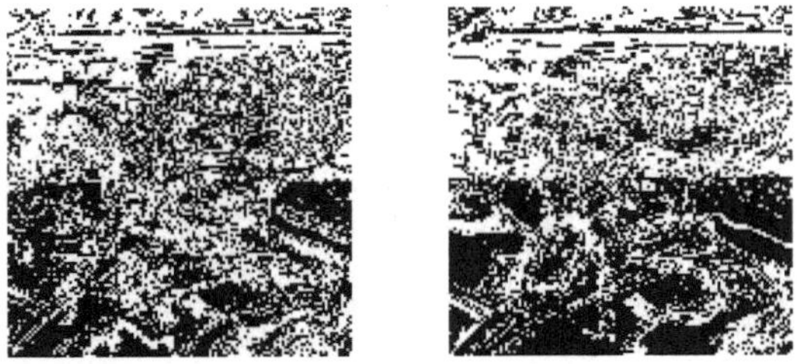

(b) $p_1 = 1.0$, $p_2 = 0.0$, $\mathrm{BCR}_1 = 67.00\%$, $\mathrm{BCR}_2 = 69.71\%$

Fig. 12.12. The two extracted watermarks under the case when one channel is total breakdown in Sec. 12.5.2, with a codebook size of $L = 512$.

algorithm, we can embed twice as much as the watermark capacity than those given in [10] and [11]. Thus, while only one watermark can be extracted using the existing algorithms, the corresponding BCR values using our algorithm are better than those in [10] and [11].

Table 12.2. Comparisons of the watermarked image quality under different channel erasure probabilities with a codebook length of $L = 512$ after considering the embedding of the two watermarks in Sec. 12.5.1.

Channel erasure probability		PSNR with our method (in dB)	PSNR with [10] (in dB)	PSNR with [11] (in dB)
p_1	p_2			
0	0	30.74	30.46	30.64
0.1	0.1	28.15	28.14	28.56
0.25	0.25	24.39	24.37	24.40
0.5	0.5	19.88	19.93	19.86
0	1	26.19	25.92	25.41
1	0	26.13	26.04	25.48

In Fig. 12.13, similar comparisons can be made by following those given in Fig. 12.11. Fig. 12.13(a) shows the extracted watermarks during error-free transmission. These are identical to those embedded in Fig. 12.8. In

Table 12.3. Comparisons of watermark robustness under different channel erasure probabilities with codebook length of $L = 512$ after considering the embedding of two watermarks in Sec. 12.5.1.

Channel erasure probability		BCR with our method (in %)		BCR with [10] (in %)	BCR with [11] (in %)
p_1	p_2	W_1'	W_2'	W_1'	W_1'
0	0	100	100	100	100
0.1	0.1	94.12	93.60	90.48	94.90
0.25	0.25	87.50	85.64	78.47	87.19
0.5	0.5	74.30	72.08	62.88	74.69
0	1	81.03	68.23	75.72	79.72
1	0	67.00	69.71	66.38	66.52

Fig. 12.13(b)–(d), they represent the results when transmitting over the lightly to heavily erased channels. The BCR values are high and the extracted watermarks are recognizable even with $p_1 = p_2 = 0.5$. When comparing these results with Fig. 12.11(b)–(d), although the BCR values are a little inferior, all the extracted watermarks are recognizable. In Fig. 12.14, when one of the channels fails, both of the first watermarks are recognizable, while the second watermarks can only be partially distinguished.

In Table 12.4 and Table 12.5, PSNR and BCR values under different erasure probabilities are indicated. Comparisons with results from [10] and [11] are also made. PSNR values in Table 12.4 show the error-resilient capabilities using MDVQ having severely erased channels. The PSNR values using our algorithm outperform others in most cases, and under the error free condition, the watermarked PSNR using our algorithm performs best. In comparison with Table 12.2, with a larger codebook length given in Table 12.4, we obtain better PSNR values. Also, the BCR values in Table 12.3 are acceptable even with heavily erased channels. Again, with our algorithm, we can embed twice as much watermark capacity than those in [10] and [11]. Only one watermark can be extracted with existing algorithms, and the corresponding BCR values with our algorithm are better than [10] and [11].

Summing up, under a wide range of channel erasure situations, the results using the multiple watermarking algorithm with MDC demonstrate both the effective transmission of watermarked images, and the robustness of the extracted watermarks. To compare with the results in Sec. 12.4.1, we also double the amount of watermark capacity embedded with our algorithm.

12.10 Conclusions

In this chapter, we propose an innovative scheme for VQ-based image multi-watermarking with multiple description coding (MDC), which is suitable for

(a) $p_1 = 0$, $p_2 = 0$, $\text{BCR}_1 = 100\%$, $\text{BCR}_2 = 100\%$

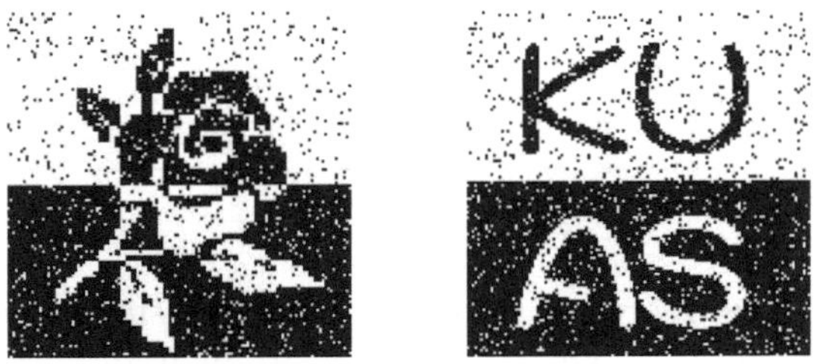

(b) $p_1 = 0.1$, $p_2 = 0.1$, $\text{BCR}_1 = 94.27\%$, $\text{BCR}_2 = 93.44\%$

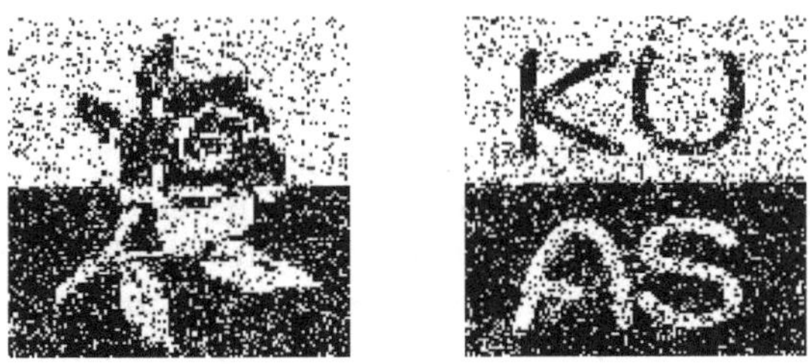

(c) $p_1 = 0.25$, $p_2 = 0.25$, $\text{BCR}_1 = 86.52\%$, $\text{BCR}_2 = 84.78\%$

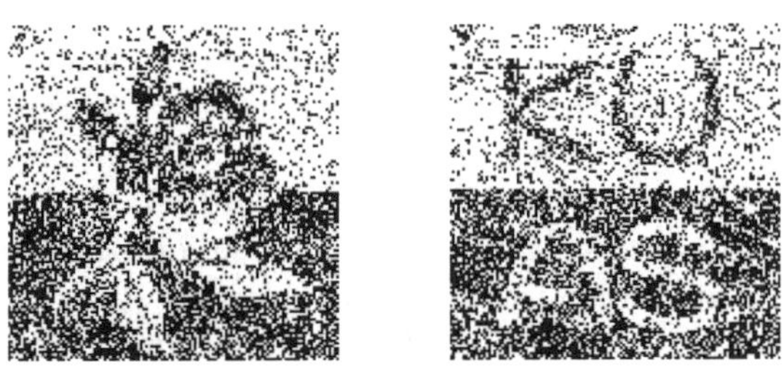

(d) $p_1 = 0.5$, $p_2 = 0.5$, $\text{BCR}_1 = 73.28\%$, $\text{BCR}_2 = 71.34\%$

Fig. 12.13. The two extracted watermarks under different channel erasure probabilities, with a codebook size of $L = 1024$.

transmission over noisy channels. We modified the MDVQ and MDSQ index assignments for watermark embedding and extraction. By incorporating this with MDC, we obtain promising results. Simulation results gave better robustness of the watermarking algorithm, and the more resilience to com-

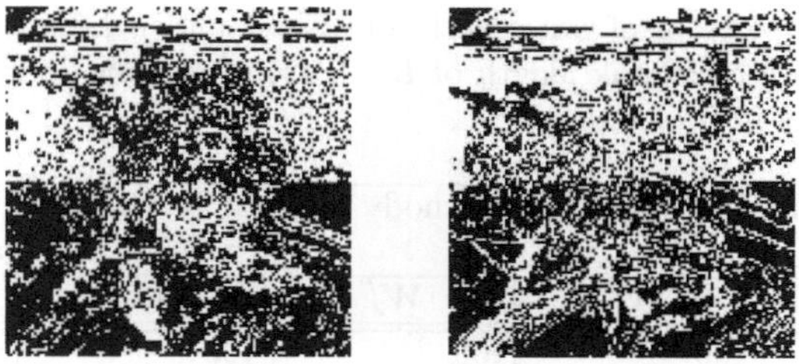

(a) $p_1 = 0.0$, $p_2 = 1.0$, $\text{BCR}_1 = 76.61\%$, $\text{BCR}_2 = 70.78\%$

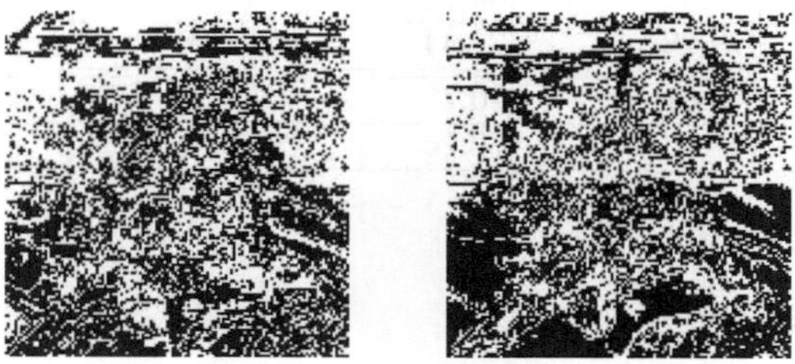

(b) $p_1 = 1.0$, $p_2 = 0.0$, $\text{BCR}_1 = 68.56\%$, $\text{BCR}_2 = 70.26\%$

Fig. 12.14. The two extracted watermarks under the case when one channel is total breakdown, with a codebook size of $L = 1024$.

Table 12.4. Comparisons of watermarked image quality under different channel erasure probabilities with a codebook length of $L = 1024$ after considering the embedding of two watermarks in Sec. 12.5.1.

Channel erasure probability		PSNR with our method (in dB)	PSNR with [10] (in dB)	PSNR with [11] (in dB)
p_1	p_2			
0	0	32.74	31.84	32.20
0.1	0.1	28.35	28.47	28.88
0.25	0.25	24.27	24.33	24.34
0.5	0.5	19.78	19.77	19.79
0	1	25.10	24.88	25.17
1	0	25.04	24.72	25.17

bat with channel noise under both lightly and heavily erased channels. Also, in comparison with existing VQ-based algorithms in the literature, our algorithm perform better than others in both the watermark imperceptibility, shown by PSNR, and the watermark robustness, shown by BCR. Therefore, our algorithm is not only innovative for research, but also suitable for practical implementation.

Table 12.5. Comparisons of watermark robustness under different channel erasure probabilities with a codebook length of $L = 1024$ after considering the embedding of two watermarks in Sec. 12.5.1.

Channel erasure probability		BCR with our method (in %)		BCR with [10] (in %)	BCR with [11] (in %)
p_1	p_2	$\boldsymbol{W}_1'$	$\boldsymbol{W}_2'$	$\boldsymbol{W}_1'$	$\boldsymbol{W}_1'$
0	0	100	100	100	100
0.1	0.1	94.27	93.44	90.77	94.76
0.25	0.25	86.52	84.78	79.06	85.77
0.5	0.5	73.28	71.34	62.66	72.42
0	1	76.61	70.78	75.89	80.94
1	0	68.56	70.26	66.66	68.13

Acknowledgement

This work was supported by National Science Council (Taiwan, R.O.C.) under Grant No. NSC 93-2219-E-009-006 and NSC 95-2221-E-390-034.

References

1. Decker, S. (2001): Engineering considerations in commercial watermarking. IEEE Communications Magazine, **39**, 128–133
2. Koenen, R.H., Lacy, J., Mackay, M., and Mitchell, S. (2004): The long march to interoperable digital rights management. Proceedings of the IEEE, **92**, 883–897
3. Pan, J.S., Huang, H.C., and Jain, L.C. (editors) (2004): Intelligent watermarking techniques. World Scientific Publishing Company, Singapore
4. Sion, R., Atallah, M., and Prabhakar, S. (2004): Rights protection for relational data. IEEE Trans. Knowledge and Data Engineering, **16**, 1509–1525
5. Katzenbeisser, S. and Petitcolas, F. (2000): Information Hiding — Techniques for Steganography and Digital Watermarking. Artech House, Norwood, MA
6. Chu, W.C. (2003): DCT-based image watermarking using subsampling. IEEE Trans. Multimedia, **5**, 34–38
7. Kang, X., Huang, J., Shi, Y.Q., and Lin, Y. (2003): A DWT–DFT composite watermarking scheme robust to both affine transform and JPEG compression. IEEE Trans. Circuits and Systems for Video Technology, **13**, 776–786
8. Ramkumar, M., Akansu, A.N. (2004): On the design of data hiding methods robust to lossy compression. IEEE Trans. Multimedia, **6**, 947–951
9. Podilchuk, C.I. and Zeng, W.J. (1998): Image-adaptive watermarking using visual models. IEEE Journal on Selected Areas in Commun., **16**, 525–539
10. Lu, Z.M. and Sun, S.H. (2000): Digital image watermarking technique based on vector quantisation. IEE Electronics Letters, **36**, 303–305
11. Pan, J.S., Wang, F.H., Huang, H.C., and Jain, L.C. (2003): Improved schemes for VQ-based image watermarking. IEEE Int'l Symposium on Consumer Electronics 2003, paper no: ISCE03011

12. Glover, F. and Laguna, M. (1997) Tabu Search. Kluwer Academic Publishers, Boston, MA
13. Li, C., Liao, X., and Yu, J. (2004) Tabu search for fuzzy optimization and applications. Information Sciences, **158**, 3–13
14. Shieh, C.S., Huang, H.C., Wang, F.H., and Pan, J.S. (2004): Genetic watermarking based on transform domain techniques. Pattern Recognition, **37**, 555–565
15. Shih, F.Y. and Wu, Y.T. (2005): Robust watermarking and compression for medical images based on genetic algorithms. Information Sciences, **175**, 200–216
16. Linde, Y., Buzo, A., and Gray, R.M. (1980): An algorithm for vector quantizer design. IEEE Trans. Commun., **28**, 84–95
17. Pan, J.S., Sung, M.T., Huang, H.C., and Liao, B.Y. (2004): Robust VQ-based digital watermarking for the memoryless binary symmetric channel. IEICE Trans. on Fundamentals, **E-87A**, 1839–1841
18. Pan, J.S., Hsin, Y.C., Huang, H.C., and Huang, K.C. (2004): Robust image watermarking based on multiple description vector quantisation. IEE Electronics Letters, **40**, 1409–1410
19. Piva, A., Bartolini, F., and Barni, M. (2002): Managing copyright in open networks. IEEE Internet Computing, **6**, 18–26
20. Waller, A.O., Jones, G., Whitley, T., Edwards, J., Kaleshi, D., Munro, A., MacFarlane, B., and Wood, A. (2002): Securing the delivery of digital content over the Internet. Electronics & Communication Engineering Journal, **14**, 239–248
21. Petitcolas, F.A.P. (2004): Stirmark benchmark 4.0. Available from: `http://www.petitcolas.net/fabien/watermarking/stirmark/`
22. Lee, C.C. and Leu, Y. (2005): Efficient data broadcast schemes for mobile computing environments with data missing. Information Sciences, **172**, 335–359
23. Goyal, V.K. (2001): Multiple description coding: Compression meets the network. IEEE Signal Processing Magazine, **18**, 74–93
24. El Gamal, A.A. and Cover, T.M. (1982): Achievable rates for multiple descriptions. IEEE Trans. Inform. Theory, **28**, 851–857
25. Zhang, Z. and Berger, T. (1987): New results in binary multiple descriptions. IEEE Trans. Inform. Theory, **33**, 502–521
26. Loo, P. and Kingsbury, N. (2003): Watermark detection based on the properties of error control codes. IEE Proceedings – Vision, Image and Signal Processing, **150**, 115–121
27. Vaishampayan, V.A. (1993): Design of multiple description scalar quantizers. IEEE Trans. Inform. Theory, **39**, 821–834
28. Görtz, N. and Leelapornchai, P. (2003): Optimization of the index assignments for multiple description vector quantizers. IEEE Trans. Commun., **51**, 336–340
29. Wang, Y., Orchard, M.T., Vaishampayan, V.A., and Reibman, A.R. (2001): Multiple description coding using pairwise correlating transforms. IEEE Trans. Image Processing, **10**, 351–366
30. Wang, Y., Reibman, A.R., Orchard, M.T., and Jafarkhani, H. (2002): An improvement to multiple description transform coding. IEEE Trans. Signal Processing, **50**, 2843–2854
31. Jo, M. and Kim, H.D. (2002): A digital image watermarking scheme based on vector quantisation, IEICE Trans. Information and Systems, **E85-D**, 1054–1056

13

Reversible Watermarking Techniques

Shao-Wei Weng[1], Yao Zhao[1], and Jeng-Shyang Pan[2]

[1] Institute of Information Science, Beijing Jiao Tong University, Beijing 100044, P.R. China
wswweiwei@126.com
yzhao@center.njtu.edu.cn
[2] National Kaohsiung University of Applied Sciences, Kaohsiung 807, Taiwan, R.O.C.
jspan@cc.kuas.edu.tw
http://bit.kuas.edu.tw/~jspan/

Summary. In this chapter, several reversible watermarking algorithms are introduced. The key idea of existing reversible watermarking techniques according to two basic classifications is generalized in this chapter. The first classification is based on Robust Spatial Additive Watermarks combined with modulo addition. The second classification is partitioned into three subsets. The first subset based on Lossless Compression Techniques contains lossless bit-plane compression methods in the spatial domain and in the Integer Discrete Wavelet Transform (IDWT) domain, the reversible RS data-embedding method, and the lossless G-LSB data-embedding method, respectively. The second subset contains the algorithm based on histogram shifting techniques. The third subset based on the value expansion techniques contains Integer Discrete Cosine Transform (IDCT) based bit-shifting method. Finally, the chapter introduces our own technique. The performance of related techniques is compared and their respective advantage and disadvantage are also analyzed in this chapter.

13.1 Introduction

Digital watermarking refers to the process of embedding some labels or signatures into digital media without introducing perceptible artifacts. It plays a vital role in the applications to copyright protection of digital media, authentication, date integrity, fingerprinting, and data hiding. However, digital watermarking usually introduces a slight but irreversible or permanent distortion to the original image. Although the distortion is generally quite small, it may not be acceptable for some applications, such as in the fields of the law enforcement, medical and military systems. It is desired to restore the original image from the watermarked image after the hidden data is retrieved due to the highly-precise requirement. The data embedding techniques, capable of reversing to the exact copy of the original image, are referred to as Reversible,

S.-W. Weng et al.: *Reversible Watermarking Techniques*, Studies in Computational Intelligence (SCI) **58**, 357–389 (2007)
www.springerlink.com

Invertible, Lossless, Distortion-Free, or Erasable Data Embedding Technique. The reversible data embedding techniques either have the desirable properties of a digital watermark, such as perceptible transparency, robustness, security, and data capacity, or have reversibility.

From the literature, most data embedding techniques cannot be completely reversed, since embedded distortion due to discarded information, quantization and integer rounding at the boundaries of the grayscale range cannot be removed. For example, by replacing the bits in the bit-planes, that is, least significant bit-plane (LSB), with watermarking bits, watermarking techniques discard all replaced bits of the bit-planes. Consequently, the bit-replacement is clearly lossy. For watermarking techniques, based on the quantization such as Vector Quantization (VQ), Quantization Index Modulation (QIM), and so on, quantization error makes that retrieved pixel values mismatch with original pixel values. Hence, there is little hope to restore the original image without distortion. For spread spectrum watermarking techniques in Discrete Cosine Transform (DCT) domain and/or Discrete Wavelet Transform (DWT) domain, round-off error and truncation error make invertible watermarking impossible. Additive, non-adaptive schemes (truncation addition) are almost lossless except for the pixels with grayscales close to 0 or 255 where truncation has occurred owing to overflow or underflow.

In all of the above mentioned embedding techniques are not suitable in some applications. Those require high-precision, such as the medical images, artworks, and so on. Some watermarking techniques have been developed in order to presented to satisfy the reversible requirement over the last a few years. All existing reversible watermarking techniques can be classified into two categories.

Type-I algorithms [1]-[4] are based on robust, spatial additive watermarks combined with modulo addition. These techniques add the payload by modulo addition to the host image during embedding process. At the decoder, the payload can be reconstructed from the watermarked image, and then it is subtracted to restore the original image. However, modulo additions would cause a disturbing visual artifact resembling a correlated salt-and-pepper noise into the watermarked image when pixel values close to the maximally allowed value are flipped to zero and vice versa. Type-I algorithms generally combine statistical approaches. For example, the patchwork algorithm with modulo additions is used to ensure correct watermark extraction. Hence, Type-I algorithms are robust for the data embedding and allow for extraction of hidden data even for the perturbed watermarked image. It can not ensure that the original image is precisely retrieved. The algorithm in [4] has certain degree of robustness against JPEG lossy compression. This is the only existing robust lossless data embedding algorithm for use against JPEG compression.

Type-II algorithms [5]-[12] can be partitioned into three offsets. The first offset based on lossless compression techniques and contains lossless bit-plane compression methods in the spatial domain [5] and in the Integer Discrete Wavelet Transform (IDWT) domain [6]. The reversible RS data-embedding method is given in [7], and the lossless G-LSB data-embedding method is given in [8]. The second offset contains the algorithm [9] and is based on histogram shifting techniques. The third offset based on the value expansion techniques contains Integer Discrete Cosine Transform (IDCT) based on a bit-shifting method in [10], and the difference expansion methods are given in [11, 12]. Type-II algorithms can not cause salt-and-pepper noise, but can achieve higher embedding capacities, albeit at the loss of the robust properties of the first category.

The chapter is organized as follows. Section 13.2 and Section 13.3 respectively introduce several existing reversible watermarking algorithms of two categories. In Section 13.4, an introduction about our proposed reversible watermarking techniques is given. Future research is discussed in Section 13.5. The performance of related techniques is compared and their respective advantages and disadvantages are also analyzed in this chapter.

13.2 Type-I Algorithms: Robust Spatial Additive Watermarks

Robust Spatial Additive Watermarks combined with Modulo Addition first appeared in a patent by Honsinger et al. [1]. It is owned by the Eastman Kodak Company. Paper [1] utilizes modulo 256 addition to embed the authentication hash to the original image. The embedding method is equivalent to the arithmetic formula $i_w = i \oplus w = 256 \cdot \lfloor \frac{i}{256} \rfloor + \bmod (i+w, 256)$, where '$\oplus$' denotes modulo 256 addition, i and w respectively indicate any pixel value and corresponding watermarking bit coming from the hash function of the original image. The symbol $\lfloor \cdot \rfloor$ denotes the truncation operation to the integer part, and i_w stands for the watermarked pixel. At the decoder, the watermarking bits are extracted from the watermarked image. Then, watermarked bits are subtracted from the watermarked pixel values to restore the original pixel values according to the operation: $i = i_w - w = i_w \oplus (-w)$. Modulo 256 addition can be represented as the following permutation: $0 \to 1,\ 1 \to 2,\ \cdots,\ 254 \to 255,\ 255 \to 0$. From the above permutation, pixel values close to the grayscale value 255 are flipped to zeros and vice versa, so watermarked image would suffer from the disturbing visual artifact resembling the salt-and-pepper noise. Macq [2] applied modulo additions and the patchwork algorithm [3] to achieve reversible data embedding. But papers [1, 2] cannot resolve the salt-and-pepper noise caused by modulo additions. De Vleeschouwer et al. [4] proposed a lossless data hiding algorithm based on the patchwork theory and effectively avoided the salt-and-pepper noise.

13.2.1 De Vleeschouwer et al.'s Method

De Vleeschouwer et al. [4] hide a binary message. That is, the watermark payload loaded into the original image using a patchwork algorithm. Each bit of the message is associated with a group of pixels. For example, a block in an image. Each group is equally divided into two pseudo-random sets of pixels. That is, zones A and B. A small constant value δ is added to the pixel values of zone A and is subtracted from the pixel values of another zone B. Since zones A and B are pseudo-randomly selected, they have close average values before embedding. After embedding, and depending on the bits embedded, their luminance values are incremented or decremented. The extracted bit is inferred from the comparison between the mean values of zone A and B.

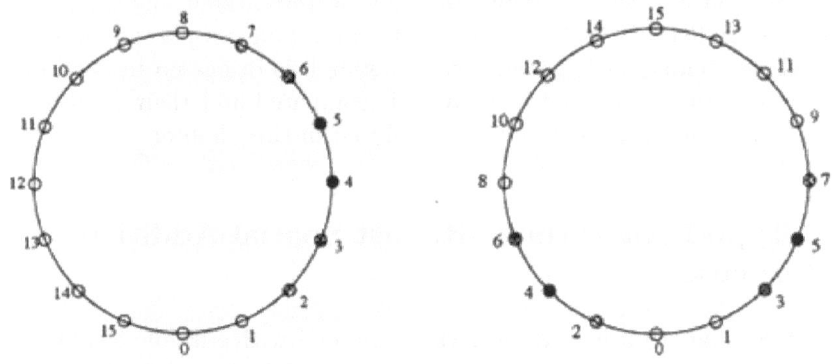

(a) Traditional modulo addition (b) Symmetric modulo addition

Fig. 13.1. Modulo additions.

The histogram of each zone is mapped to a circle. The positions on the circle are indexed by the corresponding luminance. See Fig. 13.1(a). The embedding process is summarized in Fig. 13.2. It can be observed that in most cases the vectors V_a and V_b point to the center of mass of zones A and B and are close to each other. Hence slight rotation of vectors V_a and V_b in opposite ways allows for embedding a bit of information. Vector V_a rotates either clockwise to embed a "1" or counterclockwise to embed a "0". At the receiver, the bit is inferred from the sign of the smallest angle between vectors V_a and V_b. The pixel values are obtained from the rotations of the vectors correspond to luminance shifts. The magnitude of the shift, is also called the Embedding Level. The shifts of luminance caused by sequence (a) and sequence (b) are equivalent to modulo additions and subtractions in Fig. 13.1(a). From Fig. 13.3, it is clear that modulo 256 addition or modulo 16 addition is used. Therefore this algorithm also suffers from the salt-and-pepper noise.

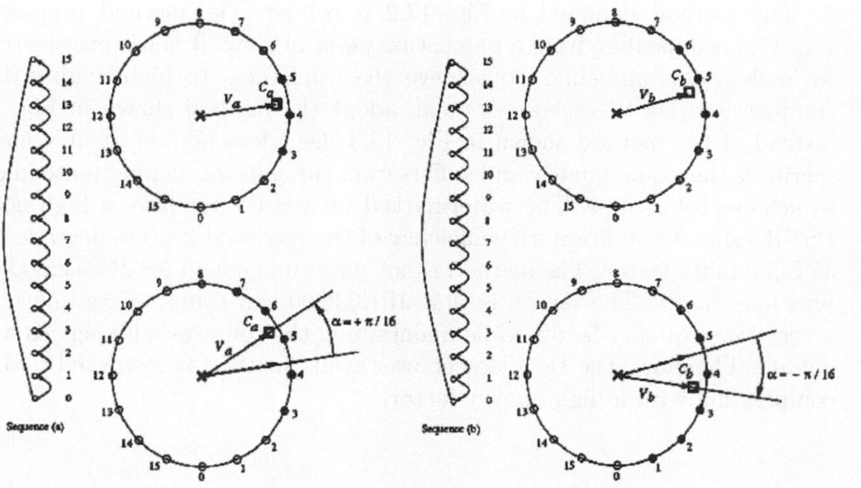

Fig. 13.2. Data embedding diagram.

Traditional modulo additions (Fig. 13.1(a)) complete an existing additive method to ensure reversibility. However, such approaches are not satisfactory. The wrapped around pixels cause a salt-and-pepper visual artifact. That is, pixels close to the maximally allowed value are flipped to zero and vice versa. Even worse, once flipped, values that should be increased or decreased are actually decreased or increased. This impacts on the average value of the zone, and consequently the inferred bit. To avoid a salt-and-pepper visual artifact, an alternative mapping of the histogram to the circle is proposed in Fig. 13.1(b). At the circle level, the embedding transform is the same. That is, a rotation in Fig. 13.3. However, at the pixel level (see sequence (a) and (b) in Fig. 13.3), no value is shifted by an outstandingly large step anymore. The transform is now free from disturbing visual artifacts such as the salt-and-pepper effect.

In Fig. 13.1(b), odd and even luminance values are spread symmetrically around the circle. Consequently, the histogram is also spread symmetrically around the circle and the center of mass is close to the vertical axis of symmetry. The positions of luminance values on the circle are chosen so that all neighbors correspond to close luminance values. It prevents the salt-and-pepper effect after rotation. We call the method the Symmetric Modulo Addition.

De Vleeschouwer et al. adopt the data embedding scheme (Fig. 13.3) to effectively avoid the salt-and-pepper noise. The vector pointing to the center of mass no longer indicates the position of the histogram on the circle. The direction of the principal axis with minimal inertia is used instead. Embedding and retrieval procedures are similar to those described previously.

The method depicted in Fig. 13.2 is robust. The method proposed in Fig. 13.3 is appealing from a perceptual point of view. It is however restricted to lossless environments. To achieve the robustness to high quality JPEG compression, De Vleeschouwer et al. adopt the method shown in Fig. 13.2, instead of the method shown in Fig. 13.3. De Vleeschouwer et al.'s method sacrifices the visual quality and suffers from the salt-and-pepper noise in order to achieve robustness. The watermarked images do not have a high enough PSNR value. In addition, the efficiency of the retrieved process degrades with JPEG quality factor. The method is not powerful enough for JPEG2000 compression images. The reason is that JPEG2000 can compress an image with a very lower quality factor while maintaining the compressed image to a high quality. Therefore, the De Vleeschouwer et al.' method is restricted to JPEG compression with a high quality factor.

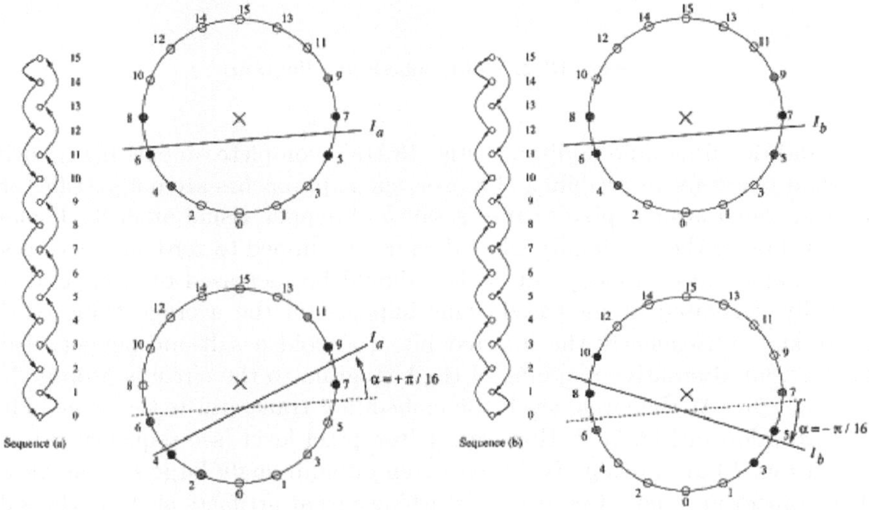

Fig. 13.3. Embedding illustration when restricted by the salt-and-pepper effect. The pixels in each zone are transformed according to sequence (a) and (b); it impacts the principal axis orientation.

13.3 Type-II Algorithms

13.3.1 Algorithms Based on Lossless Compression Techniques

Lossless Bit-Plane Compression in the Spatial Domain

Fridrich's group produced profound research on lossless data hiding techniques and developed a number of algorithms. This group [5] proposed two techniques in this area. Since the second technique is classified as belonging to the second category, we introduce two techniques here. The first technique, based on robust spatial additive watermarks, utilizes the modulo addition to embed the hash of the original image. The second technique uses the JBIG Lossless Compression Scheme [13] for losslessly compressing the bit-planes to make room for data embedding. In order to provide sufficient room for data embedding for the second technique, it is usual to compress the high level bit-plane. This mostly leads to visual quality degradation. Since the method aims at authentication, the amount of embedded data is limited.

They also describe two reversible data hiding techniques [14] for lossy compressing the JPEG image. The first technique is based on lossless compression of biased bit-streams derived from the quantized JPEG coefficients. Before introducing the first techniques, it is necessary to depict the JPEG compression process for grayscale images or colored images. All disjoint 8×8 DCT coefficient blocks of the original image are denoted as $d_k(i,j), 0 \leq i,\ j \leq 8$, where $k = 1, 2, \cdots, B$, and B is the total number of blocks in the image. In each block, all authentication coefficients are further quantized to integers with a JPEG quantization matrix in Eq. (13.1),

$$D_k(i,j) = \text{integer}_{\text{round}}\left[\frac{d_k(i,j)}{D_k(i,j)}\right]. \tag{13.1}$$

The quantized coefficients $D_k(i,j)$ are arranged in a zigzag manner and compressed using the Huffman coder. The resulting compressed stream together with a header forms the final JPEG file.

The algorithm for invertible authentication of JPEG files is generalized in five steps. We describe each step below.

(1) In the first step, the set of L authentication pairs (i_1, j_1), (i_2, j_2), $\cdots$, (i_L, j_L), in middle frequencies is determined according to the JPEG quality factor.
(2) Next, the JPEG file is read and the values of quantized DCT coefficients, $d_k(i,j),\ \ 0 < i,\ j < 8,\ \ k = 1, 2, \cdots, B$ are obtained using the Huffman decompressor.
(3) Thirdly, the hash of the Huffman decompressed stream $D_k(i,j)$ is calculated.
(4) The fourth step seeds a Pseudo-Random Number Generator (PRNG) with a secret key and follows a random non-intersecting walk through the set $E = \{D_1(i_1, j_1), \cdots, D_B(i_1, j_1),\ D_1(i_2, j_2), \cdots, D_B(i_2, j_2), \cdots, D_1(i_L, j_L), \cdots, D_B(i_L, j_L)\}$. While following the random walk, the adaptive context-free lossless arithmetic coder for the LSBs of the coefficients from E is run until there is enough space for the hash to be inserted. The set of visited coefficients is denoted as E_1, where $E_1 \subseteq E$.
(5) The final step concatenates the compressed bit-stream, the hash and inserts the resulting bit-stream into the LSBs which are the coefficients

from E_1. Huffman coding compresses all DCT coefficients $D_k(i, j)$ including those modified and stores the authenticated image as a JPEG file on a disk.

The first three steps, which are the same as Steps 1, 2, 4 in the invertible authentication, are skipped for the introduction of the integrity verification. The fourth step runs the context-free lossless arithmetic decoder for the LSBs containing the coefficients visited during the same random walk as the embedding process. Once the length of the decompressed bit-stream reaches $B+|H|$, where $|H|$ stands for the hash length, the procedure is stopped. The decompressed bit-stream is separated into the LSBs of visited DCT coefficients and the extracted candidate for hash h. The retrieved LSBs replace the LSBs of all visited coefficients to restore the original quantized DCT coefficients $d_k(i, j)$, $0 \leq i,\ j \leq 8, k = 1, 2, \cdots, B$. For authentication, the hash H of all retrieved quantized DCT coefficients is calculated. H' is compared with H. If they match, the JPEG file is authentic and the original JPEG image is obtained. If $H \neq H'$, the image is deemed non-authentic. Experimental results show that the distortion increases with the compression ratio.

Lossless Bit-Plane Compression in the IDWT Domain

Paper [6] embeds data into the middle bit-planes of the integer wavelet transform coefficients and applies histogram modification in the preprocess. This is done to prevent the overflow and underflow problem caused by modification of the wavelet modification. The method achieves a larger bias between binary 1's and binary 0's in the middle and the high bit-plane of the IDWT coefficients than that in the spatial domain. Owing to the larger bias, those bit-planes coefficients can be losslessly compressed to accommodate the more hidden data. The method is able to imperceptibly embed about 5 k to 94 kbits into a grayscale image of $512 \times 512 \times 8$. This is much more than that achieved by existing techniques.

Lossless RS Data-Embedding Method

Goljan et al. [7] presented the first lossless marking technique suitable for data embedding. They generated loss free compressible bit-streams using the concepts of invertible noise adding or flipping. Special discrimination or prediction functions were also used on small groups of pixels. The new approach is much more efficient when allowing for large payload with minimal or invertible distortion.

The details are as follows. The pixels in an image with size $M \times N$ are partitioned into non-overlapped n groups, each of which consisting of adjacent pixels $(x_1, x_2, \cdots, x_n)$. For instance, it could be a horizontal block having four consecutive pixels. A discrimination function f is established that assigns a real number $f(x_1, x_2, \cdots, x_n) \in \mathbb{R}$ to each pixel group $G(x_1, x_2, \cdots, x_n)$.

The authors use the discrimination function to capture the smoothness of the groups. For example, the 'variation' of the group of pixels $(x_1, x_2, \cdots, x_n)$ can be chosen as the discrimination function $f(\cdot)$:

$$f(x_1, x_2, \cdots, x_n) = \sum_{i=1}^{n-1} |x_{i+1} - x_i| . \tag{13.2}$$

The purpose of the discrimination function is to capture the smoothness or "regularity" of the group of pixels G. An invertible operation F with the amplitude A can be applied to the groups. It can map a gray level value to another gray level value. It is reversible since after applying it to a gray level value twice produces the original gray level value. That is, F has the property that F^2 =Identity or $F(F(x)) = x$, for all $x \in P$, where $P = 0, 1, \cdots, 255$, for an 8-bit gray-scale image. This invertible operation is called flipping F. The difference between the flipped values and the original values is A.

A suitably chosen discrimination function $f(\cdot)$ and the flipping operation F are utilized to define three types of pixel groups: Regular R, Singular S, and Unusable U.

$$\begin{array}{ll} \text{Regular groups:} & G \in R \Leftrightarrow f(F(G)) > f(G); \\ \text{Singular groups:} & G \in S \Leftrightarrow f(F(G)) < f(G); \\ \text{Unusable groups:} & G \in U \Leftrightarrow f(F(G)) = f(G). \end{array}$$

From the definitions of the R, S, and U groups, it is apparent that if G is regular, $F(G)$ is singular, if G is singular, $F(G)$ is regular, and if G is unusable, $F(G)$ is unusable. Thus, the R and S groups are flipped into each other using the flipping operation F. The unusable groups U do not change their status. In a symbolic form, $F(R) = S$, $F(S) = R$ and $F(U) = U$.

In the expression $F(G)$, the flipping function F may be applied to all or to selected components of the vector $G(x_1, x_2, \cdots, x_n)$. The noisier the group of pixels $G(x_1, x_2, \cdots, x_n)$ is, the larger the value of the discrimination function becomes. The purpose of the flipping F is to perturb the pixel values in an invertible way by a small amount thus simulating the act of "Invertible Noise Adding." In typical pictures, adding small amount of noise, or flipping by a small amount, will lead to an increase in the discrimination function rather than to a decrease. Although this bias may be small, it will enable us to embed a large amount of information in an invertible manner.

As explained above, F is a permutation that consists entirely of two-cycles. For example, the permutation F_{LSB} is defined as $0 \leftrightarrow 1$, $2 \leftrightarrow 3$, $\cdots$, $254 \leftrightarrow 255$ corresponds to flipping or negating the LSB in each gray level. The permutation corresponds to an invertible noise with a larger amplitude than two. The amplitude A of the flipping permutation F is defined as $0 \leftrightarrow 2$, $1 \leftrightarrow 3$, $\cdots$, $253 \leftrightarrow 255$. The average change of under the application of F is:

$$A = \frac{1}{|P|} \sum_{x \in P} |x - F(x)|. \tag{13.3}$$

For F_{LSB} the amplitude is 1. The other permutation from the previous paragraph has $A = 2$. Larger values of the amplitude A correspond to the action of adding more noise after applying F.

The main idea for lossless embedding is that the image by groups can be scanned according to a predefined order and losslessly compress the status of the image. — The bit-stream of R and S groups or the RS-vector with the U groups may be skipped. This may be considered as overhead needed to leave room for data embedding. It is not necessary to include the U groups, because they do not change in the process of message embedding and can be all unambiguously identified and skipped during embedding and extraction. The higher a bias between the number of R and S groups, the lower the capacity consumed by the overheads and the higher the real capacity. By assigning a 1 to R and a 0 to S they embed one message bit in each R or S group. If the message bit and the group type do not match, the flipping operation F is applied to the group to obtain a match. The data to be embedded consist of the overhead and the watermark signal.

The extraction starts by partitioning the watermarked image into disjoint groups using the same pattern as used in the embedding. They apply the flipping operation F and discrimination function f to all groups to identify the R, S and U groups. They then then extract the bit-stream from all R and S groups ($R = 1$, $S = 0$) by scanning the image in the same order as embedding. The extracted bit-stream is separated into the message and the compressed RS-vector C. The bit-stream C is decompressed to reveal the original status of all R and S groups. The image is then processed once more and the status of all groups is adjusted as necessary by flipping the groups back to their original state. Thus, an exact copy of the original image is obtained. The block diagram of the embedding and extracting procedure is given in Fig. 13.4.

Let N_R, N_S and N_U be respectively used to indicate the number of regular, singular, and unusable groups in the image. The sum of N_R, N_S and N_U is equal to $\frac{MN}{n}$ (the number of all groups). The raw information capacity for this data embedding method is $N_R + N_S = \frac{MN}{n} - N_U$ bits. However, since the compressed bit-stream C consumes a large part of the available capacity, the real capacity C_{ap} that can be used for the message is given by

$$C_{\text{ap}} = N_R + N_S - |C|, \tag{13.4}$$

where $|C|$ is the length of the bit-stream. A theoretical estimate or an upper bound C'_{ap} for the real capacity is

$$C'_{\text{ap}} = N_R + N_S + N_R \log\left(\frac{N_R}{N_R + N_S}\right) + N_S \log\left(\frac{N_S}{N_R + N_S}\right). \tag{13.5}$$

An ideal lossless context-free compression scheme (the entropy coder) would compress the RS-vector consisting of $(N_R + N_S)$ bits using $-N_R \cdot \log\left(\frac{N_R}{N_R+N_S}\right) - N_S \cdot \log\left(\frac{N_S}{N_R+N_S}\right)$ bits.

This estimate for C'_{ap} will be positive whenever there is a bias between the number of R and S groups, or when $N_R \neq N_S$. This bias is influenced by the size and shape of the group G, the discrimination function f, the amplitude of the invertible noisy permutation F, and the content of the original image. The bias increases with the group size and the amplitude of the permutation F. Smoother and less noisy images lead to a larger bias than images that are highly textured or noisy.

In a practical application, for some natural images, by defining a different discrimination function f, choosing the group size, selecting the number of the pixels that should be flipped, or selecting embedding mask $M = [A_1, \cdots, A_n]$ for example, the embedding capacity can be further improved.

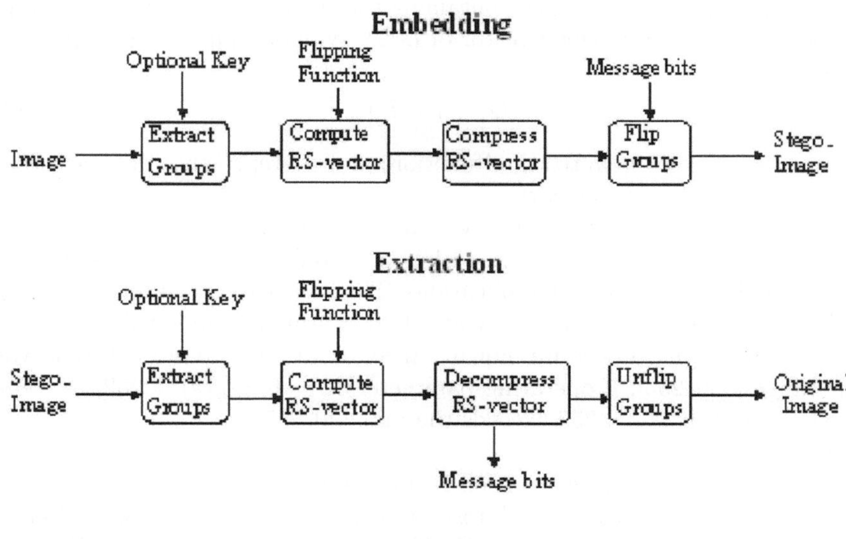

Fig. 13.4. Diagram for the distortion-free data embedding and extraction algorithm.

The method provides a high embedding capacity while introducing a very small and invertible distortion. A number of experimental results show that the highest capacity was obtained for relatively small groups where n is approximately equal to four.

Lossless G-LSB Data-Embedding Method

Celik et al. [8] presented a high capacity, low distortion reversible data hiding technique. A generalization of the least significant bit (GLSB) modification is proposed as the data-embedding method. Lossless recovery of the host signal is achieved by compressing the lowest levels instead of the bit planes of the signal. The levels chosen were those susceptible to embedding distortion and transmitting the resulting compressed bitstream as a part of the embedding payload. The CALIC compression algorithm, which uses the unaltered portions of the host signal as side information, improves the compression efficiency and, thus, the data-embedding capacity.

Generalized-LSB (G-LSB) Embedding

A generalization of LSB-embedded method, namely G-LSB, is employed by Celik et al. [8]. If the host signal is represented by a vector, G-LSB embedding and extraction can be represented as:

$$s_w = Q_L(s) + w, \tag{13.6}$$

$$w = s_w - Q_L(s_w), \tag{13.7}$$

where s_w represents the signal containing the embedded information, w represents the embedded payload vector of L-ary symbols. That is, $w_i \in \{0, 1, \ldots, L-1\}$, and

$$Q_L(x) = L \left\lfloor \frac{x}{L} \right\rfloor \tag{13.8}$$

is an L-level scalar quantization function, and $\lfloor \cdot \rfloor$ represents the operation of truncation to the integer part.

In the embedding procedure given in Eq. (13.6), for L-ary watermark symbols w_i, it is necessary for them to be converted into binary bit-stream and vice versa in some practical applications. The binary to L-ary conversion algorithm given below, can effectively avoid out-of-range sample values produced by the embedding procedure. For instance, in an 8 bpp representation where the range is $[0, 255]$, if operating parameters $L = 6$, $Q_L(s) = 252$, $w = 5$ are used, the output $s_w = 257$ exceeds the range $[0, 255]$.

The binary to L-ary conversion is presented as follows:
The binary input string h is interpreted as the binary representation of a number H in the interval $R = [0, 1)$. That is, $H = .h_0 h_1 h_2 \cdots$ and $H \in [0, 1)$. The signal is encoded using integer values between zero and $s_{\max}$.

1) Given s and $s_{\max}$, determine $Q_L(s)$ and $N = \min(L, s_{\max} - Q_L(s))$ the number of possible levels.
2) Divide R into N equal subintervals, R_0 to R_{N-1}.
3) Select the subinterval that satisfies $H \in R_n$.
4) The watermark symbol is $w = n$.
5) Set $R = R_n$ and then go to Step 1, for the next sample.

The conversion process is illustrated in Fig. 13.5. The inverse conversion process is performed by the dual of the above algorithm. This process is given below.

1) Given s and $s_{\max}$, determine $Q_L(s)$ and $N = \min(L, s_{\max} - Q_L(s_w))$ which is the number of possible levels.

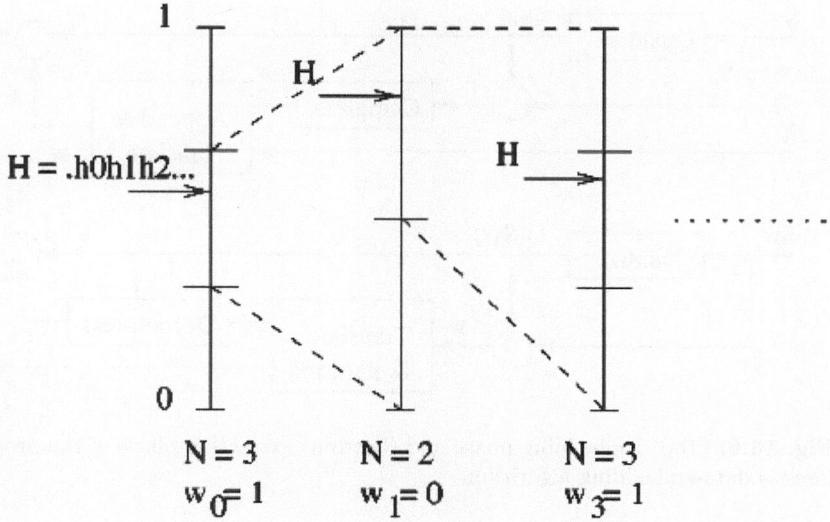

Fig. 13.5. Binary to L-ary conversion using a variant of arithmetic encoding.

2) Divide R into N equal subintervals, R_0 to R_{N-1}.
3) Set $R = R_w$, where $w = s_w - Q_L(s_w)$ is the current watermark symbol.
4) If there are remaining symbols, go to Step 1. Find shortest binary string $H \in R$.

The classical LSB modification, which embeds a binary symbol (bit) by overwriting the least significant bit of a signal sample, is a special case. Here $L = 2$. G-LSB embedding enables the embedding of a non-integer number of bits in each signal sample. Thus, it introduces new operating points along the rate- or capacity-distortion curve.

Lossless Generalized-LSB Data Embedding And Extraction

Fig. 13.6 shows a block diagram of the proposed algorithm. In the embedding phase, the host signal is quantized and the residual is obtained in Eq. (13.9). Then they adopt the CALIC lossless image compression algorithm. This has the quantized values as side information, to efficiently compress the quantization residuals in order to create high capacity for the payload data. The compressed residual and the payload data are concatenated and embedded into the host signal using the generalized-LSB modification method. The resulting bit stream is converted to L-ary symbols as mentioned above. This is then added to the quantized host to form the watermarked signal s_w in Eq. (13.6). Note that the compression block uses the rest of the host signal, $Q_L(s)$, as side-information, to facilitate better compression and higher capacity.

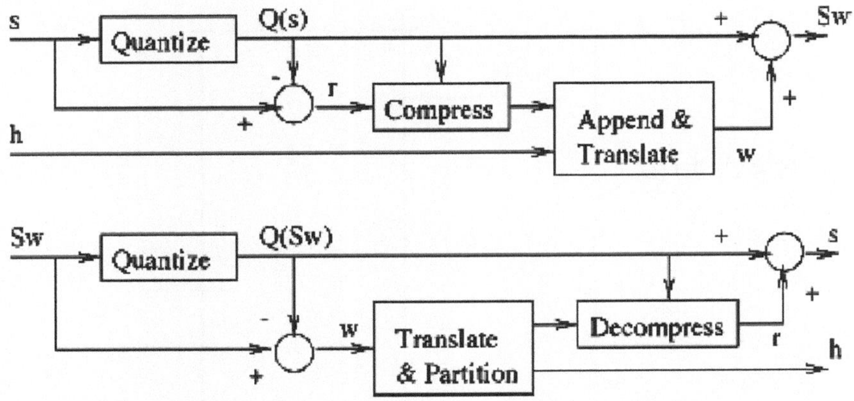

Fig. 13.6. (Top) Embedding phase and (bottom) extraction phase of the proposed lossless data-embedding algorithm.

In the extraction phase, the watermarked signal s_w is quantized and the watermark payload h which is the compressed residual and the payload data is extracted in Eq. (13.9). The residual r is decompressed by $Q_L(s_w) = s - Q_L(s)$ as side information. The original host is reconstructed by replacing the lowest levels of the watermarked signal by the residual in Eq. (13.10):

$$r = s - Q_L(s), \quad (13.9)$$

$$s = Q_L(s) + r = Q_L(s_w) + r. \quad (13.10)$$

The lossless-embedding capacity of the system is given by

$$C_{\text{Lossless}} = C_{\text{GLSB}} - C_{\text{residual}}, \quad (13.11)$$

where C_{Lossless} is the raw capacity of GLSB embedding ($C_{\text{GLSB}} = \log_2(L)$) and C_{residual} is the capacity consumed by the compressed residual. To further improving the lossless embedding capacity, Celik et al. adopt CALIC lossless image compression algorithm [13, 15]. This uses the unaltered portions of the host signal, $Q_L(s)$ as side-information, to efficiently compress the residual.

From what is reported in [8], Celik et al. applied several test images, F-16, Mandrill and Barbara to the lossless G-LSB algorithm with its selective embedding extension, Celik et al. compare the results with the RS embedding scheme [7]. The amplitude of the flipping function varied from 1 to 6. The lossless G-LSB algorithm at 100% embedding outperforms the RS embedding scheme from a capacity distortion perspective at most points except for the lowest distortion points at $A = 1$ and $L = 2$. The reason is that RS embedding modifies the pixels corresponding to the R and S groups while skipping U groups. By modifying the embedding extension from 100% to 75%, the lossless G-LSB algorithm slightly surpasses RS embedding at the lowest distortion points. From the above description, the LGLSB (Lossless G-LSB) algorithm can operate at a specified distortion value by flexibly modifying the embedding intensity, or an extension at a given level. The LGLSB also has an advantage over the RS embedding scheme in embedding capacity for a comparable distortion, computational complexity. The LGLSB algorithm can achieve embedding capacities exceeding 1bpp, while RS embedding's capacities was less than 1 bpp.

13.3.2 Algorithms Based on Histogram Shifting Techniques

Ni et al. [9] proposed a novel reversible algorithm based on histogram shifting techniques. The algorithm first finds a zero point (no pixel) and a peak point (a maximum number of pixels) of the image histogram. If zero point does not exist for some image histogram, a minimum point with a minimum number of pixels is treated as a zero point by memorizing the pixel grayscale value and the coordinates of those pixels as overhead information. Paper [9] shifts peak point towards the zero point by one unit and embeds the data in the peak point and the neighboring point. The specified embedding process is illustrated in Fig. 13.7.

Note that original peak point after embedding disappears in the histogram. Hence, to ensure the reversible restoration, the embedding algorithm needs to memorize the zero point and peak point as a part of the overhead information. The algorithm can embed a significant amount of data (5 k to 80 kbits for a $512 \times 512 \times 8$ grayscale image) while keeping a very high visual quality for all natural images. Specifically, the PSNR of the marked image versus the original image is guaranteed to be higher than 48 dB.

13.3.3 Algorithms Based on Value Expansion Techniques

Integer DCT Based Bit-Shifting Method

Yang et al.'s method [10] is based on the block 8×8 integer discrete cosine transform (DCT) domain. It applies the one-bit left shifted operation to all selected $N \leq 64$ AC coefficients, and then embeds watermarking bits in their LSBs. The parameter selection can be adjusted according to the required visual quality or embedding capacity. Yang et al. [10] first estimates the pixel values errors and then sets two thresholds (in the range of $[0, 255]$) to select suitable blocks where all pixel values must fall between two thresholds. These selected blocks are embedded with watermarking bits without concerning overflow or underflow caused by the modification of DCT coefficients. To differentiate watermarked image blocks from ineligible, or unsuitable blocks, Yang et al. [10] use additional overhead bits to record the watermarked blocks locations. These overhead bits are embedded in those blocks, which are proof against overflows and underflows after doing embedding process twice. The method is known as a Block Discrimination Method "twice-try."

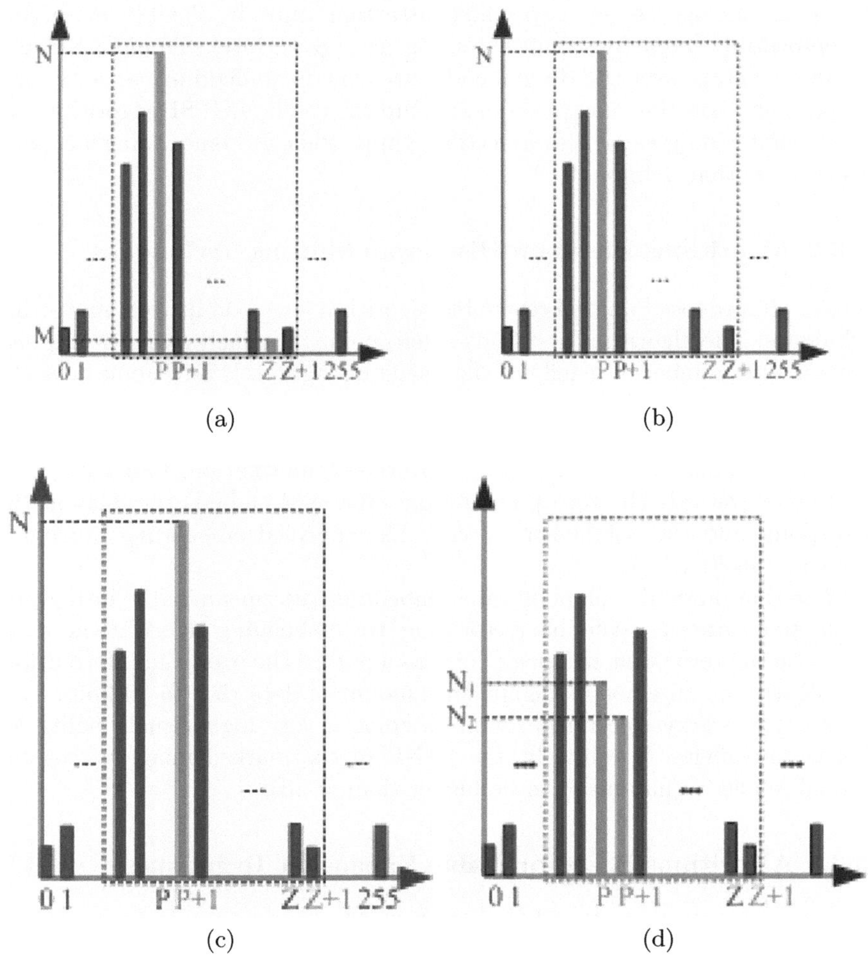

Fig. 13.7. (a) The histogram with the minimum point Z and peak point P. (b) The histogram with setting minimum point as zero point Z and peak point P. (c) Shift the points in the range of $[P, Z-1]$ one unit toward zero point Z. (d) The histogram after embedding.

At the decoder, the proposed method first identifies the twice-embedding permitted blocks and then retrieves the overhead bits recording information on the location of the other blocks used for embedding. These are known as Once-Embedding Permitted Blocks. By overhead bits, Once-Embedding Permitted Blocks is determined from the unsuitable blocks. The original DCT coefficients are retrieved by dividing watermarked DCT coefficients by 2.

From the reported information in [10], the proposed scheme shows an advantage in capacity while retaining good quality of watermarked image.

The Reversible Method Based on the Difference Expansion Method

Tian [11] presented a high-capacity approach based on expanding the pixel difference value between neighboring pixels. His method allows one bit to be embedded in every pair of pixels.

The main idea of his technique is given below. For a pair of 8 bits grayscale-valued x and y, they first compute the integer average l and difference h of x and y, where

$$l = \left\lfloor \frac{x+y}{2} \right\rfloor, \quad h = x - y. \tag{13.12}$$

The inverse transform of Eq. (13.12) is

$$x = l + \left\lfloor \frac{h+1}{2} \right\rfloor, \quad y := l - \left\lfloor \frac{h}{2} \right\rfloor. \tag{13.13}$$

The reversible integer transforms in Eqs. (13.12) and (13.13) is called Integer Haar Wavelet Transform, or the S transform. They shift h to the left one unit and append the watermarking bit b in LSB (Least Significant Bit) according to Eq. (13.14),

$$h' = 2 \times h + b. \tag{13.14}$$

This reversible data-embedding operation given in Eq. (13.14) is called the Difference Expansion (DE).

To prevent overflow and underflow problems, that is to restrict x and y in the range of $[0, 255]$, h must satisfy the condition in Eq. (13.15). Here the inverse transform is computed as,

$$|h| \leq \min\left(2 \cdot (255 - l),\ 2l - 1\right). \tag{13.15}$$

The authors classify Difference Values into four disjoint sets according to the following definitions.

(1) The first set, EZ, contains all the expandable $h = 0$ and the expandable $h = -1$.
(2) The second set, EN, contains all the expandable $h \notin EZ$.
(3) The third set, CN, contains all the changeable h which are not in $EZ \cup EN$.
(4) The fourth set, NC, contains the rest of h, which are not able to be changed.

Definition 1 *A difference value h is expandable under the integer average value l if $|2 \times h + b| \leq \min\left(2 \cdot (255 - l),\ 2l - 1\right)$ for both $b = 0$ and 1.*

Definition 2 *A Difference Value h is changeable under the integer average value l if* $\left|2 \times \left\lfloor \frac{h}{2} \right\rfloor + b\right| \leq \min\left(2 \cdot (255 - l),\ 2l - 1\right)$ *for both* $b = 0$ *and* 1.

From Definitions 1 and 2, it can be proved that:

1) A changeable difference value h remains changeable even after modifying its LSB.
2) An expandable difference value h is changeable.
3) After the DE, the expanded difference value h' is changeable.
4) If $h = 0$ or -1, the conditions for expandable and changeable are equivalent.

At the receiving end, to extract embedding data and restore the original image, the expandable, changeable, and non-changeable sets must be identified. Since an expanded difference value via the DE h' and a changeable difference value with its modified LSB are both changeable after embedding , which is mentioned above. All difference values in NC (not changeable) can be unambiguously identified during extraction using the condition in Eq. (13.15). It is necessary to know which difference value has been selected for the DE. That is, some additional information needs to be used to further identify all the expanded difference values via the DE from all the changeable values. The authors create a binary location map, which contains the location information of all selected expandable difference values, as an overhead for later reconstruction of the original image.

To achieve the payload capacity limit, they select all expandable differences that are in the range of $[-255, 255]$ for the DE, but the peak signal to noise ratio (PSNR) value is generally very low and the visual quality degradation of the watermarked image is almost perceptible. To build a balance between the PSNR value and payload size, they present two selection methods to reduce payload size which is less than the payload capacity limit, and consequently improve the PSNR value. The first method is described as follows. They select h with small magnitudes for the DE. That is, they choose a threshold value T, $h \in [-T, T]$, partition EN into EN_1 and EN_2. Using $EN_1 = \{h \in EN : |h| \leq T\}$, $EN_2 = \{h \in EN : |h| > T\}$. For a payload whose size is equal to the payload capacity limit $EN_1 = EN$, and $EN_2 = \emptyset$. For an h in $EZ \cup EN_1$, a value of '1' is assigned in the location map; for a value of h in $EN_2 \cup CN \cup NC$, a value of '0' is assigned. Hence a value of '1' indicates the selected expandable difference values.

The embedding process is generalized as follows. After creating the location map, it is compressed without loss using a JBIG2 compression or an arithmetic compression coding to form a bitstream L. For every h in $EN_2 \cup CN$, LSB (h) is stored in a bitstream C. The payload P, including an authentication hash of the original image (for example, MD5), bitstream L and bitstream C are concatenated to form final binary bitstream B. They then embed B into LSBs of one bit left-shifted versions of difference values in $EZ \cup EN_1$ and also into LSBs of difference values in $EN_2 \cup CN$. In the embedding process, the difference values in NC is kept intact.

Table 13.1. Embedding on difference values.

Category	Original Set	Original Set	Location Map Value	New Value	New Set
Changeable	EZ or EN_1	h	1	$2 \times h + b$	CH
	EN_2 or CN	h	0	$2 \times \lfloor \frac{h}{2} \rfloor + b$	
Non-Changeable	NC	h	0	h	NC

The data embedding by replacement is illustrated in Table 13.1. After all bits in B are embedded, they then apply the inverse transform in Eq. (13.13) to obtain the embedded image.

The extraction process starts by calculating the average value $\tilde{l}$ and the difference value $\tilde{h}$ of pixel pairs $(\tilde{x}, \tilde{y})$ by scanning the watermarked image in the same order used during embedding. Referring to Table 13.1, they divide pixel pairs into two sets CH (changeable) and NC (not changeable) using the condition given in Eq. (13.15). They extracts all LSBs of $\tilde{h}$ for each pair in CH to form a bitstream B which is identical to that formed during embedding. The extracted bitstream B is decompressed to restore the location map by a JBIG2 decoder. Hence, all expanded pixel pairs after the DE in CH are identified. By identifying an end of message symbol at its end for a JBIG2, bitstream C including the original LSBs of the changeable difference in $EN_2 \cup CN$ and the payload is retrieved. The original values of differences are restored as follows. For $\tilde{h}$ in $EZ \cup EN_1$, they restore the original values of $\tilde{h}$ as follows:

$$h = \left\lfloor \frac{\tilde{h}}{2} \right\rfloor . \tag{13.16}$$

For $\tilde{h}$ in $EN_2 \cup CN$, they restore the original values of according to the following Eq. (13.17).

$$h = 2 \times \left\lfloor \frac{\tilde{h}}{2} \right\rfloor + b_1, \quad b_1 \in C. \tag{13.17}$$

Finally, they apply the inverse transform given in Eq. (13.13) to retrieve the original image. They then compare the retrieved authentication hash with the hash function of the restored image. If the two hash functions match exactly, the image content is authentic and the restored image is exactly the same as the original image.

Tian implemented the DE method and tested the method on various standard grayscale images. Tian also implemented the RS lossless data-embedding method in [7] and the lossless G-LSB data-embedding method in [8] in order to compare the results among the three methods using 512×512, 8 bpp grayscale Lena. From the comparison results described in [11], Tian achieves the highest embedding capacity, while keeping the lowest distortion. Except for images with large very smooth regions, the payload capacity limit of the G-LSB method does not exceed 1 bpp. The DE method could easily embed more than 1 bpp. The payload capacity limit of the RS method is lower than both the G-LSB and the DE method. By embedding a payload of the same bit length, the embedded Lena image by the DE method is about 2 to 3 dB higher than both the G-LSB and the RS method.

13.3.4 The Reversible Method Based on the Difference Expansion Method of Vectors

Alatter [12] presented a high-capacity, data-hiding algorithm. The proposed algorithm is based on a generalized, reversible, integer transform, which calculates the average and pair-wise differences between the elements of a vector extracted from the pixels of the image. Several conditions are derived and used in selecting the appropriate difference values. Watermark bits are embedded into either the LSBs (least significant bits) of selected differences or alternatively the LSBs are one bit left-shifted versions of selected differences. Derived conditions can identify which difference is selected after embedding to ensure new vector computed from average and embedded difference has grayscale values. To ensure reversibility, the locations of shifted differences and the original LSBs must be embedded before embedding the payload. The proposed algorithm can embed $N-1$ bits in every vector with a size of $N \times 1$.

The proposed algorithm is based on a Generalized, Reversible, Integer Transform (GRIT). We will now introduce the theorem for GRIT.

Theorem 3 *For* $Du = [a, d_1, d_2, \cdots, d_{N-1}]^T$, *if* $v = \lfloor Du \rfloor$, *then* $u = \lceil D^{-1} \lfloor v \rfloor \rceil$. *$v$ and u form a GRIT pair, where D is an $N \times N$ full-rank matrix with an inverse D^{-1}, u is an $N \times 1$ integer column vector, a is the weighted average value of the elements of u, $d_1, d_2, \cdots, d_{N-1}$. These are the independent pair-wise differences between the elements of u, $\lceil \cdot \rceil$ and $\lfloor \cdot \rfloor$ respectively. It indicates round up or down to the nearest integer.*

The proof is given in Alatter [12].

Alatter generalized the algorithm based on GRIT to vectors of length of more than 3. Alatter uses an example in which $N = 4$. One possible value of D is given by

$$D = \begin{bmatrix} {a_0}/{c} & {a_1}/{c} & {a_2}/{c} & {a_3}/{c} \\ -1 & 1 & 0 & 0 \\ 0 & -1 & 1 & 0 \\ 0 & 0 & -1 & 1 \end{bmatrix}, \tag{13.18}$$

where $c = \sum_{i=0}^{N-1} a_i, 0 \le i \le 3$, and

$$D^{-1} = \begin{bmatrix} 1 - (c-a_0)/_c & -(a_2+a_3)/_c & -a_3/_c \\ 1 & a_0/_c & -(a_2+a_3)/_c & -a_3/_c \\ 1 & a_0/_c & (a_0+a_1)/_c & -a_3/_c \\ 1 & a_0/_c & (a_0+a_1)/_c & (c-a_3)/_c \end{bmatrix}. \tag{13.19}$$

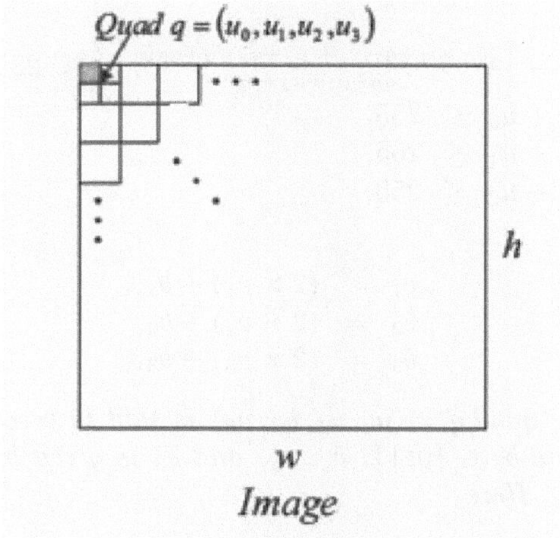

Fig. 13.8. Quads configuration in an image.

Using the above theorem, for the vector $q = (u_0, u_1, u_2, u_3)$, the appropriate GRIT may be defined as:

$$\begin{cases} v_0 = \left\lfloor \frac{a_0u_0+a_1u_1+a_2u_2+a_3u_3}{a_0+a_1+a_2+a_3} \right\rfloor, \\ v_1 = u_1 - u_0, \\ v_2 = u_2 - u_1, \\ v_3 = u_3 - u_2. \end{cases} \tag{13.20}$$

$$\begin{cases} u_0 = v_0 - \left\lfloor \frac{(a_0+a_1+a_2)v_1+(a_2+a_3)v_2+a_3v_3}{a_0+a_1+a_2+a_3} \right\rfloor, \\ u_1 = v_1 + u_0, \\ u_2 = v_2 + u_1, \\ u_3 = v_3 + u_2. \end{cases} \tag{13.21}$$

To describe the reversible algorithm in detail and unambiguously, we choose quads to introduce the embedding process and the detection process. A quad is a 1×4 vector formed from four pixel values chosen from four different locations each having the same component according to a predetermined order. Each quad is assembled from 2×2 adjacent pixel values in Alatter's algorithm (Fig. 13.8). Each pixel quad of the original image is classified into three groups according to the following definitions.

(1) The first group, contains all expandable quads having $v_1 \le T_1$, $v_2 \le T_2$, and $v_3 \le T_3$. T_1, T_2 and T_3 are predefined thresholds.
(2) The second group, S_2 contains all changeable pairs which are not in S_1.
(3) The third group, S_3 contains the rest of the pairs and these are not changeable.

Definition 4 *The quad $q = (u_0, u_1, u_2, u_3)$ is said to be expandable if for all values of b_1, b_2 and $b_3 \in \{0, 1\}$*

$$\begin{array}{lcl} 0 \le \tilde{v}_0 - \left\lfloor \frac{(a_0+a_1+a_2)\tilde{v}_1+(a_2+a_3)\tilde{v}_2+a_3\tilde{v}_3}{a_0+a_1+a_2+a_3} \right\rfloor \le 255, \\ 0 \le \tilde{v}_1 + u_0 \le 255, \\ 0 \le \tilde{v}_2 + u_1 \le 255, \\ 0 \le \tilde{v}_3 + u_2 \le 255, \end{array} \tag{13.22}$$

where

$$\begin{array}{lcl} \tilde{v}_1 &=& (2 \times v_1) + b_1, \\ \tilde{v}_2 &=& (2 \times v_2) + b_2, \\ \tilde{v}_3 &=& (2 \times v_3) + b_3. \end{array} \tag{13.23}$$

Definition 5 *The quad $q = (u_0, u_1, u_2, u_3)$ is said to be changeable if for all values of b_1, b_2 and $b_3 \in \{0, 1\}$, $\tilde{v}_1$, $\tilde{v}_2$, and $\tilde{v}_3$ is given by Eq. (13.24), and satisfy Eq. (13.22). Here*

$$\begin{array}{lcl} \tilde{v}_1 &=& 2 \times \left\lfloor \frac{v_1}{2} \right\rfloor + b_1, \\ \tilde{v}_2 &=& 2 \times \left\lfloor \frac{v_2}{2} \right\rfloor + b_2, \\ \tilde{v}_3 &=& 2 \times \left\lfloor \frac{v_3}{2} \right\rfloor + b_3. \end{array} \tag{13.24}$$

Each of v_1, v_2 and v_3 in S_1 was shifted left by one bit to form $\tilde{v}_1$, $\tilde{v}_2$, and $\tilde{v}_3$. Watermark bits b_1, b_2 and b_3 are respectively appended in the LSBs of $\tilde{v}_1$, $\tilde{v}_2$, and $\tilde{v}_3$. The conditions in Eq. (13.22) ensure that new quad which is computed using v_0, $\tilde{v}_1$, $\tilde{v}_2$, and $\tilde{v}_3$ according to the inverse transform had grayscale values. v_1, v_2 and v_3 in S_2 are the same as $\tilde{v}_1$, $\tilde{v}_2$, and $\tilde{v}_3$ with replaced LSBs with watermark bits. A changeable quad after LSB has been modified is still changeable. An expandable quad is also changeable.

The locations of all the quads in S_1 are indicated by 1's in a binary location map. The JBIG algorithm is used to compress the map to produce the bitstream B_1. The LSBs of v_1, v_2 and v_3 of all the quads in S_2 are now extracted into a bitstream B_2. The payload P, including the authentication hash (MD5) of original image, bitstream B_1 and B_2 are concatenated to form B. Finally, the bitstream B is embedded into LSBs of one-bit left-shifted versions of difference values in S_1. For any quad in S_2, a bit is embedded in the difference by replacing the LSB.

Since the embedding process is completely reversible, the algorithm can be applied to the image recursively to embed more data. However, the difference between the original image and the embedded image increases with every application of the algorithm. Fig. 13.9 depicts four different structures that can be used to permute a quad which is a 1×4 vector.

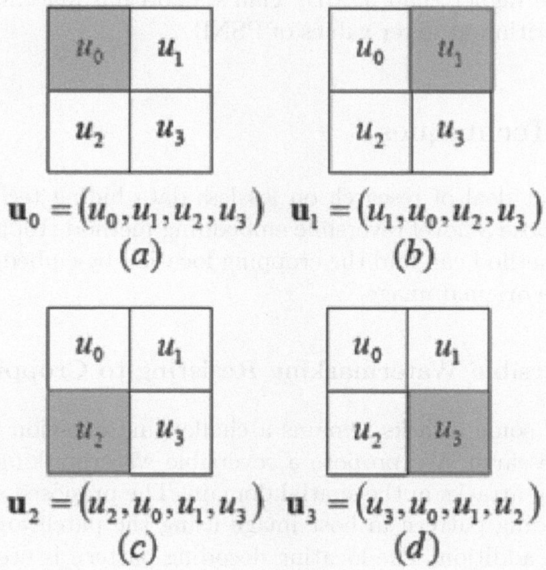

Fig. 13.9. Quads configuration in an image.

The retrieval process starts by identifying all the changeable quads in the embedded image using the conditions in Eq. (13.22). The LSBs of the difference values of all the changeable quads are collected to form a bitstream B. The JBIG algorithm is then used to decompress bitstream B to retrieve the location map. By use of the location map, all expandable quads are separated from the changeable quads. The original image can be restored by dividing each difference in the expandable quads by 2, and replacing the LSBs of each difference in the changeable quads with the retrieved original bits. The retrieved authentication hash is compared to the hash function of the restored image. If they match exactly, the image content is authentic and the restored image will be exactly the same as the original image.

Alatter tested the quad-based algorithm on several test image. These were Fruits, Lena and Baboon. The experimental results indicate that the achievable embedding capacity depends on the nature of the image. The algorithm performs much better with Fruits and Lena than with Baboon. It performs slightly better with Fruits than with Lena. With Fruits, the algorithm is able to embed 982 kB (3.74 bits/pixel) with a image quality of 28.42 dB. It is also able to embed 296 kB (0.77 bits/pixel) with the high image quality of 39.05 dB. With Baboon the algorithm is able to embed 808 kB (3.08 bits/pixel) at 20.18 dB and 130 kB (0.50 bits/pixel) at 32.62 dB.

Alatter respectively compared the performance of quad-based algorithm [12] with that of Tian's method described in [11] using grayscale Lena and Barbara images. The results indicate that quad-based algorithm outperforms Tian's at a PSNR value higher than 35 dB. Tian's algorithm marginally outperforms Alatter's algorithm at lower values of PSNR.

13.4 Our Techniques

We did a great deal of research on lossless data hiding techniques and as a result we propose a novel reversible embedding method [16] to resist cropping attack. The method can find the cropping location by embedding the locating pattern in the original image.

13.4.1 Reversible Watermarking Resisting to Cropping Attack

How to resist some attacks remains a challenging question in reversible watermarking research. We propose a reversible watermarking scheme able to resist cropping attacks in the spatial domain. The proposed scheme embeds a locating decoding pattern in host image using the patchwork algorithm and a modulo 256 addition. The locating decoding pattern is used to retrieve the cropped positions in the given watermarked image which was possibly cropped during the extraction process. The locating decoding pattern modifies a small partition of pixel values in each disjoint image block. An improved difference expansion (DE) method is proposed to embed a payload known as an authentication hash to the original image block. This introduced into the rest of the pixel values in each image block. The traditional modulo additions would cause an annoying visual artifact similar to the salt-and-pepper noise. The scheme adopts the method of keeping the flipped pixels unchanged to effectively avoid an artifact. Since we use the image ID and the block index as the input to the hash function, the scheme can efficiently resist to the collage attack. Experimental results show that the scheme can achieve good robustness against both cropping attack and collage attack.

13.4.2 The Improved Difference Expansion Method

Tian [11] classifies difference values into three disjoint sets according to the above definitions. The first set contains all selected expandable differences. The second set contains all those expandable but which are not in the first set and all the changeable differences. The third set contains the rest of the differences which are not changeable. Tian uses a location map to record the positions of those selected expandable differences in the original image. The location map is losslessly compressed and the compressed bitstream is embedded into the host image as an overhead for using the later reconstruction of the original image. The compressed location map would consume certain hiding capacity. Our method largely reduces the length of the compressed bitstream by adopting different classification method.

Class 1: A difference value h is classified as belonging to the first class under the integer average value l if for all values of $b_1 \in \{0, 1\}$, given by Eq. (13.14), h' does not satisfy the condition in Eq. (13.15).

Class 2: A difference value h is classified into the second class under the integer average value l if for all values of $b_1 \in \{0, 1\}$, given by Eq. (13.14), h' does satisfy the condition in Eq. (13.15). For all values of $b_2 \in \{0, 1\}$, h'', given by Eq. (13.25), does not satisfy the condition in Eq. (13.15),

$$h'' = 2 \times h' + b_2. \tag{13.25}$$

Class 3: A difference value h is classified into the third class under the integer average value l if for all values of $b_1 \in \{0, 1\}$, given by Eq. (13.14). The value h' does satisfy the condition in Eq. (13.15), and for all values of $b_2 \in \{0, 1\}$. The value h'', given by Eq. (13.25), satisfies the condition in Eq. (13.15).

After we embed watermark bits w into some pixel pairs of class 2, these watermarked pixel pairs can be classified as Class 2 or Class 3 in the decoding process. Those especial pixel pairs are called as the Flipping Class 2. We take an example in order to introduce the Flipping Class 2.

A pair of pixel values $(x = 194, y = 219)$ is selected from Class 2, and $(l, h) = (206, -25)$ is then obtained according to Eq. (13.12). Owing to the embedded bit $b_1 \in \{0, 1\}$, the h' via Eq. (13.14) is equal to -49 or -50. On the decoding side, the average value l and watermarked difference value h' are obtained via the integer transform Eq. (13.12). If h' is -50, h'' according to Eq. (13.25) does not satisfy the condition in Eq. (13.15). However, if h' is -49, the value h'' via Eq. (13.25) does satisfy the condition Eq. (13.15). Therefore, h' may be classified as Class 3 or Class 2 in the decoding process.

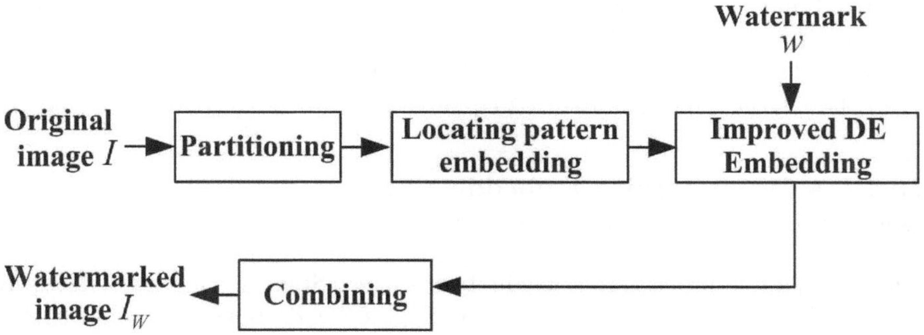

Fig. 13.10. General framework of watermark embedding scheme.

Those flipping pixel pairs are classified into the Flipping Class 2. The values h and l have certain relationships for those pixel pairs. That is, $|2 \times (2 \times h + b_1) + b_2| = \min(2 \cdot (255 - l),\ 2l - 1)$ for all values of $b_1 \in \{0, 1\}$ and $b_2 \in \{0, 1\}$.

13.4.3 The Locating Decoding Pattern

General scheme for reversible watermarking is shown in Fig. 13.10. The host image is partitioned into not-overlapping blocks with size $N \times N$ starting from top-left corner. All disjoint image blocks are denoted as $B_k(x, y)$, where $1 \leq x,\ y \leq N,\ 1 \leq k \leq n$, and n is the total number of blocks in the image. The locating decoding pattern is the size of the whole image, created by tiling, using the same basic pattern (block) of size $N \times N$. We use a one-to-one correspondence between each image block and the basic decoding pattern in x and y coordinates.

We assume that the value at each point in the locating decoding pattern is initialized to zero. Independently in the basic decoding pattern, we utilize the same random generator to determine a small partition of all N^2 points. There are a total of 100 points. These are divided into two equal sets of points, A and B. A given intensity correspond to δ value used below is respectively added to and subtracted from the values at all the points of the patches A and B. We add a small constant value δ to the values at all the points of patch and subtract the same value δ from the values at all the points of patch B. Hence, the values of all unchanged points remain zero, while the values of the changed points are δ or $-\delta$.

Some pixel values in the k-th image block, $B_k(x, y)$, having the same x and y coordinates as the points incremented or decremented by the δ value in the basic decoding pattern, correspond to add or subtract a constant value δ. This is done according to modulo 256 addition. Modulo additions would cause an annoying visual artifact resembling a correlated salt-and-pepper noise when the pixel values close to the maximally allowed value are flipped to zero and vice versa. To avoid the salt-and-pepper noise, we keep those flipping pixel values ($p \in ([0, 3] \cup [252, 255])$, $\delta = 4$), p is one pixel value) unchanged. We create a binary location map called as $pMap$ which contains the position information for all the changed pixels in the patches A and B. Symbol '1' indicates unchanged pixels and the symbol '0' denotes changed pixels of patches A and B in the $pMap$. The size of this is equal to the number of patches A and B.

13.4.4 A Watermarking Embedding Scheme Based on the Improved Difference Expansion Method

The embedding process is done in two stages. Stage 1 embeds a locating decoding pattern according to the method described above in Section 13.3.3.

The Stage 2, the embedding process is shown in Fig. 13.11. In each block, for the remnant pixels-instead of pixels selected for the locating decoding pattern, we employ an improved DE method to embed a payload. The remnant pixels are grouped into pairs of pixel values. A pair consists of two neighboring pixel values or two values with a small difference value. We apply the integer transform in Eq. (13.12) to each pair.

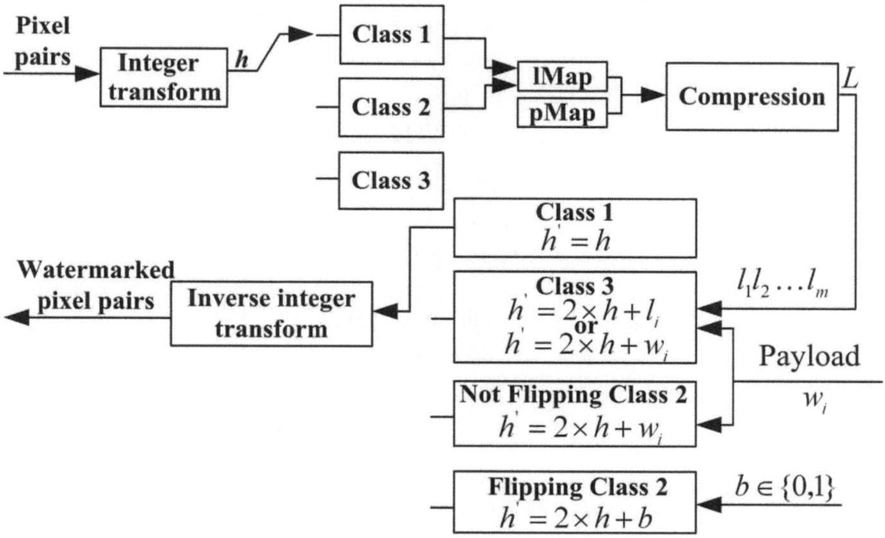

Fig. 13.11. Embedding process of the improved DE method.

According to a predefined scanning order, all the difference values are ordered as a one dimensional list $\{h_1, h_2, \ldots, h_n\}$. Then, difference values are classified into four classes according to Fig. 13.12. A location map denoted as $lMap$ is created to record the positions of Class 1, Class 2 and the Flipping Class 2. For the h in Class 1, we assign a value 1 in the $lMap$; for the value h in Class 2, we assign a value 0 in the $lMap$. $lMap$ and $pMap$ are concatenated to form a sub-bitstream l. l is losslessly compressed using arithmetic coding. The compressed sub-bitstream is denoted as the L.

In Class 1 h is kept intact. Considering h in the Flipping Class 2. If the embedded bit is 1, then h'_f via Eq. (13.14) is equal to $2 \times h + 1$, otherwise the value of h''_f is $2 \times h$. We select h'_f if h'_f does not satisfy the the condition Eq. (13.15), otherwise h''_f is selected. This ensures that the difference values in the Flipping Class 2 will be classified into the Class 2 during extraction.

All of L is embedded in the LSB space saved by the bit-shift operation over h of Class 3. Then most of real watermark bits including the hash function of image block, P, are embedded in the space saved by the bit-shift operation over the remanent h in Class 3. The remaining values of P are embedded into LSBs of the one-bit left shifted versions of h in Class 2. That is with the exception of Flipping Class 2.

Watermarking Decoding Scheme Based on the Improved Difference Expansion Method

The general framework of the watermark detection scheme is shown in Fig. 13.13. The locating decoding pattern is created by tiling with the basic

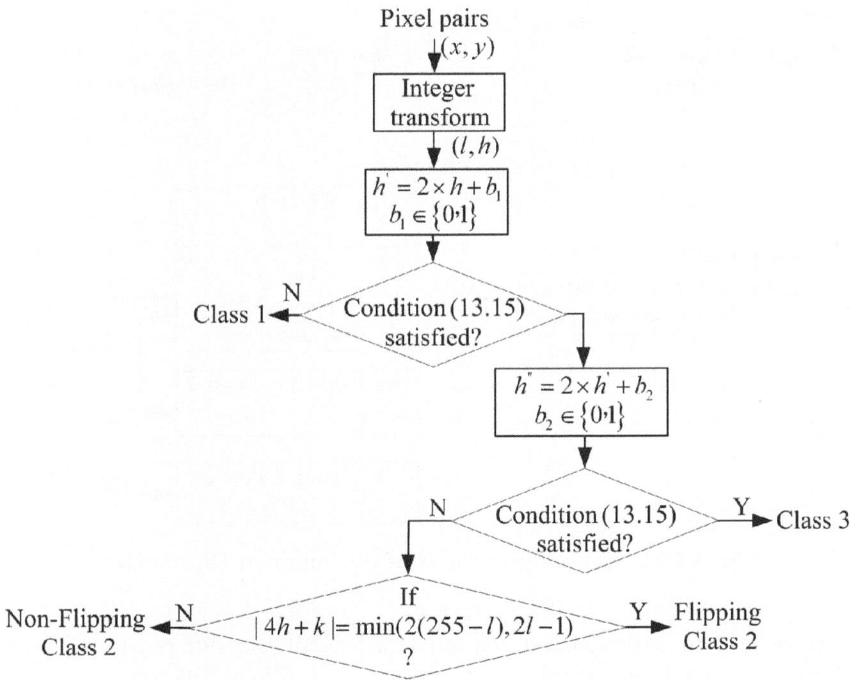

Fig. 13.12. Classification structure.

decoding pattern which has a size of $N \times N$. We obtain the height and width of the given image which may have been cropped and then compute the numbers $\left(\left\lceil\frac{\text{height}}{N}\right\rceil + 1\right) \times N$ and $\left(\left\lceil\frac{\text{width}}{N}\right\rceil + 1\right) \times N$. These calculated values are deemed to be the height and width of the locating decoding pattern.

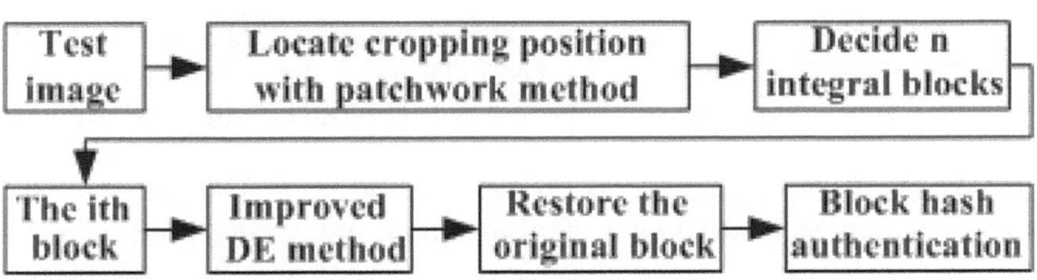

Fig. 13.13. General framework of the watermark detection scheme.

Stage 1: Locating

Align the top-left pixel of the given image with the top-left point of the locating decoding pattern. Translate the given image using the locating decoding pattern. Test all translations of the image against the locating decoding pattern. For example ensure that the top-left corner is within the top-left block $N \times N$ of the locating decoding pattern.

At each translation, evaluate $S = \sum_{i=1}^{n} (a_i - b_i)$ for the given image using the patches coordinates defined by the locating decoding pattern. In this expression, n represents the number of the pixel values selected for patch A or B during the embedding process. The values a_i and b_i respectively indicate the pixel values of a point pair in the given image. The same point pair in the locating decoding pattern is a patch pair whose values are respectively increased and decreased by δ during embedding. Determine the translation that produces the maximal S, and denote by (x'_1, y'_1) the translation parameters. The coordinates (x'_1, y'_1) indicate the deviation from the top-left pixel of the locating decoding pattern pixel. Ensure that the retrieved coordinates are in the correct cropped position. By (x'_1, y'_1), we obtain the remnant integral blocks. That is, every block of $N \times N$ size.

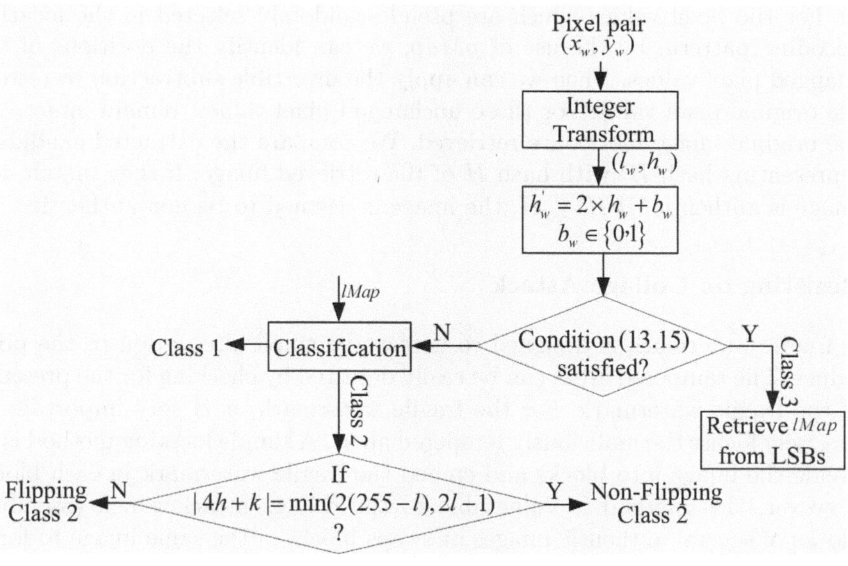

Fig. 13.14. The classification of pixel pairs during extraction.

Stage 2: Decoding and Authentication

For each integral block obtained, the remnant pixels are grouped into pairs of pixel values in each block. We then apply the integer transform given in Eq. (13.12) to each pair to calculate their average value l and difference value h. We use the same scanning order as that in embedding to place all difference values in a one dimensional list $\left\{\tilde{h}_1, \tilde{h}_2, \cdots, \tilde{h}_n\right\}$.

We can directly determine all difference values in Class 3 by using the retrieval algorithm itself without any additional information according to Fig. 13.14. We then collect the LSBs of all difference values in Class 3, and form a binary bitstream B. The bitstream B is decompressed to restore the location maps. That is, the $lMap$ and the $pMap$ by an arithmetic decoder. Hence, by $lMap$, we can differentiate between Class 1 and Class 2.

The original difference value h is restored as follows: for difference values $\tilde{h}$ in Class 1, $h = \tilde{h}$. For difference values $\tilde{h}$ in Class 2 and Class 3, $h = \left\lfloor \frac{\tilde{h}}{2} \right\rfloor$. The original pixel values computing from h and l using Eq. (13.13) are next obtained.

All watermarked bits including the hash function of the image blocks are obtained by using the expression $w = (\tilde{h} - 2 \times \lfloor \frac{\tilde{h}}{2} \rfloor)$ for Class 2 and Class 3. This can be done for any value of $k \in \{0, 1, 2, 3\}$, provided the inequations $|4 \times h + k| > \min(2 \times (255 - l), 2 \times l - 1)$ satisfy, h in Class 2. This is classified as the Flipping Class 2. Accordingly, the calculated binary numbers obtained using the above expression are useless and discarded.

For the pixel values which are pseudo-randomly selected in the locating decoding pattern, by the use of *pMap*, we can identify the positions of the changed pixel values. Then we can apply the invertible subtraction to restore the original pixel value. For those unchanged pixel values, remain intact. All the original image blocks are retrieved. We compare the extracted candidate representing hash H' with hash H of the retrieved image. If they match, the image is authentic. If $H' \neq H$, the image is deemed to be non-authentic.

Resisting on Collage Attack

A fragile watermark is designed to detect any small alternation to the pixel values. The tampered areas can be easily detected by checking for the presence of the fragile watermark. For the fragile watermark, it is very important to precisely locate the maliciously tempered areas. A simple locating method is to divide the image into blocks and embed the fragile watermark in each block. However, this method is vulnerable to the collage attack which assembles blocks of several authentic images or swaps blocks of the same image to forge a new authentic image.

Our scheme, based on a block-wise fragile watermark, also suffers from the collage attack. The attackers simulate our embedding method for another arbitrary, interconnected image and visibly copy a portion of its watermarked image to our watermarked image. During detection, since the retrieved hash matches with the hash function of the restored fake image block, our method is defeated. To resist collage attack, we utilize the method, proposed by Holliman et al. [17]. The method resolves this problem by adding the image ID and block index to the input of hash function.

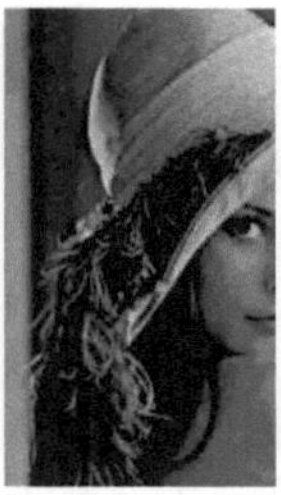

(a)
The cropped version of the watermarked image ($\delta = 4$)

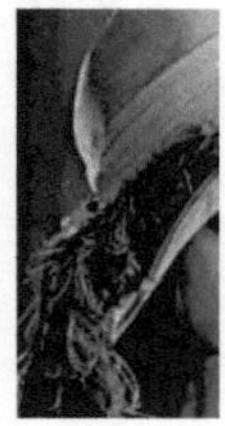

(b)
The restored image block corresponding to (a)

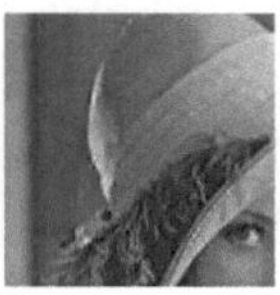

(c)
The cropped version of the watermarked image ($\delta = 8$)

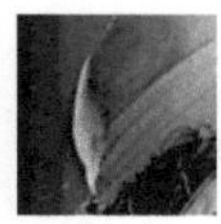

(d)
The restored image block corresponding to (c)

Fig. 13.15. The cropped watermarked image and the retrieved image.

In Fig. 13.15, generally δ is equal to 4. If the size of the cropped image is very small, for example the size being not larger than 32×32. To find the correct cropped position, we can for example select $\delta = 8$ in Fig. 13.15.

In the practical application, the watermarked image can suffer from collage attack. We use the image ID and the block index as the input to the hash function. The scheme can efficiently resist collage attack. Fig. 13.16 shows that our method can efficiently resist collage attack.

This chapter presents a detailed investigation on the development of all existing lossless data hiding techniques. The mechanism, the merits and the drawbacks of these techniques are discussed. In this chapter we introduce our own method for reversible watermarking.

13.5 The Future Research

High-capacity lossless data-embedding algorithms still provide an active research foreground. Robust lossless data-embedding algorithms have attracted considerable attention from researchers in recent years. Reversible algorithms such as JPEG compression are capable of retrieving watermarking information even if the watermarked images under attack. Shi et al. [18] note that robust lossless data hiding algorithms may find wide applications in semi-fragile authentication of JPEG2000 compressed images. Future research work

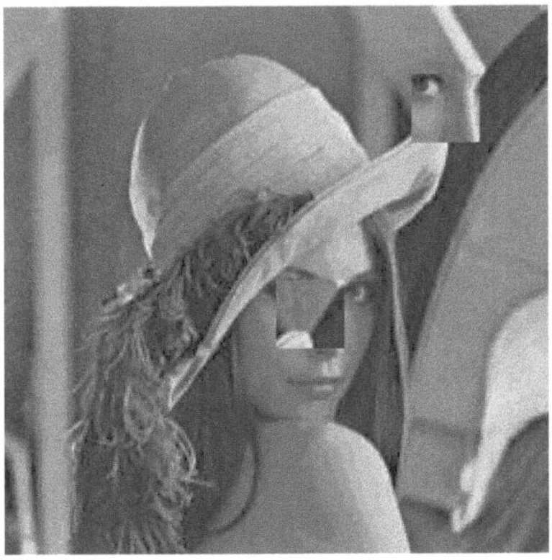

(a)
The tampered image by swapping two blocks of the same image

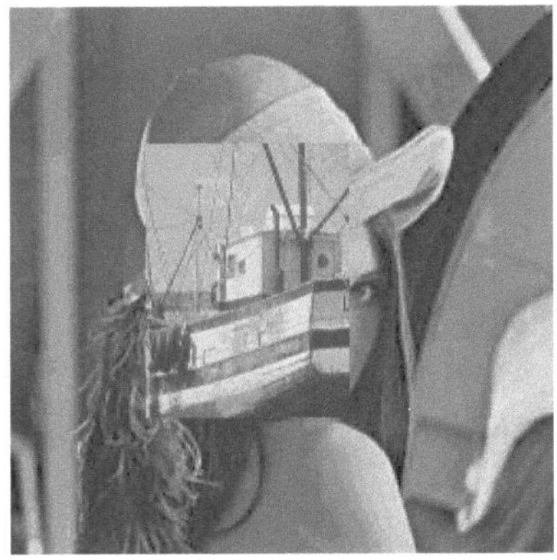

(b)
The tampered image by copying a portion of another image

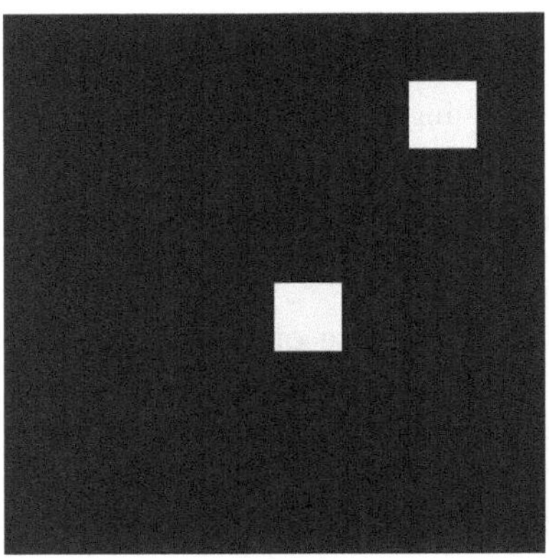

(c)
The result of fragile detection corresponding to (a)

(d)
The result of fragile detection corresponding to (b)

Fig. 13.16. The tampered image and the result of using fragile detection.

on reversible watermarking techniques still continue to be restricted in two aspects. That is, robustness and the provision of high-capacity.

References

1. Honsinger, C., Jones, P., Rabbani, M., and Stoffel, J. (1999): US Patent, No. US6278791
2. Macq, B. and Deweyand, F. (1999): Trusted headers for medical images. DFG VIII-D II Watermarking Workshop

3. Bender, W., Gruhl, D., and Morimoto, N. (1997): Techniques for data hiding. IBM Systems Journal, **35**, 313–336
4. De Vleeschouwer C., Delaigle, J.F., and Macq, B. (2001): Circular interpretation on histogram for reversible watermarking. IEEE International Multimedia Signal Processing Workshop, 345–350
5. Fridrich, J., Goljan, M., and Du, R. (2001): Invertible authentication. Proc. SPIE, Security and Watermarking of Multimedia Contents, **3971**, 197– 208
6. Xuan, G., Zhu, J., Chen, J., Shi, Y., Ni, Z., and Su, W. (2002): Distortionless data hiding based on integer wavelet transform. IEE Electronics Letters, **38**, 1646–1648
7. Goljan, M., Fridrich, J., and Du, R. (2001): Distortion-free data embedding for images. 4th Information Hiding Workshop, LNCS, **2137**, Springer-Verlag, 27–41
8. Celik, M., Sharma, G., Tekalp, A.M., and Saber E. (2002): Reversible data hiding. Proc. of the International Conference on Image Processing 2002, 157–160
9. Ni, Z., Shi, Y., Ansari, N.,and Su, W. (2003): Reversible data hiding. Proc. IEEE ISCAS'03, **2**, II-912–II-915
10. Yang, B., Schmucker, M., Funk, W., and Busch, C. (2004): Integer DCT-based reversible watermarking for images using companding technique. Proc. SPIE, Security and Watermarking of Multimedia Content, **5306**, 405–415
11. Tian, J. (2002): Reversible watermarking by difference expansion. Proceedings of Workshop on Multimedia and Security, 19–22
12. Alattar, A.M. (2004) Reversible watermark using difference expansion of quads. in Proc. IEEE Int. Conf. Acoustics, Speech, and Signal Processing (ICASSP'04), **3**, 377–380
13. Wu, X. and Memon, N. (1997): Context-based, adaptive, lossless image codec. IEEE Trans. Commun., **45**, 437–444
14. Fridrich, J., Goljan, M. and Du, R. (2001): Invertible authentication watermark for JPEG images. Proc. ITCC 2001, 223–227
15. Wu X. (1997) Lossless compression of continuous-tone images via context selection, quantization, and modeling. IEEE Trans. Image Process., **6**, 656–664
16. Weng, S., Zhao, Y., and Pan, J.-S. (2006): Cropping resistant lossless watermarking based on improved DE method. INFORMATICA International Journal, submitted
17. Holliman, M. and Memon, N. (2002): Counterfeiting attacks on oblivious blockwise independent invisible watermarking schemes. IEEE Trans. on Image Proceesing, **9**, 432–441
18. Shi, Y.Q., Ni, Z., Zou, D., Liang, C., and Xuan G. (2004): Lossless data hiding: fundamentals, algorithms and applications. Proc. of the 2004 International Symposium on Circuits and Systems, ISCAS '04, **2**, pp. II-33–II-36

A

Programs Relating to Topics of This Book

A.1 Messages from the Editors

Authors from five chapters in this book contributed their executables and/or source codes relating to the topics of their chapters. These programs are gathered in the CD attached to this book. Please contact authors in the chapters cited below for further discussions.

A.2 The Programs

These programs are put in five directories in the attached CD. They are briefly described as follows.

A.2.1 Programs Relating to "Bit-Level Visual Secret Sharing Scheme for Multi-Secret Images Using Rotation and Reversion Operations"

Authors in Chapter 4 offered their source codes and executables relating to their topics. These codes are offered in the attached CD under the directory:

```
\IMDH\Demo\Ch04\
```

A.2.2 Programs Relating to "Adaptive Data Hiding Scheme for Palette Images"

Authors in Chapter 5 offered their source codes and executables relating to their topics. These codes are offered in the attached CD under the directory:

```
\IMDH\Demo\Ch05\
```

A.2.3 Programs Relating to "Steganographic Methods Focusing on BPCS Steganography"

Authors in Chapter 8 offered their executables relating to their topics. These codes are offered in the attached CD under the directory:

\IMDH\Demo\Ch08\

Some explanations of their codes have been described in Sec. 8.7 of this book.

A.2.4 Programs Relating to "Multipurpose Image Watermarking Algorithms and Applications"

Authors in Chapter 11 offered three sets of their executables relating to their topics. These codes are offered in the attached CD under the directory:

\IMDH\Demo\Ch11\

The users' manuals are also provided in the CD under the same directory.

A.2.5 Programs Relating to "Reversible Watermarking Techniques"

Authors in Chapter 11 offered their source codes and executables relating to their topics. These codes are offered in the attached CD under the directory:

\IMDH\Demo\Ch15\

A.3 Conclusion

The editors are grateful for these authors who contributed their valuable research materials. Interested readers are suggested to check these programs.

Subject Index

ADSL network, 51
annotation, 317
arithmetic coding, 15, 20–22, 26, 27, 46, 51, 69, 77, 210, 363, 364, 369, 374, 386
attack, 126, 128–130, 134, 138, 152, 199, 207, 214, 215, 301, 304, 307, 311, 313, 319, 325, 326, 346, 380
authentication, 103, 123, 124, 145, 148, 149, 151, 153, 287, 288, 304, 308, 314, 357, 363, 364, 374, 375, 378, 380

bandwidth, 18, 27, 36, 40, 48, 51, 52, 55
bar code, 261–264, 269–271, 279, 282, 284
  1-dimensional, 269
  2-dimensional, 269, 282
  3-dimensional, 271
base layer, 44, 45, 64, 66, 67, 76
Bhattacharyya coefficient, 239
Bit Correct Rates (BCR), 342–344, 346–354
bit rate, 4, 14, 25, 36, 37, 41, 43–46, 48, 50, 62, 67, 69, 165, 169, 171, 183, 185, 210, 211
bit-error rate (BER), 160, 172, 176–181, 183–185
bit-plane, 84, 86, 88, 89, 92, 94, 95, 149, 150, 189, 193, 194, 199, 201, 203, 210, 211, 213, 357–359, 362–364, 367
bitstream, 29, 34, 37–39, 42, 44, 55, 68, 73, 79, 113, 116, 210, 212, 233, 235, 246, 250, 251, 256, 363, 364, 366, 368, 369, 374, 378, 380, 386
blocking artifact, 23
BMP, 104, 194, 196, 220, 221, 223, 225, 228
Boolean, 237
buffer, 37, 38
buffer management, 63

camera-phone, 262
  D901iS, 262
  J-SH04, 262
capacity, 7, 8, 52, 103–105, 112, 114, 116–121, 128, 142, 144–147, 189, 190, 194–197, 206, 209, 221, 222, 225, 226, 326, 351, 358, 359, 366–371, 373–376, 379, 380
CDROM, 13
central limit theorem, 192
channel coding, 327
chrominance, 25, 27, 35, 40
clustering, 103–105, 109, 117, 119, 120, 291
codebook, 85, 86, 95, 98, 152, 214, 291, 293–301, 303, 305, 307, 308, 329, 331, 333–335, 338, 339, 342, 344, 345, 347–354
codeword, 105, 291, 292, 294, 295, 297, 300
coding efficiency, 63, 64
ColorCode, 271
communication channel, 195
complexity, 23, 36, 37, 45, 48, 50, 63, 90, 95, 190–194, 199–201, 203,

206–209, 212, 213, 221, 225, 315, 371
compression, 3, 5, 13, 15–18, 34, 40, 144, 149–151, 159, 172, 225, 288, 291, 301, 305, 311, 313, 319, 326, 358, 359, 362–364, 368–370, 374
  lossless, 5, 17, 144, 145, 149–151, 359, 363, 364, 369, 370, 374
    CALIC, 368–370
  lossy, 5, 17, 358, 363
compression ratio, 15, 17, 21, 28, 29, 37, 48, 291, 364
conjugation, 191, 192, 194, 204, 206, 208
content adaptive binary arithmetic coding (CABAC), 51
content-based image retrieval (CBIR), 313
context-adaptive bit-plane coding, 56
copy protection, 287, 288
copyright notification, 287, 288
copyright protection, 123, 124, 157, 287, 288, 290, 308, 313, 314, 317, 325, 327, 332, 333, 357
correlation, 129, 140–142, 147, 173, 175–177, 180, 181, 274
cost function, 29
covariance, 237
cryptography, 288, 313
cubic spline algorithm, 138

data hiding, 3, 6, 103–105, 108, 123, 124, 129, 153, 272, 357–359, 362, 367, 376, 380, 387
data tracing, 123
database, 198, 252, 256, 264, 288, 289, 313, 317–320
DE, *see* difference expansion (DE)
decryption, 85, 88–90, 92, 94–96, 98–100, 288
Delaunay Triangulation, 133
descriptor, 235
differential pulse code modulation (DPCM), 20, 25, 31, 32, 38, 40
digital broadcasting, 157
digital rights management (DRM), 325
digital signature, 148, 357
digital television, 13
digital television broadcasting, 43
Digital Versatile Disk (DVD), 13, 14, 43, 51, 157, 159
discrete cosine transform (DCT), 8, 15, 18, 22–29, 32–35, 37, 38, 41–47, 57, 62, 140, 147, 213–219, 226, 287, 288, 290, 308–311, 317, 326, 358, 363, 364, 371, 372
  forward transform, 23
  inverse transform, 23
  two dimensional, 23
discrete Fourier transform (DFT), 23, 130, 131, 287, 290, 326
discrete wavelet transform (DWT), 8, 130, 132, 210, 287, 290, 308, 326, 358
distance, 105, 134–136, 239, 291, 313
  Euclidean distance, 327
distortion, 15, 17, 25, 28, 127, 129, 133, 134, 136, 138–140, 142, 143, 147, 149, 150, 152, 153, 160, 292, 301, 342, 358, 364, 367, 371, 375
  central distortion, 327, 329–331
  side distortion, 327, 329, 332
dithering, 84

embedded block coding with optimized truncation (EBCOT), 74
  3-D, 74
embedded zero-block coding (EZBC), 74
encryption, 85, 86, 88–90, 92, 95, 98, 100, 103, 189, 288, 308, 313
End of the Block (EOB), 26
energy, 22
enhancement layer, 44, 45, 64, 66, 69, 70, 72, 76
entropy coding, 15, 18–20, 26, 31, 41, 46, 62, 73, 366
error concealment, 45, 47, 328, 335, 338
error resilience, 210, 327, 328, 346, 348, 351
error resilient coding, 326, 327
error resilient transmission, 325, 326, 332, 333, 335
error-prone channel, 55
event detection, 233–236, 243, 244, 256
evolutionary algorithm, 326
exclusive-or (XOR), 194, 216, 218, 293, 295, 297

expectation-maximization (EM) algorithm, 181, 182
EZW, 210

false alarm, 246
false-negative, 137, 171
false-positive, 137
feature, 234, 277, 279, 280, 288, 289, 313, 317, 320
feature extraction, 278, 279, 282, 314, 316
feature retrieval, 280
fingerprinting, 123, 293, 308, 357
fitness function, 342
fractal transform, 17
frame, 14
frame buffer, 62
frame difference, 28–30
frequency domain, 158

Gaussian, 233, 235, 236, 243, 310, 311, 313
Geographical Information System (GIS), 123, 124, 127, 152
GIF, 104
Gifshuffle, 104
Gray code, 205
group of pictures (GOP), 35, 37, 58, 64, 70, 72, 250

H.120, 40, 41
H.261, 27, 40–42, 46, 51
H.262, 40, 41, 50, 51
H.263, 13, 27, 40, 41, 46, 51, 56, 64
H.263 2000, *see* H.263++
H.263+, 46, 51
H.263++, 46, 50, 51
H.264, 27, 40, 41, 48, 50–52, 55, 58, 60, 68, 72, 77
H.26L, 50
H.26x, 17, 18, 40
Haar integral, 315
Hamming distance, 299
hash, 124, 145–151, 363, 364, 374, 375, 378, 380
  MD5, 145–147, 151
HDTV, 43
heterogeneous network, 55
Hidden Markov Model, 234
histogram, 181, 192, 199, 201, 203, 214–218, 316, 359–361, 371, 372
Huffman code tree, 20
Huffman coding, 15, 20, 21, 26, 27, 151, 363, 364
Huffman table, 27
human visual system (HVS), 15, 16, 20, 23–25, 47, 84, 94, 97, 161, 189, 190, 288, 309

image coding standard, 23
image hiding, 103, 104
image processing, 159
image recognition, 261–263
ImageBridge, 272
index assignment, 329–338, 340, 352
integer discrete cosine transform (IDCT), 140, 147, 357, 359, 371
integer discrete wavelet transform (IDWT), 357, 359, 364
integer Haar wavelet transform, 373
integrity verification, 287
intellectual property right, 5
interleaving, 318
International Electro-technical Commission (IEC), 40
International Standards Organization (ISO), 40
International Telecommunication Union – Telecommunication (ITU-T), 40, 46, 50
  Video Coding Experts Group (VCEG), 40, 43, 48, 50
Internet, 3–5, 40, 41, 46, 50, 55, 123, 157, 189, 190, 196, 262, 265, 268, 270, 287, 288, 309, 311
ISDN channel, 41
ISO-IEC
  Moving Picture Experts Group (MPEG), *see* MPEG
ITU, 56, 79

JAN (Japan Article Number) code, 269, 270
JBIG, 363, 378, 379
JBIG2, 374, 375
joint video team (JVT), 50
JPEG, 17, 18, 25, 27, 189, 196, 198, 213, 214, 216, 218–221, 225, 226,

228, 292, 293, 300–302, 307, 311, 313, 319, 321, 358, 362–364
quality factor, 362, 363
quality factor (QF), 214, 215, 218, 301, 302, 307, 313, 319, 321
JPEG2000, 17, 27, 74, 78, 189, 210–213, 362
EBCOT algorithm, 210
JPG, *see* JPEG
just noticeable distortion (JND), 7

Karhunen-Loéve transform (KLT), 17, 23
key, 83, 90, 92, 94–96, 100, 103, 136, 195, 198, 204, 221, 223, 224, 292, 293, 295–297, 318, 363
key management, 83

Lagrange cost, 68
Lagrange optimization, 68
leaky prediction, 70, 71
learning rate, 237
least significant bit (LSB), 8, 142, 144–146, 149, 152, 204, 205, 209, 214, 358, 363–365, 371, 373–376, 378, 379, 386
lifting scheme, 59
bidirectional prediction, 60
prediction filter, 59
update filter, 59
lossy channel, 326
lossy compression, 210
luminance, 25, 27, 35, 40, 44, 104, 105, 111, 158, 160–163, 166, 167, 173, 317, 338, 360, 361

map object, 124, 142
point, 125, 129, 134–137, 140
polygon, 125, 142
polyline, 125, 131, 135, 142
masking effect, 161
MD5, 374, 378
mean, 141, 143, 145, 146, 173, 237, 290, 293, 316
mean absolute difference (MAD), 29
mean square error (MSE), 15
memory bandwidth, 63
metadata, 198
MiLuLa, 279, 281
mobile channel, 4
mobile communication, 51
mobile network, 51
3GPP, 51
3GPP2, 51
mobile phone, 261, 263, 264, 266–268, 270, 272, 277, 278, 284
mobile phone camera, 261–263, 266, 269, 270, 272–274, 276–279, 281, 284
Monte-Carlo method, 315
morphological filtering, 236–238
most significant bit (MSB), 8
motion compensated embedded zero block coding (MC-EZBC), 74
motion compensated frame difference, 28–30
motion compensated temporal filtering (MCTF), 56, 58–64, 69, 70, 72–75
motion compensation, 14, 18, 32, 34–38, 41, 43, 60, 63
overlapped block motion compensation, 46
motion estimation, 29–32, 37, 38, 73, 158, 160, 161, 165, 166
block matching, 29, 31, 161–163
diamond search, 31
four-step search, 31
full search, 31
hexagon-based search, 31
three-step search, 31
two dimensional logarithmic search, 31
motion flow, 233, 235, 236, 246, 250–254, 256
motion picture, 43, 157–159, 161, 168, 183, 186
motion prediction, 18
motion vector, 29, 31, 32, 37, 38, 44, 46, 66, 75, 158, 161–164, 186, 233, 235, 250–252, 256
moving picture, 42
MP3, 42
MPEG, 17, 18, 36, 40, 41, 43, 48, 50, 55–57, 73, 79, 159, 161, 162, 165, 167, 172, 186, 233, 235, 246, 250, 256
VidWav, 73, 75–77
MPEG-1, 13, 27, 40–43, 46, 51

MPEG-2, 13, 14, 27, 40, 41, 43–46, 50, 51, 56, 64, 165, 167, 168, 170, 171, 183, 185, 256
MPEG-4, 27, 40, 41, 46–48, 50, 51, 55, 56, 64
  Advanced Video Coding (AVC), 40, 48, 50, 51, 55, 58, 60, 68, 72, 77
  fine granularity scalability (FGS), 27
MSE, 16, 125
multimedia, 3, 5, 13, 41, 47, 48, 51, 104, 124, 126, 140, 256, 262, 287, 288, 311, 326
  continuous, 4
  discrete, 4
  image, 3
  sound, 3
  video, 3
multimedia representation, 3
multimedia retrieval, 287, 288
multimedia signal processing, 3
multiple description coding (MDC), 325, 327–329, 332, 334–337, 339, 342, 346, 347, 351, 352
  multiple description scalar quantization, 329, 331, 332
  multiple description scalar quantization (MDSQ), 328–330, 332, 334–338, 352
  multiple description transform coding (MDTC), 328
  multiple description vector quantization (MDVQ), 328, 332, 333, 335, 348, 351, 352

noisy channel, 326, 327
normal distribution, 173, 176, 180–182, 192
  mean, 173, 180, 181
  variance, 174, 180, 181
normalized correlation, 131
Normalized Hamming Similarity (NHS), 299–307, 311–313
NTSC, 40, 41

object, 37, 47–49
  video, 37, 47–49
object deformation, 161, 163, 164, 168, 170
object movement, 161, 163, 168, 170

optimization, 325, 326
ownership, 325–327, 335
ownership verification, 314

packet loss, 45
PAL, 13, 40, 41
palette, 119, 120
palette image, 103, 104, 119
  color palette, 104, 106, 108, 109
  image data, 103, 104, 106, 108, 109, 111–113, 115–117, 120
PaperClick Code, 278
patchwork algorithm, 160
Pattobi-by-MiLuLa, 281
payload, 145, 147, 358, 360, 364, 369, 370, 374, 380
PDF, 196
peak signal to noise ratio (PSNR), *see* PSNR
peak-signal-noise ratio (PSNR), *see* PSNR
pixel domain, 158
PNG, 196, 198, 220, 221, 223, 225, 228
precision tolerance, 125, 133, 134, 136, 137, 143, 146, 149, 150, 153
predicted frame, 33
  B-frame, 33, 34, 36–38, 250
  I-frame, 33, 36–38, 41, 250
  P-frame, 33, 34, 37, 38, 41, 250
predictive coding, 14, 18–20, 46
  adaptive, 20
  bi-directional prediction, 33, 34, 36, 46
  forward prediction, 33, 34, 36
  Inter coding, 14, 18, 19, 28, 34, 41, 42
  Intra coding, 18, 19, 28, 29, 32–38, 41, 42, 46, 50
print-to-web linking, 261–270, 272–274, 276–278, 280–284
  with a retrieve server, 264, 265, 268
  without a retrieve server, 263, 264
probability density function, 180, 182
pseudo noise sequence (PNS), 129–131
pseudo random, 136, 167, 173, 175, 183, 360
pseudo-random number generator (PRNG), 363
PSNR, 15, 16, 27, 63, 69, 117–119, 121, 125, 153, 184, 212, 218, 298, 299,

307, 321, 342–344, 346, 348, 350, 351, 353, 362, 371, 374, 380

QR (quick response) code, 261, 262, 269, 270, 273, 282, 284
quality, 7, 8, 15, 16, 25, 27, 37, 40, 41, 43, 45, 48, 51, 62, 63, 67, 68, 70, 85, 103, 105, 108, 117, 118, 120, 152, 153, 157–161, 167–172, 184, 186, 189, 193, 204, 213, 225, 262, 273, 277, 299, 301, 308, 311, 314, 319, 325, 326, 344, 345, 362, 363, 371, 373, 374, 379
quantization, 37, 41, 210
quantization index modulation (QIM), 214–216, 218, 310, 358

rate control, 25, 36, 37, 210
rate-distortion, 62, 63, 78, 211, 369
real-time, 70, 233–236, 240, 243, 245, 246
recognition, 277–279, 282
redundancy, 14, 18, 19, 28, 34, 41, 43, 64
  coding, 14
  psychovisual, 15
  spatial, 14, 18, 34, 41
  statistical, 14
  temporal, 14, 18, 19, 34, 41
redundant coding, 172
region of interest (ROI), 160, 210–212
retrieval, 233, 287–289, 311, 313, 317, 320
  query-by-example (QBE), 233, 235, 255
  query-by-sketch (QBS), 233, 235, 253, 255–258
  video retrieval, 233
retrieve server, 272, 278, 280
reversible data hiding, 140, 141, 147, 152, 363
root-mean-square (RMS) error, 27
run length coding, 14, 18, 25–27, 35, 37

salt-and-pepper noise, 358–362, 380, 382
scalable video coding (SVC), 44, 45, 55–60, 62, 63, 66, 69, 70, 73, 75, 77–79
  AVC-based, 56–58, 72, 73, 75, 77–79
  closed-loop, 62, 63
  hierarchical B picture, 60, 64, 72
  inter-layer prediction, 64–66
  JSVM, 77
  motion scalability, 74
  open-loop, 62, 63, 77, 78
  SNR scalability, 43, 55, 56, 58, 66, 70–72, 74
    coarse granularity scalability (CGS), 66, 67, 69
    fine granularity scalability (FGS), 66, 68–70
  spatial scalability, 43, 55, 56, 58, 64, 70–72, 74
  temporal scalability, 43, 55, 56, 58, 64, 70–73
    barbell-lifting, 73
  update step, 63
  wavelet-based, 56, 72, 79
SDTV, 13, 31, 51
secret, 84, 86, 92, 94–97, 99, 100, 103, 104, 106, 108, 109, 113, 115–117, 136, 189, 194, 195, 199, 201, 204–208, 211, 212, 296
secret sharing, 83, 84, 86
secure, 219, 293
security, 83, 90, 95, 104, 124, 189, 318
set-top box, 157
shadow, 83, 90–92, 94–96
Source Input Format (SIF), 43
spatial domain, 359, 362, 364, 380
SPIHT, 210
spread spectrum, 130, 131, 172, 358
  direct sequence spread spectrum, 130
standard deviation, 237
steganalysis, 217, 219
steganography, 6, 103, 105, 189, 190, 194–198, 203, 209, 211–213, 215, 216, 218, 219
  bit-plane complexity segmentation (BPCS), 189, 194–200, 203–206, 208, 209, 211–213, 220, 222, 224, 225, 228
Stirmark, 8, 304, 311, 326, 346
streaming, 40, 46, 55
sub-band, 76
subband, 68, 132, 210
subjective evaluation, 164, 165, 167

sum of absolute difference (SAD), 31, 162
Super Video CD, 45
surveillance system, 233, 234, 243–246, 256, 258
  compressed domain, 233, 235, 236, 256
  spatial domain, 233, 235, 256
  video-based, 233, 234, 256
synchronization, 35, 131

tabu search, 325–327, 336, 341–343
threshold, 7, 84, 105–107, 109, 116–120, 129, 131, 135–139, 164, 167, 170, 174, 176, 177, 190, 193, 194, 199, 200, 204, 206, 208, 209, 212, 213, 217, 221, 225, 240, 243, 253, 290, 291, 293, 304, 371, 374
tracking, 234
trajectory, 59, 63, 233–235, 239, 240, 242–244, 246–249, 252, 253, 255, 256
transform coding, 14, 22
transmission channel, 25

URL, 262–265, 267, 268, 270, 272, 278, 279, 282, 284

variable bit rate coding (VBR), 45
variable length coding, 20, 26, 35, 37, 38, 44
  3-D, 46
variance, 290, 307, 309, 316
vector map, 123–125, 127, 133, 139, 140, 142, 147, 149, 152, 153
vector quantization (VQ), 17, 41, 105, 113, 287, 290–294, 296–298, 300, 301, 303, 305, 307, 308, 325, 326, 332, 333, 335, 339, 344–346, 351, 353, 358
  generalized Lloyd algorithm (GLA), 291
  index constrained vector quantization (ICVQ), 295, 297
  iterative clustering algorithm, 291
  LBG algorithm, 298
  multistage, 290, 294, 305
video, 157
Video CD, 13, 41–43
video coding, 13, 52
video coding standard, 13, 14, 23, 34, 35, 38–41, 46, 47
  core experiments, 40
  picture type, 35
    B-Picture, 36
    I-Picture, 35, 36
    P-Picture, 36
  simulation software, 39
  test model, 40
  verification model, 39
video communication, 38
video compression, 13, 40
video conferencing, 40, 41, 46, 50
Video Home System (VHS), 41, 43
video processing, 157, 159, 160, 172, 176, 186
Video Quality Experts Group (VQEG), 16
video telephony, 40
visual cover model, 125
visual secret sharing, 83–86, 100
  $(2,2)$-VSS, 85–88, 90, 94, 95, 98, 99
  $(2,5)$-VSS, 100
  (t,n)-VSS, 84, 85, 95–97

Walsh-Hadamard transform (WHT), 17, 23
watermarking, 5, 6, 123–127, 130, 131, 133, 135, 136, 139, 145, 147, 148, 150, 152, 153, 157, 159, 160, 165–170, 172, 174, 190, 261–263, 272–274, 277, 279, 282, 287, 288, 290–293, 295–309, 311–314, 317, 319, 320, 325, 326, 333, 335, 336, 342, 344, 346, 357, 358, 360, 371, 376, 380–382, 384, 386, 387
  blind, 127, 131, 132, 290, 297, 308, 311
  cocktail, 290
  color domain, 274, 275
  detection, 6, 131, 136, 138, 158–160, 167, 170–176, 179, 184, 186, 275, 276, 290, 384, 388
  embedding, 5, 8, 103, 105, 106, 108, 109, 113, 116–121, 124, 125, 129–131, 133–135, 140, 144, 145, 150, 158–161, 165, 166, 168–174, 176, 183, 186, 194, 195, 197, 201,

203, 206, 215, 220–222, 224–226, 228, 272, 275, 279, 290, 292, 293, 295–299, 305, 307–309, 314, 318, 325, 327, 332–337, 339, 342–345, 350–354, 357, 358, 360–364, 366–376, 378–381, 385
extraction, 5, 108, 115–117, 127, 130, 131, 134, 140, 144, 145, 148, 149, 151, 172, 195, 208, 220–222, 225, 272, 274–276, 279, 290, 293, 296, 297, 300–308, 311–313, 319, 325, 332–335, 337, 338, 340, 342–353, 358, 366–368, 370, 374, 375, 380, 385
forgery, 6
fragile, 5, 6, 129, 147–149, 151–153, 195, 287–290, 292, 300, 307, 386, 388
frequency domain, 274
imperceptibility, 159, 161–165, 169, 186, 273, 326
imperceptible, 5
insertion, 5
invisibility, 134, 138
invisible, 288, 289, 309, 311–314
multiple, 289, 290
multipurpose, 287–290, 307, 311, 314, 317, 320
non-blind, 130, 131, 133
oblivious, 290
perceptible, 5
removal, 6
reversible, 148, 152, 153, 357, 358, 371, 373, 376, 378, 380, 382, 387
difference expansion (DE), 373–376, 380, 382, 383
robust, 5, 6, 127, 129, 130, 133, 138, 139, 152, 160, 172, 206, 209, 273, 274, 276, 287–290, 293, 295, 296, 298–303, 305, 306, 308, 311, 314, 317, 358, 359, 362, 363, 380
semi-fragile, 6, 287–290, 295, 297–306, 308, 314
spatial domain, 127, 133, 139, 147, 153, 274, 275
special design, 274, 276
transform domain, 127, 133, 139, 152, 153
video watermarking, 157–160, 186
visible, 288, 289, 308, 309, 311, 312
wavelet, 47, 55, 56, 59, 75, 132, 210, 212, 314
(5, 3), 59–61
Haar, 60
weighting factor, 182
wireless channel, 55

zigzag scanning, 15, 18, 25, 26, 35, 37, 43, 45

MIX
Papier aus verantwortungsvollen Quellen
Paper from responsible sources
FSC® C105338

If you have any concerns about our products,
you can contact us on
ProductSafety@springernature.com

In case Publisher is established outside the EU,
the EU authorized representative is:
Springer Nature Customer Service Center GmbH
Europaplatz 3, 69115 Heidelberg, Germany

Printed by Libri Plureos GmbH
in Hamburg, Germany